Y0-BXW-920

Royal Society of Medicine
International Congress and Symposium Series
Editor-in-Chief: H.-J. C. L'Etang

Number 74

Clobazam: Human Psychopharmacology and Clinical Applications

*Proceedings of an International Symposium
held in York from
30th November to 2nd December, 1983*

Royal Society of Medicine
International Congress and Symposium Series

Number 74

Clobazam:
Human Psychopharmacology and
Clinical Applications

Edited by
I. HINDMARCH,
P. D. STONIER, and
M. R. TRIMBLE

1985

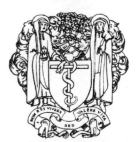

Published by
THE ROYAL SOCIETY OF MEDICINE
1 Wimpole Street, London

ROYAL SOCIETY OF MEDICINE

1 Wimpole Street, London W1M 8AE

Distributed by

OXFORD UNIVERSITY PRESS
Walton Street, Oxford OX2 6DP

London New York Toronto
Delhi Bombay Calcutta Madras Karachi
Kuala Lumpur Singapore Hong Kong Tokyo
Nairobi Dar es Salaam Cape Town
Melbourne Auckland

and associated companies in
Beirut Berlin Ibadan Mexico City Nicosia

Oxford is a trade mark of Oxford University Press

Copyright © 1985 by

ROYAL SOCIETY OF MEDICINE

British Library Cataloguing in Publication Data

Clobazam : human psychopharmacology and clinical
applications : [proceedings of an international
symposium in York from November 30th to
December 2nd, 1983]—
(International congress and symposium series,
ISSN 0142–2367; no. 74)
1. Clobazam   2. Psychopharmacology
I. Hoechst UK   II. Hindmarch, I.   III. Stonier,
P.D.   IV. Trimble, Joseph, E.   V. Royal Society
of Medicine   VI. Series
616.89'18   RC483.5.C5

ISBN 0–19–922013–1

Printed in Great Britain by Latimer Trend & Company Ltd, Plymouth

Contributors

CHAIRMEN

Dr M. Parsonage,
27 Clarendon Road, Leeds, UK

Prof. O. J. Rafaelsen,
University of Copenhagen, Psychochemistry Institute, Rigshospitalet, Blegdamsvej 9, DK-2100 Copenhagen, Denmark

Prof. A. C. P. Sims,
Department of Psychiatry, St. James's University Hospital, Leeds, UK

Prof. Dr. P. Wolf,
Freie Universität Berlin, Universitätsklinikum Charlottenburg, Spandauer Damm 130, 1000 Berlin 19.

CONTRIBUTORS

Dr G. Beaumont,
11 Dorchester Road, Hazel Grove, Stockport, UK

Prof. T. G. Bolwig,
Psykiatrisk afd, Rigshospitalet, Blegdamsvej 9, DK-2100 Copenhagen, Denmark

Dr N. Callaghan,
Neurology Department, Cork Regional Hospital, Wilton, Cork, Eire

Prof. J. P. Cano,
Institut National de la Santé et de la Recherche Médicale, Faculté de Pharmacie, 27 Boulevard J. Moulin, 13385 Marseille Cedex 5, France

Dr Ph. Coassolo,
Institut National de la Santé et de la Recherche Médicale, Faculté de Pharmacie, 27 Boulevard J.-Moulin, 13385 Marseille Cedex 5, France

Dr. E. M. R. Critchley,
Department of Neurology, Royal Preston Hospital, Preston, UK

Miss C. Cull,
Department of Neuropsychiatry, National Hospitals for Nervous Diseases, Queen Square, London, UK

Dr M. A. Dalby,
Neurological University Clinic, Aarhus City Hospital, Aarhus, Denmark

Dr I. B. Davies,
> *Charterhouse Clinical Research Unit, Boundary House, 91–93 Charterhouse Street, London, UK*

Dr P. Dawson,
> *Wharfedale General Hospital, Otley, W. Yorks, UK*

Dr C. I. Dellaportas,
> *117A Beaufort Street, Chelsea, London, UK*

Dr C. Disayavanish,
> *Department Psychiatry, Faculty Medicine, Chiang Mai University, Chiang Mai, Thailand*

Dr M. Feely,
> *Department of Medicine, The Martin Wing, The General Infirmary, Leeds, UK*

Dr L. Ferreira,
> *Rua Diogo Cao, 1 279–1–E. 4200 Oporto, Portugal*

Dr A. Gjerris,
> *University of Copenhagen, Psychochemistry Institute, Rigshospitalet, Blegdamsvej 9, DK–2100 Copenhagen, Denmark*

Dr T. Goggin,
> *Clinical Investigation Unit, Neurology Department, Cork Regional Hospital, Wilton, Cork, Eire*

Dr M. Gringras,
> *MGB Clinical & Drug Research, 23 Station Road, Cheadle Hulme, Stockport, Cheshire, UK*

Miss C. Harrison,
> *Human Psychopharmacology Research Unit, University of Leeds, Leeds, UK*

Dr I. Hindmarch,
> *Human Psychopharmacology Research Unit, University of Leeds, Leeds, UK*

Dr D. Koeppen,
> *Klinische Forschung, Hoechst AG, 6230 Frankfurt (Main) 80, West Germany*

Dr H. Kruse,
> *Department of Pharmacology, Hoechst AG, 6230 Frankfurt (Main) 80, West Germany*

Dr A. A. Martin,
> *Lancaster Moor Hospital, Quernmore Road, Lancaster, UK*

Dr. A. Moffett,
> *EEG Department, The London Hospital, Whitechapel, London, UK*

Dr F. Noel,
> *Laboratoires Diamant, Tour Roussel-Nobel, Cedex 3, 92080 Paris la Defense, France*

Dr J. Oxley,
Chalfont Centre for Epilepsy, Chalfont St. Peter, Gerrards Cross, Buckinghamshire, UK

Dr A. C. Parrott,
Institute of Naval Medicine, Alverstoke, Gosport, Hampshire, UK

Dr P. Plouin,
Laboratoire d'Explorations Fonctionelles du Systeme Nerveux, Hopital St. Vincent de Paul, 74 Avenue Denfert-Rochereau, F-75674 Paris Cedex 14, France

Prof. B. Saletu,
Psychiatrische Uniklinik Wien, Pharmakopsychiatrische Abt, A-1000 Vienna, Austria

Dr D. F. Scott,
EEG Department, The London Hospital, Whitechapel, London, UK

Dr P. D. Stonier,
Medical Department, Hoechst UK Ltd, Salisbury Road, Hounslow, Middlesex, UK

Mr Z. Subhan,
Human Psychopharmacology Research Unit, University of Leeds, Leeds, UK

Dr D. J. Thompson,
Airedale General Hospital, Skipton Road, Steeton, Keighley, West Yorks, UK

Dr M. R. Trimble,
Department of Neuropsychiatry, National Hospitals for Nervous Diseases, Queen Square, London, UK

Contents

Benzodiazepines, Psychiatry and Epilepsy

A Review of Clobazam Studies in Epilepsy

Preface

This symposium is a logical development of the First International Symposium on Clobazam (Killarney, 1979) and the Second International Symposium on the drug which was held in York in 1981. The Killarney meeting demonstrated the clinical efficacy of clobazam as an anxiolytic and emphasized the distinct differences between the chemistry and pharmacology of clobazam, the first 1,5-benzodiazepine, and conventional 1,4 derivatives. The first York Symposium established the drug's efficacy in clinical use and illustrated the potential application of clobazam in the management of epilepsy, particularly the treatment of resistant cases.

Part 1 of this monogaph contains several papers illustrating the differences which exist between clobazam and traditional treatments for anxiety. Compared with conventional 1,4-benzodiazepines clobazam has little effect on memory and information processing systems (Mr Subhan); pharmaco-EEG and psychometric assessments (Professor Saletu and Dr Hindmarch) and, in combination with an antidepressant (nomifensine), car driving and related skills (Dr Stonier). Dr Davies has shown differences between clobazam and diazepam, and their desmethyl metabolites, on performance measures in the clinical pharmacological laboratory, and these differences between 1,4- and 1,5-benzodiazepines are, arguably, reflected in the clinical studies of Drs Gringras and Beaumont, Miss Harrison and Dr Disayavanish.

The critical use of anxiety rating scales was advocated by Dr Gjerris and, in a preliminary communication not reported here, Professor Bolwig illustrated the utility of flutter fusion thresholds as a measure of sedation produced by psychotropics. Dr Parrott highlighted the way in which the action of clobazam, or any psychotropic, could be modified by personality and other psychological factors.

Preliminary results (Dr Thompson) show that clobazam is as effective as relaxation therapy in the treatment of anxiety, and Dr Dawson suggests that nocturnal administration of clobazam might have potential clinical application in the management of post-myocardial infarct patients (not published).

In studies of abuse of benzodiazepines, Dr Ferreira suggests that those which bind most strongly to the benzodiazepine receptors might have the greatest liability for abuse. Such findings have important implications for the management of chronic anxiety states and those patients wishing to stop benzodiazepine therapy.

Those involved in the care of patients with epilepsy know that a percentage of them, even with carefully monitored anticonvulsant therapy using existing highly effective anticonvulsants, fail to achieve control of seizures. In some of them, the persistence of their fits brings a total destruction of their ability to lead an ordinary life, and with each crisis a reminder to them and their relatives that they have this terrible condition. New treatments are continually being sought, and the journals are currently full of potential anticonvulsant compounds at various stages of development. It is, therefore, of interest that, amongst drugs already available, there are some that clearly may have therapeutic potential in epilepsy but, for various reasons, their use in this condition has not been recognized. One particular group is the benzodiazepines, and one particular compound, the 1,5-benzodiazepine, clobazam.

Several authors in their introductory comments to their papers in Part 2 allude to the earlier use of benzodiazepines in epilepsy. However, it is a truism that, aside from the well known use of, for example, diazepam as an intravenous compound in status epilepticus, and the acceptance of clonazepam in the management of some childhood epilepsies, generally benzodiazepines have not been established as of therapeutic value in this condition. It is recognized that tolerance to the antiepileptic effect soon occurs in many patients and that side-effects and intoxication, particularly in patients receiving polytherapy, may be a problem. However, in spite of this there are persistent reports in the literature of a percentage of patients responding successfully to the anticonvulsant effect of benzodiazepines, and in some patients this effect clearly continues for a long period of time.

The early experimental work with clobazam suggested this drug may have some potential in patients who are resistant to conventional therapy. The animal literature led to the suggestion that it was a highly effective anticonvulsant compound. Further, it seemed that the therapeutic ratio of the drug was different from other available benzodiazepines, and that the dose which produced side-effects was greater than that which led to therapeutic benefit. In this monograph some of the early literature on clobazam and epilepsy has been reviewed by Dr Kruse. Early clinical trials were completed, mainly open studies, but later some authors attempted double-blind assessments. This literature is assessed briefly by Dr Koeppen. It is clear from this analysis that not all patients respond to clobazam, but most authors who have used the drug felt it had value in a nucleus of chronic patients in whom alternative treatments had proved unsuccessful. Further, side-effects did not appear to be so great when compared to the use of other benzodiazepines for this condition. Thus, a literature has arisen on the adjunctive therapy of chronically-resistant patients with epilepsy with clobazam. This stimulated several groups to do further work with this compound.

Most of the papers in this monograph are related to recent investigations assessing the clinical value of clobazam in epilepsy. Several clinical reports provide up to date comments on the experience of several researchers. The main thrust of the trials has been towards the use of clobazam, particularly in relatively low doses, given as a single night-time administration to chronic patients. Further, some specific aspects of the relationship betwen clobazam and epilepsy are investigated, for example, in the chapter from Dr Plouin in which electroencephalographic criteria are reported, or in the work from Drs Scott and Moffett, in which both EEG and psychologi-

cal tests have been monitored under clobazam treatment.

Its use in certain special situations, for example, catamenial epilepsy, is raised by Dr Feely and others, and the pharmacokinetic parameters are analysed in considerable detail by authors such as Professor Wolf, Dr Bun and colleagues, Dr Cocks and co-workers and Drs Goggin and Callaghan. Its standing in relationship to some other benzodiazepines, both with regards to its effect on cognitive functions and as an anticonvulsant generally, are discussed by Dr Trimble and Miss Cull, and Dr Trimble outlines some of the fascinating interlinks between psychiatry and epilepsy, to emphasize how the discovery of the benzodiazepine receptor, and the common use of benzodiazepines in both a neurological condition (epilepsy) and a psychiatric condition (anxiety), furthers our knowledge in this fascinating interface.

It is hoped that this monograph will stimulate others to look for compounds already on the shelves, readily available for administration to patients, which may prove to be effective anticonvulsants, even if only for a small number who, at the present time, are unable to lead satisfactory lives because of their seizures. It may also stimulate further work with clobazam, and increase the general knowledge and acceptance of the potential for benzodiazepines to be useful drugs for the management of this condition.

I. Hindmarch, P. D. Stonier, and
M. R. Trimble.
Leeds and London, 1985.

PART 1

Psychopharmacology and Anxiolytic Activity

The Psychopharmacology of Clobazam

I. HINDMARCH

Human Psychopharmacology Research Unit, Department of Psychology,
University of Leeds, Leeds, UK

Introduction

One of the basic assumptions of the psycho-pharmacologist is that psychoactive drugs, in general, will manifest their activity by changing some behavioural variables. By measuring the change in behavioural state brought about by the administation of a particular psychotropic agent it is possible to delineate and profile the psychoactivity of that drug.

In order to make the measurement of change of behavioural state of psychological relevance, it is necessary to view the drug-induced changes of behaviour within the framework of a model of the action of the brain and central nervous system. The action of the CNS of interest to psychopharmacologists is the mode and manner of its function when processing sensory information and formulating motor sequences as behavioural responses to the novel environmental situation perceived via the sensory systems.

It has been possible to identify (Hind-march, 1980) valid psychometric tests which can reliably measure the action of psychotropic drugs on aspects of the sensory, motor and central function of information processing, and also gauge their interactive effects on sensori-motor and psychomotor activity.

The vast majority of traditional anti-anxiety therapies (barbiturates, chloral hydrate, bromides, meprobamate) have promoted sedation as their prime therapeutic action. Early 1,4-benzodiazepines—loraze-pam, diazepam, chlordiazepoxide—and later drugs of similar profile (clorazepate, praze-pam, ketazolam), are also sedative agents. Sedation reduces the overall activity of the nervous system and the patient becomes detached from the environmental stimulation producing the anxiety and is tranquillized. Such sedative therapy, in reducing the capacity of the CNS to sense and respond to stimulation from the milieu, does not permit the individual to utilize his own cognitive systems to come to terms with the cause and origins of his anxiety. Removal of the sedation, via withdrawal of the sedative agent, is

accompanied in most cases by a return of the anxiety. Sedation can be regarded as an unwanted effect in the treatment of anxiety states for, as well as actually hindering the recovery of the patient, such lethargy, drowsiness and impaired psychomotor activity can place ambulant patients at risk of accident in home, work and road traffic situations as well as interfering with short-term memory and related cognitive functions.

The psychopharmacological profile of clobazam has to be established by determining its effects on aspects of sensori-motor, CNS and "working memory" functions. The profile established by considering the drug's effects on the various cognitive systems and sub-systems will help determine the tolerability and safety of the drug in clinical use and the extent to which clobazam, a 1,5-benzodiazepine, differs from conventional 1,4-benzodiazepines in its anxiolytic and sedative activity.

Clobazam and other benzodiazepines compared on tests of sensori-motor activity

There are many sensitive tests of sensory processing ability which can discriminate drugs. For example using the number of spontaneous reversals of the Necker cube as an index of sensory performance Wittenborn et al. (1979) were able to show that the pattern of acquisition was impaired by 5 mg diazepam but not by 10 mg clobazam. The authors also found a complex vigilance task to discriminate between clobazam and diazepam, with the latter drug reducing performance. Salkind et al. (1979) found that digit symbol substitution (DSST) performance, a test of sensory perceptual speed, was improved in patients following clinical dose regimens of 10 mg clobazam t.d.s. In contrast to the lack of effects of clobazam on DSST and other tests of sensory function, 20 mg chlordiazepoxide (Shaffer et al., 1963; Besser and Steinberg, 1967) and diazepam 10 and 17–28 mg (Jäättela et al., 1971; Shira, 1978) have been shown to impair DSST performance. Furthermore 1 and 2·5 mg lorazepam produce a significant impairment of letter cancellation performance (File and Bond, 1979) and 5 and 10 mg diazepam impair letter search and cancellation tests as well as reducing the velocity of saccadic eye movements (Jones et al., 1978; Lawton and Cahn, 1963; Aschoff et al., 1975). 15 mg potassium clorazepate, a pro-drug for N-desmethyldiazepam, has much the same disruptive capacity on sensory activity as diazepam and it impairs sensory identification tests (Hindmarch and Parrott, 1979).

Steiner-Chaskel and Lader (1981) showed that 1 h after an acute dose of 10 mg diazepam there was a significant impairment of DSST performance in contrast to the enhancement of DSST ability found following 10 mg clobazam.

Although there are few published trials, patient studies of DSST, letter cancellation tests and related measures of sensory processing activity have also discriminated between clobazam and other benzodiazepines (Wittels and Stonier, 1981). The lack of DSST impairment following treatment of anxious patients with clobazam is in contrast to the impairments found following diazepam and N-desmethyldiazepam.

It is perhaps difficult to isolate a purely motor activity from its sensory or CNS precursors. However, some assessments require a predominantly motor response mode and have been used to discriminate between benzodiazepines. Clobazam (10 mg) was found to improve performance on a balance beam (Wittenborn et al., 1979) while stabilometer and body sway measures were not impaired following 20 mg clobazam (Hindmarch, 1979; Taeuber et al., 1979). The lack of effect of clobazam on motor activity has also been shown at doses up to and including 30 mg using motor reaction time as the response measure (Gudgeon and Hickey, 1981; Siegfried et al., 1981). Such findings are in marked contrast to the overall impairment of motor activity produced by 10 mg chlordiazepoxide (Hindmarch, 1979), 2·5–28 mg diazepam (Hart et al., 1976; Uhlenhuth et al., 1977; Mattila et al., 1978; Shira, 1978), and 1–4 mg lorazepam (Hedges et al., 1971; Harry and Richards, 1972; Ogle et al., 1976; File and Bond, 1979; Siegfried et al., 1981).

Most of the habitual behaviour of patients involves sensori-motor coordination, which probably accounts for the popularity of psychomotor tests to assay drug activity, because not only do valid tests act as analogues of everyday situations but they are relevant to the daily performance of ambulant patients.

Gudgeon and Hickey (1981) found significant impairments of complex reaction time following 10–30 mg diazepam, while clobazam showed an impairment only after acute doses of 30, 40 or 60 mg. Nicholson (1981) found that 20 mg clobazam had no effect on the performance of a visuo-motor task, whereas 10 mg diazepam was associated with a significant impairment up to 4 h after an acute dose.

Following 20 mg clobazam, Steiner-Chaskel and Lader (1981) found instances of enhanced performance on a card sorting task, in contrast to the impairment produced by 10 mg diazepam. Also, Siegfried et al. (1981) were unable to distinguish between the performance of subjects following placebo or 30 mg clobazam on a choice reaction time task, while at the same time demonstrating the significant impairment on task performance produced by 3 mg lorazepam.

The results with patient populations are most consistent with these laboratory findings and demonstrate the distinct difference between clobazam, in not affecting performance of a complex sensori-motor task and other, 1,4-benzodiazepines, which impair psychomotor function. Card sorting and/or complex reaction time have been significantly impaired in anxious patient populations, following subchronic treatment with diazepam, lorazepam and N-desmethyldiazepam (Wittels and Stonier, 1981). However, Radmayr (1980), found that clobazam had no effect on the complex reaction time of neurotic outpatients, and Hill et al. (1981) were also unable to find any deterioration of a complex reaction time task following two weeks of repeated nocturnal doses of 20 or 40 mg clobazam in a group of anxious general practice patients.

Clobazam and other benzodiazepines compared on tests of overall CNS function

By far the most widely used test of CNS arousal is the critical flicker fusion threshold

(CFF) due to its ease of use and its high correlation with other measures of CNS performance and alertness (Parrott, 1982a). A review of the effects of benzodiazepines on this measure has shown (Hindmarch, 1982) that 10 mg chlordiazepoxide, 5–22·8 mg diazepam, 15 mg medazepam, 20–40 mg oxazepam and 0·5–2·5 mg lorazepam all produce a significant depression of CFF. When 10 mg clobazam t.d.s. for five days was compared to 5 mg diazepam t.d.s. and 10 mg chlordiazepoxide t.d.s. for a similar period of time on CFF, it was found (Hindmarch, 1979) that both 1,4-benzodiazepines produced an overall sedative depression of the CFF threshold while at no point during the five-day treatment did clobazam exhibit any sedative effect. Gudgeon and Hickey (1981) concluded in a dose ranging comparison of clobazam 10, 20, 30, 40 and 60 mg against diazepam 5, 10, 15, 20, 30 mg and placebo, that there is a significantly greater lowering of CFF per unit dose for diazepam than clobazam and found no evidence of sedation following acute doses of up to 20 mg clobazam. Parrott (1982b) reviewing the effects of clobazam on CFF, showed that acute doses up to 20 mg did not produce any significant CFF changes. Repeated doses of 20 mg produced a significant elevation of CFF. Acute doses of 30–60 mg clobazam produced a reduction in CFF values which, however, vanished after repeated dosing. The overall lack of sedation found following repeated doses of clobazam clearly differentiate the drug from other 1,4-benzodiazepines used as anxiolytics. There is a clear separation of the anxiolytic and the sedative potential of clobazam evidenced in the clinical studies of Hill *et al.* (1981) and Ponciano *et al.* (1981), where CFF levels were measured in anxious patients. There was an overall augmentation of CFF levels in both these studies which were concordant with improvements in anxiety measured on clinical ratings by both physician and patient.

CFF is an objective measure of the overall state of CNS alertness which has been shown (Parrott, 1982b) to correlate with other, subjective, measures of alertness and sedation. Patients "feelings" of tiredness, drowsiness, lethargy and an overall inability to remain alert and attentive are often reported following conventional 1,4-benzodiazepines. Diazepam 5 and 10 mg produced "drowsiness", as rated on 10 cm visual analogue ratings scales, whereas 10 and 20 mg clobazam had no effect (Steiner-Chaskel and Lader, 1981). Following treatment with ketazolam 30 mg, significant evidence of tiredness, drowsiness and a lack of alertness was found on subject completed analogue rating scales, whereas clobazam 20 mg had no effect which distinguished it from placebo (Robinson *et al.*, 1981).

Anxious patients in general practice have been shown (Hill *et al.*, 1981) to have an improved CFF concordant with ratings of less drowsiness, less tiredness and increased alertness following a sub-chronic treatment with clobazam 20 mg nocte for two weeks.

The lack of subjective feelings of sedation following medication with clobazam is further evidence to suggest basic differences in the pharmacodynamics of 1,4- and 1,5-benzodiazepines.

Clobazam and other benzodiazepines compared on tests of car driving and vehicle handling ability

Antianxiety agents might interfere with the complex psychomotor skills of everyday living by producing sedation and impairment of cognitive, perceptual and motor function. Skills like car driving are important to maintain in ambulant patients as an impairment of such habitual behaviour might lead to domestic or work problems which could exacerbate the subjects' perceived anxiety.

Clobazam has already been shown to differ from 1,4-benzodiazepines, like lorazepam and diazepam, in its lack of detrimental action on laboratory analogues of complex psychomotor functions, such as reaction time and critical flicker fusion threshold.

Tests of "on-the-road" car driving ability have been performed with clobazam and the laboratory findings have been replicated in a "real-life" situation of car handling skills. Biehl (1979) found that in real traffic conditions 10 mg diazepam significantly impaired brake reaction time in comparison to 20 mg clobazam and placebo. Hindmarch *et al.* (1977) also found that clobazam 20 mg nocte for six nights had no discernible effect on car handling tests of reverse parking, steering, width estimation and garaging. In contrast to the lack of effect on car driving found following clobazam 10 mg t.d.s. for three days, lorazepam 1 mg t.d.s. for three days (an equipotent clinical dose) was found to significantly impair braking, parking, three-point turning and steering abilities.

Other 1,4-benzodiazepines are as potent as lorazepam in destroying the basic dimensions of "on-the-road" car handling skills. Chlordiazepoxide 10 mg × 5 significantly impaired reversing and overtaking gap judgements (Betts *et al.*, 1972), diazepam 5–20 mg/day impaired the overall car driving performances of anxious outpatients (de Gier *et al.*, 1981), medazepam 5–30 mg/day caused patients to make more technical driving errors (Moore, 1977), and temazepam 20 mg significantly impaired gap judging ability (Betts and Birtle, 1982).

Silverstone (1974) has pointed out that actual car driving performance is difficult to control in "on-the-road" tests and many authors have, therefore, used simulated, as opposed to "real-life" driving, to measure the effects of antianxiety benzodiazepines. Berry *et al.* (1974) were unable to show any change in brake reaction time following either clobazam 10 mg or placebo, but a significant impairment followed the administration of diazepam 10 mg. Diazepam has also been shown to increase the frequency of a collision, to impair decision making and speed/position control and to cause patients to ignore traffic rules (Linnoila and Mattila, 1973; Linnoila and Hakkinen, 1974; Ziedmand *et al.*, 1979). Chlordiazepoxide 20 mg has also been shown to impair simulated driving tests (Kielholz *et al.*, 1967).

Clobazam and other benzodiazepines compared on amnestic properties

The amnestic properties of 1,4-benzodiazepines like diazepam and lorazepam, coupled with their pronounced sedative activity, make them ideal drugs for pre-operative medication where sedation and loss of memory for unpleasant procedures like endoscopy and dental surgery is required (Brown *et al.*, 1978; Clarke *et al.*, 1970; Gregg *et al.*, 1974).

However, amnesia in ambulant anxious patients can pose problems. A disruption of the ability to process information adequately because of amnesia can lead to a delay in therapeutic response and, because of the widespread disruption of cognitive systems due to disorders of memory, cause problems with the handling of everyday information, especially in elderly patients and those of reduced intellectual capacity.

1,4-Benzodiazepines in general are powerful amnestic agents. More specifically amongst the antianxiety agents chlordiazepoxide 5 mg (Liljequist *et al.*, 1979), diazepam 10 and 20 mg (Haffner *et al.*, 1973; Ghoneim *et al.*, 1975) and lorazepam 1–3 mg (Dundee and George, 1976; Heisterkamp and Cohen, 1975; Siegfried *et al.*, 1981), have been shown to possess powerful amnestic action. On the other hand, clobazam 20 mg has been shown to be free from any effect on memory although some impairment on some memory tests with clobazam 40 and 60 mg has been reported (Subhan, 1981). These later results show that a clear separation of untoward amnestic effect from no amnestic activity can be obtained simply by manipulating the dose regimen. Doses up to 30 mg clobazam are free from amnestic properties.

The difference between clobazam 10 mg t.d.s. and lorazepam 1 mg t.d.s. for four weeks in a group of elderly anxious patients on a test of short-term "working" memory is well illustrated in the clinical study of Paes de Sousa *et al.* (1981), where the significant impairment of patients memory produced by lorazepam is not to be found in those patients treated with clobazam.

The psychopharmacological profile of clobazam

Although there are difficulties in making a summary of all the published data comparing clobazam with other benzodiazepines due to differences in methodology, dose/treatment regimens, tests employed and patient populations studied, there are general differences to be observed between the psychopharmacological profile of clobazam and other benzodiazepines.

The lack of any untoward sedative, amnestic or disruptive effects of clobazam on the various tests of psychomotoric activity reviewed here is obvious with respect to the comparator derivatives shown in Table 1. It is interesting that a lack, or presence, of a particular psychopharmacological effect is not wholly dependent on the pharmacokinetic assessment of elimination half-life— although such variables might be important measures with respect to other clinical requirements such as dose regimen and treatment frequency.

Psychopharmacological measures have clinical relevance in that they are analogues of

Table 1

Psychopharmacological profile of benzodiazepines used as anti-anxiety agents: a comparison of clinical-equivalent doses

	CRT	CFF	Car driving	Memory	Sedation
Diazepam[a]	—[b]	—[b]	—[b]	—[b]	—[b]
Chlordiazepoxide	—[b]	—[b]	—[b]	—[b]	—[b]
Lorazepam	—[b]	—[b]	—[b]	—[b]	—[b]
Bromazepam	—	×	ND	ND	—
Clobazam	×	+	+	×	+
Oxazepam	—	ND	ND	ND	—

[a]clorazepate, prazepam, ketazolam and medazepam as pro-drugs for diazepam and/or its active metabolite N-desmethyldiazepam can be regarded as possessing the same profile as diazepam.
[b]Statistical significance at $P \leqslant 0.05$.
—, Impairment with respect to placebo; ×, no change with respect to placebo; +, improvement with respect to placebo; ND, no published data.

the situations ambulant patients encounter during their daily routine. An impairment of basic sensori-motor, CNS or information processing skills can have important clinical consequences. The results presented here clearly distinguish the 1,5-benzodiazepine clobazam from conventional 1,4-derivatives. Laboratory studies have been confirmed in the clinical situation with anxious patients. The psychopharmacological profile of clobazam, with its lack of sedation, lack of amnesia and lack of detrimental effects on car driving and psychomotor performance, achieves clinical relevance in the management of ambulant anxious patients and delineates clobazam as a unique substance in contrast to the conventional sedative, amnestic, performance impairing 1,4-benzodiazepine tranquillizers.

Summary

The psychopharmacological profile of clobazam, established by its effects on sensori-motor, CNS and memory functions, is reviewed. Laboratory studies have been confirmed in the clinical situation with anxious patients. The profile of clobazam with its lack of sedation, lack of amnesia and lack of impairment on car driving and psychomotor performance achieves clinical relevance in the management of ambulant anxious patients and is contrasted to the conventional sedative, amnestic performance impairing 1,4-benzodiazepine tranquillizers.

References

Aschoff, J.C., Becker, W., and Weinert, D. (1975). Computer analysis of eye movements: evaluation of the state of alertness and vigilance after sulpiride medication. *Journal of Pharmacologie Clinique* 11 (2), 93–97.

Berry, P.A., Burtles, R., Grubb, D.J., and Hoare, M.V. (1974). An evaluation of the effects of clobazam on human motor coordination, mental activity and mood. *British Journal of Clinical Pharmacology* 1, 346.

Besser, G.M., and Steinberg, H. (1967). L'interaction du chlordiazepoxide et du dexamphetamine chez l'homme. *Therapie* 22, 977–990.

Betts, T.A., and Birtle, J. (1982). Effect of two hypnotic drugs on actual car driving performances. *British Medical Journal* 285, 852.

Betts, T.A., Clayton, A.B., and Mackay, G.M. (1972). Effects on four commonly-used tranquillisers on low-speed driving performance tests. *British Medical Journal* 4, 580–584.

Biehl, B. (1979). Studies of clobazam and car-driving. *British Journal of Clinical Pharmacology* 7, 85S–90S.

Brown, J., Lewis, V., Brown, M.W., Horn, G., and Bowes, J.B. (1978). Amnesic effects of intravenous diazepam and lorazepam. *Experientia* **34**, 501.

Clarke, P.R.F., Eccersley, P.S., Frisby, J.P., and Thornton, J.A. (1970). The amnesic effects of diazepam (Valium). *British Journal of Anaesthesia* **42**, 690–697.

Dundee, J.W., and George, D.A. (1976). The amnesic action of diazepam, flunitrazepam and lorazepam in man. *Acta Anaesthesia Belgica* **27**, 3–11.

File, S.E., and Bond, A.J. (1979). Impaired performance and sedation after a single dose of lorazepam. *Psychopharmacology* **66**, 309–313.

Gier, de J., Hart, B.J., Nelemans, F.A., and Bergman, H. (1981). Psychomotor performance and real driving performance of outpatients receiving diazepam. *Psychopharmacology* **73**, 340–344.

Ghoneim, M.M., and Mewaldt, S.P. (1975). Effects of diazepam and scopolamine on storage, retrieval and organisational processes in memory. *Psychopharmacology* **44**, 257–262.

Gregg, J.M., Ryan, D.E., and Levin, K.H. (1974). The amnesic actions of diazepam. *Journal of Oral Surgery* **32**, 657.

Gudgeon, A.C., and Hickey, B.J. (1981). A dose-range comparison of clobazam and diazepam: 1. Tests of psychological functions. *Royal Society of Medicine International Congress and Symposium Series* **43**, 1–5.

Haffner, J.F.W., Mørland, J., Setekleiv, J., Strømsaether, C.E., Danielsen, A., Frivik, P.T., and Dybing, F. (1973). Mental and Psychomotor effects of diazepam and alcohol. *Acta Pharmacologica et Toxicologica* **32**, 161.

Harry, T.V.A., and Richards, D.J. (1972). Lozazepam—a study in psychomotor depression. *British Journal of Clinical Practice* **26**, 371–373.

Hart, J., Hill, H.M., Bye, C.E., Wilkinson, R.T., and Peck, A.W. (1976). The effects of low doses of amylobarbitone sodium and diazepam on human performance. *British Journal of Clinical Pharmacology* **3**, 289–298.

Hedges, A., Turner, P., and Harry, T.V.A. (1971). Preliminary studies on the central nervous system effects of lorazepam, a new benzodiazepine. *Journal of Clinical Pharmacology* **16**, 423–427.

Heisterkamp, D.V., and Cohen, P.J. (1975). The effect of intravenous premedication with lorazepam (Ativan), pentobarbitone or diazepam on recall. *British Journal of Anaesthesia* **47**, 79–81.

Hill, A.J., Walsh, R.D., and Hindmarch, I. (1981). Tolerability of nocturnal doses of clobazam in anxious patients in general practice. *Royal Society of Medicine International Congress and Symposium Series* **43**, 133–140.

Hindmarch, I. (1979). Some aspects of the effects of clobazam on human performance. *British Journal of Clinical Pharmacology* **7** (1), 77S–82S.

Hindmarch, I. (1980). Psychomotor function and psychoactive drugs. *British Journal of Clinical Pharmacology* **10**, 1189–1209.

Hindmarch, I. (1982). Critical flicker fusion frequency (CFFF): The effects of psychotropic compounds. *Pharmacopsychiatria* **15** (Suppl. 1), 44–48.

Hindmarch, I., and Parrott, A.C. (1979). The effects of repeated nocturnal doses of clobazam, dipotassium clorazepate and placebo on subjective ratings of sleep and early morning behaviour and objective measures of arousal, psychomotor performance and anxiety. *British Journal of Clinical Pharmacology* **8**, 325–329.

Hindmarch, I., Hanks, G.W., and Hewett, A.J. (1977). Clobazam, a 1,5-benzodiazepine derivative and car driving ability. *British Journal of Clinical Pharmacology* **4**, 573–578.

Jäättela, A., Männistö, P., Paatero, H., and Tuomisto, J. (1971). The effects of diazepam or diphenhydramine on healthy human subjects. *Psychopharmacologia (Berlin)* **4**, 235–246.

Jones, D.M., Lewis, M.J., and Spriggs, T.L.B. (1978). The effects of low doses of diazepam on human performance in group administered tasks. *British Journal of Clinical Pharmacology* **6**, 333–337.

Kielholz, P., Goldberg, L., Obersteg, I., Poeldinger, W., Ramseyer, A., and Schundt, P.

(1967). Strassenverkehr, tranquilizer und alkohol. *Deutsche Mediz. Wochen* **92**, 1525–1531.

Lawton, M.P., and Cahn, B. (1963). The effects of diazepam and alcohol on psychomotor performance. *Journal of Nervous and Mental Disorders* **136**, 550–554.

Liliequist, R., Palva, E., and Linnoila, M. (1979). Effects on learning and memory of two weeks treatment with chlordiazepoxide lactam, N-desmethyldiazepam, oxazepam and methyloxazepam, alone or in combination with alcohol. *International Pharmacopsychiatry* **14**, 190–195.

Linnoila, M., and Hakkinen, S. (1974). Effects of diazepam and codeine alone and in combination with alcohol on simulated driving. *Clinical Pharmacology and Therapeutics* **15**, 368–373.

Linnoila, M., and Mattila, M.J. (1973). Drug interaction on psychomotor skills related to driving: Diazepam and alcohol. *European Journal of Clinical Pharmacology* **5**, 186–194.

Mattila, M.J., Palva, E., Seppälä, T., and Ostrovskaya, R.U. (1978). Actions and interactions with alcohol of drugs on psychomotor skills: Comparison of diazepam and gamma-hydroxybutyric acid. *Archives of Internal Pharmacology and Therapeutics* **234** (2), 236–246.

Moore, N.C. (1977). Medazepam and the driving ability of anxious patients. *Psychopharmacology* **52**, 103–106.

Nicholson, A.N. (1981). Studies of the effects of 1,4- and 1,5-benzodiazepines on sleep in man. *Royal Society of Medicine International Congress Symposium Series* **43**, 67–72.

Ogle, C.W., Turner, P., and Markomihelakis, H. (1976). The effects of high doses of oxporenolol or propranolol on pursuit rotor performance, reaction time and critical flicker frequency. *Psychopharmacologia (Berlin)* **46** (3), 295–299.

Paes de Sousa, M., Figuiera, M-L., Loureiro, F., and Hindmarch, I. (1981). Lorazepam and clobazam in anxious elderly patients. *Royal Society of Medicine International Congress and Symposium Series* **43**, 13–21.

Parrott, A.C. (1982a). Critical Flicker Fusion Threshold and their relationship to other measures of alertness. *Pharmacopsychiatria* **15** (1), 39–43.

Parrott, A.C. (1982b). The effects of clobazam upon CFF. *Drug Development Research* (Suppl.) **1**, 57–66.

Ponciano, E., Relvas, J., Mendes, F., Lameiras, A., Vaz Serra, A., and Hindmarch, I. (1981). Clinical effects and sedative activity of bromazepam and clobazam in the treatment of anxious out-patients. *Royal Society of Medicine International Congress and Symposium Series* **43**, 125–131.

Radmayr, E. (1980). Clobazam and diazepam in the treatment of neurotic out-patients. *Therapiewoche* **30**, 117.

Robinson, R., Gudgeon, A.C., and Hindmarch, I. (1981). Oxazolam, ketazolam and clobazam compared with placebo on tests of psychomotor function. *Royal Society of Medicine International Congress and Symposium Series* **43**, 60–65.

Salkind, M.R., Hanks, G.W., and Silverstone, J.T. (1979). Evaluation of the effects of clobazam, 1,5-benzodiazepine, on mood and psychomotor performance in clinically anxious patients in general practice. *British Journal of Clinical Pharmacology* **7**, 113S–118S.

Shaffer, J.W., Freinek, W.R., Wolf, S., Foxwell, N.H., and Kurland, A.A. (1963). A controlled evaluation of chlordiazepoxide in the treatment of convalescing alcoholics. *Journal of Nervous and Mental Disorders* **137**, 494–507.

Shira, R.B. (1978). A technique for investigating the intensity and duration of human psychomotor impairment after intravenous diazepam. *Oral Surgery* **45** (4), 493–502.

Siegfried, K., Koeppen, D., Taeuber, K., Badian, M., Malerczyk, V., and Sittig, W. (1981). A double-blind comparison of the acute effects of clobazam and lorazepam on memory and psychomotor functions. *Royal Society of Medicine International Congress Symposium Series* **43**, 13–21.

Silverstone, T. (1974). Drugs and driving. *British Journal of Clinical Pharmacology* **1**, 451–454.

Steiner-Chaskel, N., and Lader, M.H. (1981). Effects of single doses of clobazam and diazepam on psychological functions in normal subjects. *Royal Society of Medicine International Congress and Symposium Series* **43**, 23–32.

Subhan, Z. (1981). A dose-range comparison of clobazam and diazepam: II. Effects on memory. *Royal Society of Medicine International Congress and Symposium* **43**, 7–120.

Taeuber, K., Badian, M., Brettel, H.F., Royen, Th., Rupp, W., Sittig, W., and Uihlein, M. (1979). Kinetic and dynamic interaction of clobazam and alcohol. *British Journal of Clinical Pharmacology* **7**, 92S–97S.

Uhlenhuth, E.H., Turner, D.A., Purchatzke, G., Gift, T., and Chassan, J. (1977). Intensive design in evaluating anxiolytic agents. *Psychopharmacology* **52**, 79–85.

Wittels, P.Y., and Stonier, P.D. (1981). The effects of benzodiazepines of psychomotor performance in patients. *Royal Society of Medicine International Congress Symposium Series* **43**, 111–118.

Wittenborn, J.R., Flaherty, C.F., McGough, W.E., and Nash, R.J. (1979). Psychomotor changes during the initial day of benzodiazepine medication. *British Journal of Clinical Pharmacology* **7** (1), 69S–76S.

Ziedman, K., Smiley, A., and Moskowitz, H. (1979). Effects of drugs on driving: driving simulator tests of diazepam and secobarbital. Proceedings of Human Factors Society, 23rd Annual Conference, Boston, USA, pp. 259–262.

Comparison of N-Desmethylclobazam and N-Desmethyldiazepam: Two Active Benzodiazepine Metabolites

I. B. DAVIES,* J. McEWEN,† A. W. PIDGEN, J. ROBINSON, and P. D. STONIER

*Department of Clinical Pharmacology, Hoechst UK Ltd,
Walton Manor, Milton Keynes, Buckinghamshire, UK*

Introduction

Clobazam, a 1,5-benzodiazepine, impairs psychomotor performance less than equipotent anxiolytic doses of diazepam, a 1,4-benzodiazepine (Hindmarch, 1979). The major metabolites of clobazam and diazepam are the products of N-1 desalkylation reactions which are N-desmethylclobazam (norclobazam) and N-desmethyldiazepam (nordiazepam) (Volz et al., 1979; Fulton et al., 1981). Norclobazam and nordiazepam are active metabolites (Fielding and Hoffmann, 1979; Greenblatt et al., 1981a) and accumulate in man after multiple dosing of the parent compounds (Rupp et al., 1979; Greenblatt et al., 1981a; Volz et al., 1979) so that norclobazam or nordiazepam may be responsible for some of the effects seen after long-term administration of clobazam or diazepam, respectively. The separation of anxiolytic from psychomotor-impairing effects may be greater for norclobazam than for clobazam (Fielding and Hoffmann, 1979). Therefore, it seemed important to compare the effects of norclobazam with nordiazepam upon psychomotor performance.

Subjects and Methods

Six normal subjects (3 F, age 23–42, weight 50–60 kg) were given, blind, single morning (08:00 h) doses of norclobazam (30 mg) or nordiazepam (15 mg) or lactose placebo on three occasions each two weeks apart. Each dose was given with water (200 ml) after subjects had fasted from 24:00 h the night before. The study was carried out in a balanced crossover, Latin square design.

The following tests were done at 0, 1, 2, 3, 6 and 8 h after dosing: visual analogue self-rating scales of drowsiness (VASD) and concentrating ability (VASC) (Bond and Lader, 1972), critical flicker fusion test of vigilance (CFF) (Hindmarch, 1975) using two ascending and two descending thresholds, maze drawing test of coordination (drawing a line with the dominant hand between two lines printed on paper like the Gibson maze—(Gibson, 1965) (M-test) and finger tapping on a morse code key (FTT) (testing the dominant hand), digit symbol substitution test (DSST) of cognitive ability (Wechsler Adult Intelligence Scale). Each subject was familiarized with each test before the study.

Evaluation of results was by analysis of variance to determine differences between drugs, subjects and treatment sequences (after testing for normality of distribution with Shapiro-Wilk's test), and then by multiple pairwise comparisons with Duncan's multiple comparison test. Statistically significant results were taken as those with $P < 0.05$.

The study was approved by the local Ethics Committee and was carried out according to the Declaration of Helsinki. Each subject gave informed written consent.

Results

Visual Analogue Scales (VASD, VASC)

Scores on the visual analogue scale for drowsiness (VASD) did not differ between norclo-

*Present address: Charterhouse Clinical Research Unit, St Bartholomews Hospital, London, UK.
†Present address: Drug Development Scotland Ltd, Ninewells Hospital and Medical School, Dundee, UK.

bazam and placebo at any stage (Fig. 1). However, subjects became drowsy after 1 h with nordiazepam, which differed statistically from placebo and norclobazam at 1, 3 and 6 h ($P < 0.05$, 0·01 and 0·01, respectively) (Fig. 1A). Norclobazam had no effect on subjects' concentrating ability but nordiazepam significantly decreased concentrating ability at 1 and 3 h after dosing ($P < 0.05$, < 0.01 respectively, Fig. 1B).

Coordination tests

There was a trend, although not statistically significant, for nordiazepam to cause more errors in the maze drawing test than placebo or norclobazam between 2–4 h after dosing (Fig. 2A). Norclobazam did not differ significantly from placebo, but at 8 h significantly less errors were made in the maze test after norclobazam ($P < 0.05$, Fig. 2A). There was no difference between norclobazam and nordia-

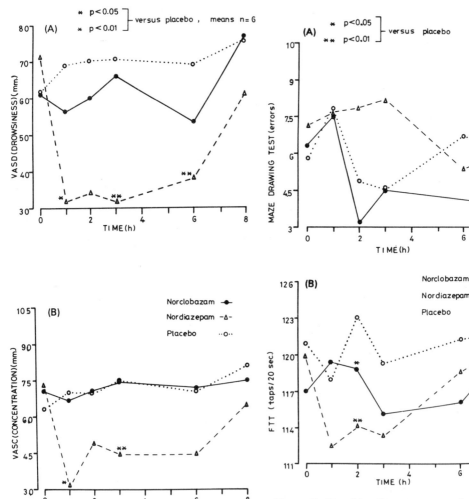

Figure 1. Visual analogue scales for (A) drowsiness (VASD) and (B) concentrating ability (VASC) after norclobazam, (●), nordiazepam (△) or placebo (○). Values are means * and ** $P < 0.05$ or < 0.01 for norclobazam or nordiazepam relative to placebo.

Figure 2. Number of errors or numbers of taps made in 20 s respectively in (A) maze drawing and (B) finger tapping tests for norclobazam, nordiazepam and placebo (symbols as for Fig. 1). Values are means. At 1 h an asterisk is omitted for nordiazepam because nordiazepam was significantly different from norclobazam ($P < 0.05$) but not from placebo (see text).

zepam in the time needed to complete the maze test, but both drugs increased the time needed relative to placebo at 1 h (nordiazepam only, $P<0.05$), 2 h (norclobazam only, $P<0.01$) and 6 h (both norclobazam and nordiazepam, $P<0.01$) (Table 1).

Nordiazepam rapidly impaired finger tapping—at 1 and 2 h nordiazepam was significantly different from norclobazam ($P<0.05$, Fig. 2B) (however, at 1 h nordiazepam was not statistically different from placebo) and nordiazepam showed a trend to greater impairment than norclobazam up to 3 h after dosing. However, at 2 h norclobazam impaired performance relative to placebo ($P<0.05$) though not as much as nordiazepam (Fig. 2B). The trend to worse performance with both norclobazam and nordiazepam persisted until 8 h after dosing.

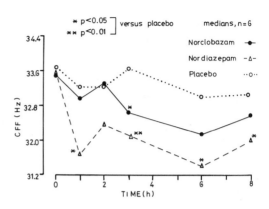

Figure 3. Critical flicker fusion threshold (CFF) after treatment with norclobazam, nordiazepam or placebo (symbols as for Fig. 1). Values are medians.

Table 1

Time to complete maze test

Time (h)	Placebo	Norclobazam	Nordiazepam
0	28·1±5·1	30·7±6·9	30·6±8·0
1	27·6±6·3	28·1±5·2	30·7±7·1*
2	27·8±5·5	32·1±7·8**	29·9±7·7
3	25·7±4·8	29·5±7·9	28·7±8·6
6	25·9±5·4	31·4±9·3**	30·7±9·0**
8	26·1±4·6	28·1±7·2	26·1±7·9

Values mean ± S.D. in s.
* or **, $P<0.05$ or 0·01 relative to placebo.
Time 0 control value before drugs given.

Critical Flicker Fusion (CFF)

Norclobazam did not differ from placebo in its effect on CFF although norclobazam caused significant impairment of CFF threshold at 2 h ($P<0.05$, Fig. 3); there was a trend for median CFF values to be lower after norclobazam relative to placebo between 4–8 h. In contrast, nordiazepam caused marked decrease of CFF threshold at 1 h and at each time point (except for 2 h) nordiazepam was significantly different from placebo; furthermore, the CFF threshold was still decreased 8 h after dosing with nordiazepam (Fig. 3).

Digit Symbol Substitution Test (DSST)

Norclobazam and nordiazepam did not differ

from placebo in the number of digit symbol substitutions made at 2 min intervals (Fig. 4A). Although no statistically significant differences were found, there was a strong trend from 2 to 6 h for a greater number of errors with nordiazepam than placebo or norclobazam (Fig. 4B). The number of errors with norclobazam closely paralleled those with placebo throughout the study and both norclobazam and nordiazepam matched placebo for errors at 8 h.

Discussion

Benzodiazepine dosage

This study compared the effect of nordiazepam, 15 mg with norclobazam 30 mg. These doses were chosen because, although a direct comparison has not been made between these active N-desmethyl metabolites, it is likely that these are equipotent doses for anxiolytic effect as suggested by data for the parent compounds and clorazepate, which is hydrolysed in the gastrointestinal tract to yield nordiazepam and is essentially a "pro-drug" for nordiazepam (Fulton et al., 1981; Greenblatt et al., 1981a).

Clorazepate, and by inference nordiazepam, has a similar pharmacological profile to diazepam and is equipotent or superior as an anxiolytic (Fulton et al., 1981). Clobazam 20 mg or 30 mg was shown to be equivalent to clorazepate 15 mg (Wallis et al., 1979). In

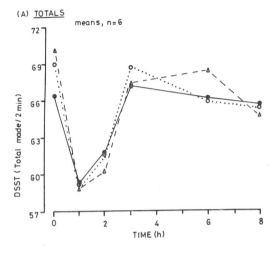

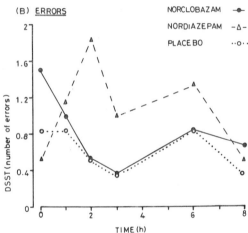

Figure 4. Total number of digit symbol substitutions made per 2 min (Fig. 4A) and number of errors (Fig. 4B) after norclobazam, nordiazepam and placebo (symbols as in Fig. 1). All values are means.

Norclobazam, nordiazepam and psychomotor performance

Nordiazepam produced greater drowsiness and more impairment of concentrating ability and CFF response than norclobazam (Figs 1, 3). Therefore, volunteers were subjectively more drowsy and less vigilant after norclobazam than after nordiazepam. These findings are similar to those for the parent compounds (Hindmarch, 1979). The separation of psychomotor-impairing from anxiolytic effects may be greater for norclobazam than clobazam (Fielding and Hoffmann, 1979), and in normal subjects the sedative and mood-lowering potency of nordiazepam may be greater than diazepam (Dasberg, 1975); these features may contribute to the differences observed between norclobazam and nordiazepam.

Norclobazam and nordiazepam both increased the time taken to complete the maze drawing test, but the effects of nordiazepam may have been worse because nordiazepam caused significantly more errors than after norclobazam (Table 1, Fig. 2). Nordiazepam seemed slightly worse in impairment of finger tapping than norclobazam (Fig. 2). It is difficult to separate the sedative effects of benzodiazepines and their metabolites from those on coordination. The greater sedative effects of nordiazepam may have caused the increased number of errors in the maze test. Muscle relaxation may also have contributed to impaired coordination; it is likely that the muscle relaxant effects of nordiazepam are greater than those of norclobazam because both metabolites have similar pharmacological profiles to their parent compounds (Fulton *et al.*, 1981; Fielding and Hoffmann, 1979) and the muscle relaxant effects of clobazam and diazepam, respectively, are known to be weak and strong (Fielding and Hoffmann, 1979; Fulton *et al.*, 1981; Steiner-Chaskel and Lader, 1981). Interestingly, at 8 h, norclobazam significantly decreased the number of errors made in the maze test compared with placebo (Fig. 2). Improvement in the Gibson maze and other performance tests have been found with the parent drug clobazam (Steiner-Chaskel and Lader, 1981).

Norclobazam, nordiazepam and cognitive function

Norclobazam and nordiazepam did not

general the clobazam–diazepam dose ratio for equi-anxiolytic effect is 2:1 (Sittig *et al.*, 1981; refs in Koeppen, 1979). Therefore, the dose ratio of 2:1 for norclobazam:nordiazepam was chosen in this study with a 30 mg dose of norclobazam since this dose has been commonly used clinically (Koeppen, 1979). However, in animals, norclobazam may be less potent than clobazam (Fielding and Hoffmann, 1979).

affect the number of digit symbol substitutions made (Fig. 4A), but there was a trend for an increased number of errors with nordiazepam (Fig. 4B). These results parallel those of previous studies in normal subjects, where clobazam enhanced DSST performance (Steiner-Chaskel and Lader, 1981) and in patients (Koeppen, 1979).

Clinical significance of properties of norclobazam and nordiazepam

After multiple doses of clobazam or diazepam their major metabolites in man, norclobazam and nordiazepam, accumulate, so that at steady state, norclobazam concentrations may be up to eight times clobazam plasma concentrations (Rupp et al., 1979) and nordiazepam plasma concentrations equal to those of the parent drug (Aucamp, 1982). Therefore, it is likely that the active N-desmethyl metabolites contribute to the effects of long-term administration of clobazam and diazepam; the situation seems more important with nordiazepam for its sedative properties may be greater than for diazepam (Dasberg, 1975), but even if norclobazam is less potent than clobazam (Fielding and Hoffmann, 1979) the greater plasma concentrations of norclobazam at steady state (Rupp et al., 1979) may make the overall pharmacodynamic effects of norclobazam significant. The greater psychomotor-impairing properties of nordiazepam than norclobazam found in this study are, therefore, likely to be reflected in the clinical use of clobazam and diazepam. The greater potential for psychomotor-impairing effects of nordiazepam than norclobazam is likely to be of special importance to patients taking other central nervous system depressants simultaneously, and in elderly patients in whom effects of sedative drugs give cause for concern (Royal College of Physicians, 1984) and in whom elimination of N-desalkylbenzodiazepines is impaired (Greenblatt et al., 1981b).

Summary

N-desmethylclobazam (norclobazam) and N-desmethyldiazepam (nordiazepam) are the active, major metabolites which accumulate in man after repeated doses of clobazam and diazepam, respectively. Therefore, we compared the effects of single, morning doses of norclobazam (30 mg) and nordiazepam (15 mg) with lactose placebo given on three occasions, in a balanced crossover, to six normal subjects. At 0, 1, 2, 3, 6 and 8 h after dosing the following tests were done, visual analogue self-rating scales for drowsiness (VASD) and concentrating ability (VASC), critical flicker fusion (CFF) test of vigilance, maze drawing (M) and morse code key finger tapping tests of coordination in the dominant hand. Greater sedation with nordiazepam relative to norclobazam or placebo were shown with VASC and VASD from 1 to 6 h. Both drugs increased the time needed to complete the M-test, but FTT impairment was worse with nordiazepam (1–4 h) than norclobazam (impairment by norclobazam only at 3 h). Nordiazepam impaired CFF from 1 to 8 h but norclobazam only at 3 h. Neither drug changed numbers or errors in substitutions in DSST although there was a tendency for more errors after nordiazepam. In conclusion this study showed that at the doses used, like the parent compounds the N-desmethyl metabolites have different effects on psychomotor performance, nordiazepam causing greater impairment, and this is likely to be important in the relative clinical effects of multiple doses of clobazam or diazepam.

References

Aucamp, A. K. (1982). Aspects of the pharmacokinetics and pharmacodynamics of benzodiazepine with particular reference to clobazam. *Drug Development Research Supplement* **1**, 117–126.

Bond, A. J. and Lader, M. H. (1972). Residual effects of hypnotics. *Psychopharmacologia* **25**, 117.

Dasberg, H. H. (1975). Effects and plasma levels of N-desmethyldiazepam after oral administration in normal volunteers. *Psychopharmacologia* (Berlin) **43**, 191–198.

Fielding, S. and Hoffman, I. (1979). Pharmacology of anti-anxiety drugs with special reference to clobazam. *British Journal of Clinical Pharmacology* **7** (Suppl. 1), 7S–16S.

Fulton, A., Maguire, K. P., Norman, T. R. and Wurm, J. M. E. (1981). Benzodiazepine pharmacokinetics, plasma levels and clinical responses. In "Psychotropic Drugs. Plasma Concentrations and Clinical Response" (G. D. Burrows and T. K. Norman, eds), pp. 361–400. Marcel Dekker Inc., New York.

Gibson, H. B. (1965). "Manual of Gibson Spinel Maze." University of London Press, London.

Greenblatt, D. J., Shader, R. I., Divoll, M. and Harmatz, J. S. (1981a). Benzodiazepines: a summary of pharmacokinetic properties. *British Journal of Clinical Pharmacology* **11**, 11S–16S.

Greenblatt, D. J., Divoll, M., Puri, S. K. *et al.* (1981b). Clobazam kinetics in the elderly. *British Journal of Clinical Pharmacology* **12**, 631–636.

Koeppen, D. (1979). Review of clinical studies on clobazam. *British Journal of Clinical Pharmacology* **7**, 139S–150S.

Hindmarch, I. (1975). A sub-chronic study of the subjective quality of sleep and psychological measures of performance on the morning following night-time medication with temazepam. *Arzneimittel-Forschung* **26**, 2113.

Hindmarch, I. (1979). Some aspects of the effects of clobazam on human psychomotor performance. *British Journal of Clinical Pharmacology* **7** (Suppl. 1), 77S–82S.

Royal College of Physicians (1984). Medication for the elderly. A report of a working party. *Journal of the Royal College of Physicians of London* **18**, 7–17.

Rupp, W., Badian, M., Christ, O., Hadjú, P., Kulkarni, R.D., Taeuber, K., Uihlein, M., Bender, R. and Vanderbeke, O. (1979). Pharmacokinetics of single and multiple doses of clobazam in humans. *British Journal of Clinical Pharmacology* **7**, 51S–57S.

Sittig, W., Badian, M., Rupp, W. and Taeuber, K. (1981). The effect of clobazam and diazepam on computer EEG vigilance and psychomotor performance. In "Clobazam", (I. Hindmarch and P. D. Stonier, eds), pp. 39–40. International Congress and Symposium Series, Number 43. Royal Society of Medicine, London.

Steiner-Chaskel, N. and Lader, M. H. (1981). Effects of single doses of clobazam and diazepam on psychological functions in normal subjects. In "Clobazam", (I. Hindmarch and P. D. Stonier, eds), pp. 23–32. International Congress and Symposium Series, Number 43. Royal Society of Medicine, London.

Volz, M., Christ, O., Kellner, H. M. *et al.* (1979). Kinetics and metabolism of clobazam in animals and man. *British Journal of Clinical Pharmacology* **7** (Suppl. 1), 41S–50S.

Wallis, T. D., Valle-Jones, J. C., Craven, J. R., Hanks, G. W. and Stonier, P. D. (1979). Single daily dose treatment of anxiety with clobazam or potassium clorazepate. *British Journal of Clinical Pharmacology* **7** (Suppl. 1), 123S.

Weschler, D. (1955). "Weschsler Adult Intelligence Scale." The Psychological Corporation, New York. UK Distributor, NFER-Nelson Publishing Co., Windsor.

The Effect of Clobazam on Search in Short-term Memory

Z. SUBHAN

Human Psychopharmacology Research Unit, Department of Psychology,
University of Leeds, Leeds, UK

Introduction

The ability of certain benzodiazepines to cause amnesia when used for surgical premedication is well documented and a disruption of memory function has been reported for diazepam (Clarke *et al.*, 1970), lorazepam (Heisterkamp and Cohen, 1975) and flunitrazepam (Dundee and George, 1976). Recently, however, interest has focused on the impairment of memory caused by benzodiazepines used for their hypnotic or anxiolytic effects rather than as premedicants in surgery. Amnestic effects have been reported for flunitrazepam (Bixler *et al.*, 1979), triazolam, flurazepam, and lorazepam (Roth *et al.*, 1980).

Clobazam is a member of the 1,5 group of benzodiazepines which differ from conventionally obtained 1,4 derivatives in having the nitrogen atoms of the heterocyclic ring in the 1,5 as opposed to the 1,4 positions. Clobazam has already been shown to have potent anti-anxiety activity (Koeppen, 1981) with relatively fewer side-effects of sedation, drowsiness and impaired performance than comparative 1,4-benzodiazepines like diazepam, lorazepam and bromazepam (Gudgeon and Hickey, 1981; Hindmarch and Gudgeon, 1980).

The effects of clobazam on aspects of human memory function have been investigated in several studies. Paes de Sousa *et al.* (1981) compared clobazam (10 mg t.d.s.) and lorazepam (1 mg t.d.s.) on a test of object recall in an elderly (mean age of 77 years) patient population. Clobazam was found to have no effect on the ability for short term recall whereas lorazepam produced an obvious and significant impairment of immediate memory. Similarly, Subhan (1981) investigated acute dose effects of clobazam (10, 20, 30, 40 and 60 mg) and diazepam (5, 10, 15, 20 and 30 mg) on a memory span for digits test, and observed a significant impairment following all doses of diazepam but only after

high doses (40, 60 mg) of clobazam, suggesting differential effects of clobazam (1,5-benzodiazepine) and diazepam (1,4-benzodiazepine) on memory. Siegfried *et al.* (1981) employed tests of anterograde amnesia in a further study comparing clobazam (30 mg) and lorazepam (3 mg) and found lorazepam to significantly impair memory for learning material presented at the time of maximum drug effect (2·5 h post-administration). There was no significant amnesia due to clobazam.

The aim of the present study was to investigate the effects of clobazam on search processes in short-term memory (STM) using a novel technique based on the reaction time (RT) method in memory research.

Subjects and Methods

Twelve female volunteers aged between 24 and 40 years were admitted to the study. All were in good physical health and without a history of cardiac, renal, hepatic, gastric or mental illness. Actual or possible pregnancy, concurrent medication (excluding the contraceptive pill) or other treatment from a physician precluded participation. Caffeine containing beverages and alcohol were not permitted for the duration of the study and subjects were not allowed to drive.

Treatments

Each subject acted as her own control and received clobazam 30 mg and placebo presented in matching capsules. AMI/CHLOR (combination of amitriptyline 25 mg and chlordiazepoxide 10 mg) was included as an active control, as it has been shown to impair performance on a wide range of psychomotoric and cognitive tests (Hindmarch, 1979; Hindmarch *et al.*, 1980).

Design

Acute doses of one of the three treatments were given to subjects on the morning of test days (i.e. 09:30 h). The order of treatments was randomized and balanced with a one-week washout period allowed between each test day. Subjects were assessed on the memory scanning test (described below) 2·5 h following medication. Data were collected under a double-blind sealed code technique.

Assessments

High speed scanning ability and retrieval from short-term memory (STM) were assessed using the varied set procedure (Figs 1 and 2) described by Sternberg (1969, 1975). A microcomputer ("Apple II") and video monitor (Hitachi, model VM 906 AE/K)

used in conjunction with a BASIC computer programme facilitated presentation of test material, measurement of reaction time (RT) and recording of results.

Subjects were required to memorize series of one, two or three digits (positive set) presented sequentially at a 1·2 s/digit rate. Two seconds after the last digit in the set was displayed an auditory warning signal (750 ms duration) was sounded followed by a single test (probe) digit. Subjects responded by pressing one of two keys: "yes" (positive response) if the test digit was contained in the memorized list, and "no" (negative response) if it was not. In accordance with the varied set procedure, a new positive set alternating randomly over trials between one, two and three digits was presented. Each subject was instructed to respond as rapidly as possible without making errors and completed 18 "practice" trials and a further 48 "experimental" trials. The inter-trial interval was 3 s. Within the 48 trials there were an equal number of positive and negative probes. Since the proportion of incorrect responses was minimal, only correct responses were used in the analyses.

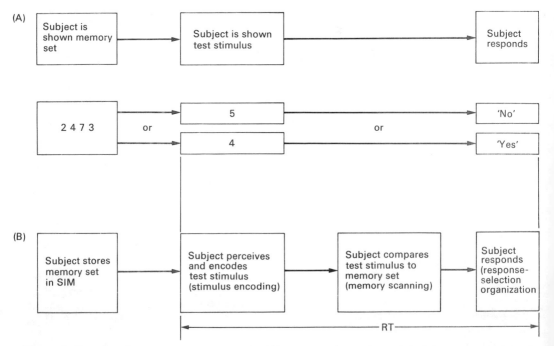

Figure 1. Sternberg's memory scanning test. (A) Events of a typical trial; (B) proposed mental events during scanning (from Klatzky, 1980).

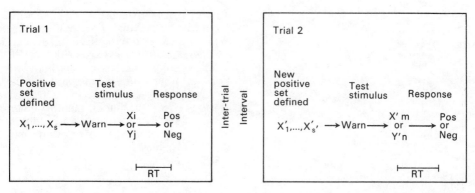

Figure 2. Memory scanning: varied set procedures. Y represents an item in the negative set. Primes are used in representing trial 2 of the varied-set procedures to show that both the items in the positive set (X₁ ... Xₛ) and its size(s) may change from trial to trial (from Sternberg, 1969).

Results

Results were analysed by means of one- and two-way randomized block analyses of variance (Kirk, 1968). Planned comparisons of means were achieved, post hoc, using 95% confidence intervals.

Analysis of the memory scanning data revealed a significant increase in overall RT (Fig. 3) following treatment with AMI/ CHLOR when compared to placebo ($F = 52\cdot3$; $df = 2,18$; $P < 0\cdot0001$, for drug main effect), and Fig. 4 shows mean RTs of the combined data from positive and negative trials as a function of memory set size. Best-fitting straight lines presented are those obtained by the method of least squares. Further analysis (Z-test) of the slopes and intercepts (Fig. 4) revealed the slope of the function that relates RT and memory set size function significantly different ($P < 0\cdot05$) for the AMI/CHLOR condition when compared to placebo.

There were no significant differences in RT between clobazam 30 mg and placebo.

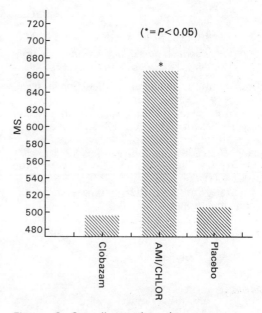

Figure 3. Overall reaction time on memory scanning test 2·5 h following treatment. * Significant difference from placebo.

Discussion

The effects of AMI/CHLOR on overall RT for the memory scanning task are clear with a significant increase in response latency observed 2·5 h following treatment.

Sternberg (1969) proposed that the reaction process in such a task occurs in a series of at least three additive stages. Assuming that the subject has the memory set stored in short-term memory (STM), the subject must first perceive and encode the test stimulus (stimulus encoding), then that stimulus is compared to members of the memory set (memory scanning or serial comparison) and, finally, a response is made on the basis of those comparisons (response selection organization). The observed RT may also be fitted with a straight line (Darley *et al.*, 1973)—the slope of that line is an estimate of serial comparison time and the intercept of

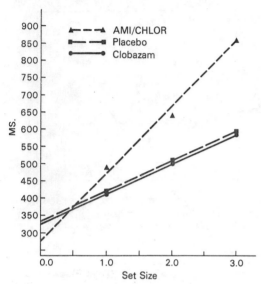

Figure 4. Reaction time as a function of memory set size 2·5 h following treatment.

both stimulus encoding and response selection organization times.

The effect of memory set size on placebo and clobazam 30 mg RT reflected an average increase of 87·6 and 85·8 ms respectively for each digit added to the positive set. In comparison, RT's increased 194·4 ms for the AMI/CHLOR condition. These data are commensurate with the significant slope difference seen in Fig. 4.

Although the question which component, encoding or response, is affected, cannot be answered here (because their effects are not separable by the analysis used), the effects of AMI/CHLOR on the serial comparison stage of the reaction process are evident.

The present results are consistent with reports of other studies demonstrating the 1,5-benzodiazepine clobazam to be free or deleterious effects on human memory (Siegfried *et al.*, 1981; Subhan, 1981; Paes de Sousa *et al.*, 1981) in contrast to conventional 1,4-benzodiazepines.

Summary

Twelve healthy volunteers received clobazam 30 mg, AMI/CHLOR (amitriptyline 25 mg, chlordiazepoxide 10 mg), and placebo according to a randomized, double-blind crossover design. Subjects then completed a Sternberg memory scanning test 2·5 h following treatment.

Search in short-term memory was found to be significantly impaired following treatment with AMI/CHLOR when compared to placebo, and results suggested a localized effect on the drug on the serial comparison stage of the reaction process.

There were no significant changes in memory test performance following treatment with clobazam.

References

Bixler, E.O., Scharf, M.B., Soldatos, C.R., Mitsky, D.J., and Kales, A. (1979). Effects of hypnotic drugs on memory. *Life Sciences* **25**, 1379–1388.

Clarke, P.R.F., Eccersley, P.S., Frisby, J.P., and Thornton, J.A. (1970). The amnesic effect of diazepam (Valium). *British Journal of Anaesthesia* **42**, 690–697.

Darley, C.F., Tinklenberg, J.R., Hollister, T.E., and Atkinson, R.C. (1973). Marihuana and retrieval from short-term memory. *Psychopharmacologia (Berlin)* **29**, 231–238.

Dundee, J.W., and George, D.A. (1976). The amnesic action of diazepam, flunitrazepam and lorazepam in man. *Acta Anaesthesia Belgica* **27**, 3–11.

Gudgeon, A.C., and Hickey, B.J. (1981). A dose-range comparison of clobazam and diazepam: 1. Tests of psychological functions. *Royal Society of Medicine International Congress Symposium Series* **43**, 1–5.

Heisterkamp, D.V., and Cohen, P.J. (1975). The effect of intravenous premedication with lorazepam (Ativan), pentobarbitone or diazepam on recall. *British Journal of Anaesthesia* **47**, 79–81.

Hindmarch, I. (1979). Some aspects of the effects of clobazam on human psychomotor performance. *Br. J. clin. Pharmac.* **7** (Suppl. 1), 775.

Hindmarch, I., and Gudgeon, A.C. (1980). The effects of clobazam and lorazepam on aspects of psychomotor performance and car handling ability. *British Journal of Clinical Pharmacology* **10**, 145–150.

Hindmarch, I., Parrott, A.C., and Stonier, P.D. (1980). Nomifensine, Clobazam and Hoe 8476. Effect on aspects of psychomotor performance and cognitive ability. *Royal Society of Medicine International Congress and Symposium Series* **25**, 47–54.

Kirk, R.E. (1968). "Experimental Design. Procedures for the Behavioural Sciences." Wadsworth Publishing Company, California, USA.

Klatsky, R.Z. (1980). "Human Memory." Freeman: San Francisco.

Koeppen, D. (1981). Clinical experience with clobazam 1968–1981. *Royal Society of Medicine International Congress Symposium Series* **43**, 193–198.

Paes de Sousa, M., Figuiera, M-L., Loureiro, F., and Hindmarch, I. (1981). Lorazepam and clobazam in anxious elderly patients. *Royal Society of Medicine International Congress and Symposium Series* **43**, 120–123.

Roth, T., Hartse, K.M., Saab, P.G., Piccione, P.M., and Kramer, M. (1980). The effects of flurazepam, lorazepam and triazolam on sleep and memory. *Psychopharmacology* **70**, 231.

Siegfried, K., Koeppen, D., Taeuber, K., Badian, M., Malercyzyk, V., and Sittig, W. (1981). A double-blind comparison of the acute effects of clobazam and lorazepam on memory and psychomotor functions. *Royal Society of Medicine International Congress and Symposium Series* **43**, 13–21.

Sternberg, S. (1969). Memory Scanning: Mental processes revealed by reaction time experiments. *American Scientist* **57**, 421–457.

Sternberg, S. (1975). Memory Scanning: New findings and current controversies. *Quarterly Journal of Experimental Psychology* **27**, 1–32.

Subhan, Z. (1981). A dose-range comparison of clobazam and diazepam: II. Effects on memory. *Royal Society of Medicine International Congress and Symposium Series* **43**, 7–12.

On Differences Between 1,5- and 1,4-Benzodiazepines: Pharmaco-EEG and Psychometric Studies with Clobazam and Lorazepam

B. SALETU, J. GRÜNBERGER, P. BERNER and D. KOEPPEN*

Section of Pharmacopsychiatry, Psychiatric University Clinic of Vienna, Vienna, Austria and
*Klinische forschung, Hoechst AG, D-6230 Frankfurt am Main 80, W Germany

Introduction

Ever since the introduction of benzodiazepines in the early 1960s, their therapeutic use has increased strikingly. Although this has been criticized as thoughtless overmedication, benzodiazepine treatment is today acknowledged as effective, safe and inexpensive (Greenblatt and Shader, 1978). One of the reasons for the high prescription rate is the broad spectrum of therapeutic action of benzodiazepines including anxiolytic, muscle-relaxant, sedative/hypnotic and anticonvulsive effects. On the other hand, relatively early efforts started to develop compounds with a more selective action in regard to these four different properties. For instance, it was thought to be useful to have daytime tranquilizers or anticonvulsants without pronounced sedative/hypnotic or muscle relaxant action. The different pharmacodynamic effects may be due to the degree of binding of benzodiazepines to different receptor subtypes (Schacht and Baecker, in preparation). As is known, in 1977 Braestrup and Squires and Möhler and Okada discovered the benzodiazepine receptors in the brain, which opened the possibility to explain the efficacy of benzodiazepines via binding to specific receptor sites of anxious patients who are supposed to have a lack of putitive endogenous ligands for these receptors. Furthermore, benzodiazepines differ also in regard to their action on other neurotransmitter systems, which may be related to their differing therapeutic effects. For example, a recent study showed that clobazam (a 1,5-benzodiazepine) was more active than diazepam (a 1,4-benzodiazepine) in reducing serotoninergic activity and less active in reducing catecholaminergic activity; while GABA-ergic activity was increased more by diazepam than by clobazam (Hsieh, 1982).

The present double-blind, placebo-controlled study focuses on pharmacodynamic differences between 1,4- and 1,5-benzodiazepines as evaluated by means of quantitative pharmaco-EEG and psychometric analyses (Saletu, 1976; Saletu and Grünberger, 1979; Saletu et al., 1981; Grünberger, 1977; Grünberger and Saletu, 1980)—with special reference to the amnestic effects. The latter have been described after 1,4-benzodiazepines mostly after intravenous or intramuscular administration in the field of anaesthesiology. However, Liljequist and Mattila (1979), McKay and Dundee (1980) and Wilson (1973) also showed amnestic effects after oral application. Since benzodiazepines are mainly prescribed as oral medication for anxious outpatients, the welcomed therapeutic amnestic effect in anaesthesia may turn into an unwanted side effect in ambulatory therapy. All amnestic effects have uniformly been reported on 1,4-benzodiazepines.

Clobazam is a 1,5-benzodiazepine. Previous studies have shown that clobazam does not, or only minimally, impair memory functions in animals (Hock and Kruse, 1982; Giurgea, in press) and humans (Siegfried et al., 1981; Subhan, 1981; Thompson and Trimble, 1981; Paes de Sousa et al., 1981). Furthermore, vigility and psychomotor functions have not been impaired at therapeutic doses of clobazam (Borland and Nicholson, 1974; Hindmarch and Gudgeon, 1980; Wittenborn et al., 1979). The objective of the following study was to compare the 1,5-benzodiazepine clobazam to a standard 1,4-benzodiazepine (lorazepam) at two dose levels with respect to their effects on the central nervous system (CNS) and vigilance (as determined by means of the computer-assisted spectral-analysed EEG), further on different aspects of human behaviour (including cognitive, amnestic, psychomotor and thymopsychic functions), as well as on the autonomic nervous system (ANS) and safety measures (including Romberg test variables).

Method

Subjects and medication

Ten healthy normal volunteers (5 males and 5 females) aged 21–30 years (mean 25 years), weighing 58–82 kg (mean 71 kg) and ranging in height from 163 to 182 cm (mean 175 cm) were included in the double-blind, placebo-controlled crossover study. In random order (Latin square design) they received single oral doses of placebo, 20 mg and 30 mg clobazam as well as 2 mg and 3 mg lorazepam, at weekly intervals. These acute benzodiazepine doses correspond to the daily dose prescription. The subjects were not allowed to take any psychoactive drug three weeks before and/or during the period of the study. They received small snacks at intervals of 2 h in order to avoid a decrease of vigilance induced by heavy meals. The study was performed in accordance with the Declaration of Helsinki as revised by the World Medical Assembly at Tokyo. An informed written consent was obtained.

Measurements and evaluations

Blood samplings, EEG recordings, psychometric tests and evaluation of blood pressure, pulse rate and side effects were carried out before as well as 2, 4, 6 and 8 h after oral drug administration (09:00 h).

a. Blood level determination

An indwelling catheter was placed in an antecubital vein and kept patent by a "saline heparin lock". Venous blood samples were collected in heparinized plastic tubes and immediately centrifuged. Thereafter, plasma was frozen and kept at −20°C until analysis by means of gas chromatography (Hajdu *et al.*, 1980). The major clobazam metabolite *N*-desmethylclobazam was also determined (sensitivity 0·018 ng/ml).

b. Quantitative EEG investigations

A 3 min vigilance-controlled EEG (V-EEG)

was recorded by means of an 8-channel Beckmann R-611 polygraph (high frequency response: 100 Hz; time constant: 0·3 s; frequency: 0·5–100 Hz) with the subjects lying relaxed with eyes closed in an electrically-shielded room. Electrodes were attached according to the international 10/20 system to the scalp. During the V-EEG recordings the technician tried to keep the subjects alert; as soon as drowsiness patterns appeared in the EEG the subjects were aroused by the technician. Four leads (01-Cz, 02-Cz, P3-Cz, P4-Cz) were recorded on a Hewlett-Packard 9068 tape recorder (cut-off frequency: 212 Hz; tape speed: 1 7/8 in/sec) and analysed off-line by an Intertechnique Plurimat S computer system utilizing power spectral density programs. The latter permits analysis of 5 s samples summarized to 20 s samples resulting in 38 measurements: the dominant frequency (in Hz), the relative (REL) and absolute (ABS) power of the dominant frequency; total power (T); the absolute and relative power in 13 different frequency bands. Further, the centre-of-gravity frequencies (centroids) (C) and their deviations (D) of the combined delta and theta (DT), alpha (A) and beta (B) bands as well as of the total activity (T). The sampling rate was 200 Hz. Each 20 s epoch with muscle movements or eye artifacts was excluded from statistical analysis.

c. *Psychometric tests* included the alphabetical cross-out test (AD-test = Alphabetischer Durchstreichtest) of Grünberger (1977) for evaluation of attention (total score), concentration (errors in percent of the total score) and the attention variability (difference between extreme scores); the psychomotor activity test (Feinmotoriktest) of Grünberger (1977) and tapping; the reaction time (in ms) as determined on the Viennese reaction-apparatus and the errors occurring in the test; complex reaction as assessed on the Wiener Determinationsgerät of Schuhfried; critical flicker frequency (CFF, descending threshold); the von Zerssen mood scale (von Zerssen Befindlichkeitsskala) (1970) for evaluation of mood; a semantic differential polarity profile for changes in affectivity; the Pauli test (total score and errors %) and microprocessor-assisted measurements of the pupillary diameter and skin conductance level (SCL) (Stöhr *et al.*, 1982). Mnestic tests included short-term memory (numerical memory) as well as long-term memory in regards to anterograde and retrograde amnesia. For the assessment of anterograde amnesia a word association test was used. The presentation of 10 word-groups took place 2 h after oral administration (at the expected time of maximum blood levels), while subjects were asked to recall at 4, 6 and 8 h. For the assessment of retrograde amnesia a card recognition test was utilized; the presentation was done before oral administration of the drug, while the recall took place 4, 6 and 8 h after oral administration.

d. *Safety data* included heart rate, blood pressure and the Romberg test. The latter included the evaluation of standing time with eyes closed for a period of up to 2 min; gait deviations (in cm) during walking on a given line of 10 m in length as well as gait speed as measured in seconds necessary to complete the 10 m walking distance on the aforementioned line.

Pulse rate, systolic and diastolic blood pressure (sitting position) and side effects were also evaluated.

e. *Statistical analyses* included MANOVA, 3-way ANOVA, the Newman-Keuls test, the *t*-test, Friedman's rank analysis of variance and the multiple Wilcoxon test.

Results

Blood levels

Determination of blood levels by means of gas chromatography demonstrated for the 2nd, 4th, 6th and 8th hour after 20 mg clobazam the following mean levels and standard deviations: 0·3111 (0·0626), 0·2297 (0·0618), 0·1964 (0·0399) and 0·1778 (0·0383) μg/ml, respectively; after 30 mg clobazam 0·3504 (0·1549), 0·3530 (0·0806), 0·2901 (0·0726), 0·2595 (0·0599) μg/ml, respectively; after 2 mg lorazepam 0·0161 (0·0036), 0·0161 (0·0048), 0·0147 (0·0046), 0·0199 (0·0032) μg/ml, respectively; after 3 mg lorazepam 0·0239 (0·0088), 0·0230 (0·0054), 0·0220 (0·0041) and 0·0260 (0·0106) μg/ml, respectively. Blood level peaks were reached after 20 mg clobazam in all but one subject in the 2nd hour (and in one subject in the 4th hour); after 30 mg clobazam in half of the subjects in the 2nd and 4th hours respectively; after 2 mg

lorazepam in half of the subjects in the 2nd and in the other half in the 4th hour; while 3 mg lorazepam peak plasma levels were seen in six out of ten subjects in the 2nd hour. Thus, blood levels showed in most of the subjects a fast rise and peak in the 2nd hour with only a slight decline until the 8th hour. No *N*-desmethylclobazam could be detected in the blood samples (sensitivity $\geqq 0·018$ μg/ml).

Pharmaco-EEG profiles

Two-way analyses of variance (ANOVA) demonstrated in 12, 10, 24 and 30 out of 38 computer-assisted, spectral-analysed EEG variables showed significant ($P < 0·05–0·01$) changes after 20 mg clobazam, 30 mg clobazam, 2 mg lorazepam and 3 mg lorazepam, respectively, while after placebo there was not even in one variable a significant alteration. Significant differences between the five substances were observed in 13, 20, 23 and 21 variables at 2, 4, 6 and 8 h after oral drug administration, respectively.

In detail, *20 mg clobazam* produced an increase in beta activity (especially in the 16–20 Hz band), a decrease of alpha activity, a slowing of the alpha centroid as well as an acceleration of the centroid of the total activity compared with placebo (Fig. 1). The alpha attenuation reached the level of statistical significance ($P < 0·05$, Newman-Keuls test). The beta augmentation was seen throughout the whole recording day and was significant in the 4th hour. The slowing of the alpha centroid reached the level of statistical significance in the 8th hour.

30 mg Clobazam induced the same type of changes as described above compared with placebo (Fig. 2). The beta augmentation was significant at any time, the alpha attenuation in the 2nd hour ($P < 0·05–0·01$, Newman-Keuls test). The acceleration of the centroid of the total activity reached the level of statistical significance in the 6th hour.

2 mg Lorazepam produced highly significant ($P < 0·05–0·01$, Newman-Keuls test) changes as compared with placebo, characterized by an increase of beta activity in all frequency ranges, decrease of alpha activity, and—indicating hypnotic/sedative properties of the drug—an increase of delta activity (Fig. 1). In addition, there was a slowing of the centroid of the combined delta and theta activity throughout the total recording ses-

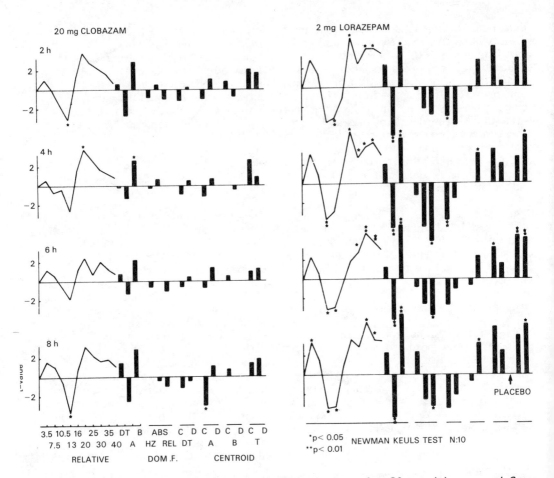

Figure 1. Computer-assisted spectral-analysed EEG changes after 20 mg clobazam and 2 mg lorazepam as compared with placebo (N:10). 38 computer EEG measurements are shown in the abscissae, differences between drug-induced and placebo-induced changes in these measurements are shown in the ordinate and expressed in terms of t-values. Placebo is represented in the 0 line. Both compounds produce an increase of beta activity, decrease of alpha activity, and an acceleration of the centroid of the total activity. However, only lorazepam augments delta activity and slows the centroid of the combined delta and theta activities.

sion, reaching the level of significance (Newman-Keuls test) in the 2nd and 4th hours. Further, there was an acceleration of the centroid of the beta activity as well as of the total activity (significant in the 6th hour). The deviation of the centroid of the total activity increased as well in the 4th to the 6th hour ($P < 0.05$–0.01, Newman-Keuls test). There was also a significant increase in the deviation of the alpha centroid in the 4th and in the 8th hour, while the relative power of the dominant frequency decreased significantly in the 4th through the 8th hour ($P < 0.05$).

3 mg Lorazepam induced, as compared with placebo, the same type of changes as 2 mg (Fig. 2). The beta augmentation was even more pronounced than after 2 mg as was the acceleration of the centroid of the total activity and the decrease of the centroid of the slow activity.

While both the 1,4- and the 1,5-benzodiazepine showed an anxiolytic profile characterized by an increase of beta activity, decrease of alpha activity and acceleration of the centroid of the total activity, slow activity was augmented markedly only by lorazepam—which indicates hypnogenic/sedative properties of this drug. The latter is also

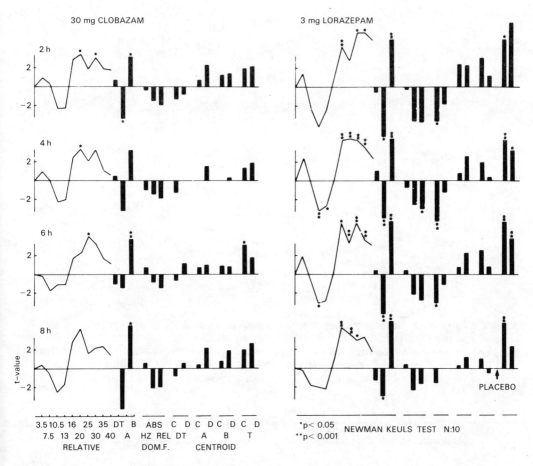

Figure 2. Computer-assisted spectral-analysed EEG changes after 30 mg clobazam and 3 mg lorazepam as compared with placebo (N:10).

reflected by changes in the *centroid of the combined delta and theta activity* (Fig. 3), which shows a trend towards an increase after placebo, no changes or only a slight decrease after 20 and 30 mg clobazam and a marked decrease after 2 mg and even a more marked decrease after 3 mg lorazepam. While clobazam does not differ significantly from placebo in regard to behaviour of slow activity, highly significant differences were observed between 2 and 3 mg lorazepam and placebo in the 2nd, 4th and 6th hours (Fig. 3). Moreover, both doses of clobazam differed significantly from both doses of lorazepam in regard to the combined delta and theta activity.

Dose/treatment and time-efficacy relations based on EEG changes

Dose/treatment efficacy calculations based on the Friedman's rank ANOVA and multiple Wilcoxon test of sign-free changes in all EEG variables demonstrated 3 mg lorazepam as the most CNS-effective compound followed by 2 mg lorazepam, 30 mg clobazam, 20 mg clobazam, while the least changes were observed after placebo (Table 1). Both active compounds differed from placebo as well as from each other (Table 1).

Time-efficacy relations based on the Friedman's rank ANOVA and multiple Wilcoxon test considering sign-free placebo-corrected

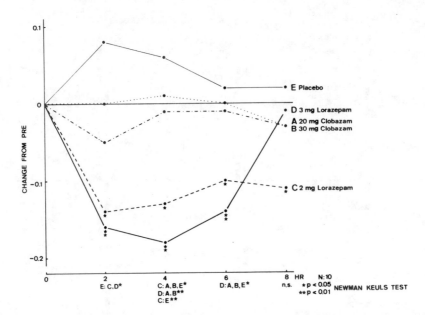

Figure 3. Changes in the centroid of the combined delta and theta activity after clobazam, lorazepam and placebo (N:10). Time is shown in the abscissa, changes of the centroid of the slow activity as compared with baseline are indicated in the ordinate. A significant slowing of the centroid is dose-dependently observed after lorazepam, while clobazam and placebo induce only minimal changes or even a slight acceleration.

Table 1

Means and standard deviations of blood levels after clobazam and lorazepam
(µg/ml)

Time-efficacy

Dose \ Time (h)	2	4	6	8	χ^2_{FR}	Multiple Wilcoxon
A 20 mg clobazam	89·5	74	73	63·5	6·95	2:8**
B 30 mg clobazam	106·5	59	68·5	66	27·43**	2:4,6,8**
C 2 mg lorazepam	93	65	79	63	11·68**	2:4,8**
D 3 mg lorazepam	85·5	90	70·5	54	15·93**	2:6,* 2:8,** 4:8**

Dose/treatment-efficacy

Time (h) \ Dose	A 20 mg clobazam	B 30 mg clobazam	C 2 mg lorazepam	D 3 mg lorazepam	E Placebo	χ^2_{FR}	Multiple Wilcoxon
2	70·5	96·5	108·5	122	52·5	42·6**	A:B,* B,D:E,** B:D* A,E:C,** A:D**
4	65·5	81·5	119·5	129	54·5	57·65**	A,B:C,** B,C,D:E** A,B:D**
6	73	75	123·5	122·5	57	50·83**	A,B:D,** C,D:E,** A,B:D**
8	78·5	84	122	119	46·5	52·34**	A,B:C,** A,B,C,D:E,** A,B:D**

* P < 0·05; ** P < 0·01.

changes in all EEG variables showed the most pronounced and encephalotropic effects of both compounds in the 2nd or 4th hours (Table 1).

Psychometric findings

a. *Attention*
Attention as evaluated by means of the alphabetical cross-out test of Grünberger demonstrated highly significant inter-drug differences in the 3-way ANOVA ($F_c = 25 \cdot 13$, $P < 0 \cdot 01$) (Fig. 4). Detailed analysis of changes after each single substance demonstrated after placebo and 20 mg clobazam no signifi-

and in the 8th hour than all but 30 mg clobazam (Fig, 4). Both lorazepam doses were significantly different from placebo as was 30 mg clobazam, but not 20 mg clobazam.

b. *Concentration*
Concentration as evaluated by means of the percentage of errors in the alphabetical cross-out test of Grünberger (1977) demonstrated highly significant inter-drug differences in the 3-way ANOVA ($F_c = 19 \cdot 55$, $P < 0 \cdot 01$) (Fig. 5). While after placebo and the two clobazam doses a trend towards an improvement was seen in concentration, a marked and signifi-cant (4th and 6th hours) increase of errors

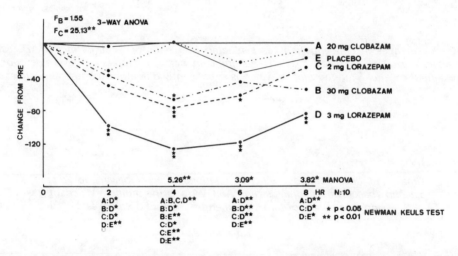

Figure 4. Changes in attention (as evaluated by means of the total score in the AD-test of Grünberger) after clobazam, lorazepam and placebo (N:10). Time is shown in the abscissa, changes in attention are indicated in the ordinate. While after placebo and 20 mg clobazam no changes occurred, there was a slight decrease in attention after 30 mg clobazam, while a marked and highly significant decrease occurred after 2 mg and especially after 3 mg lorazepam.

cant alterations in attention. After 30 mg clobazam attention declined significantly in the 4th hour, after 2 mg lorazepam in the 4th and 6th hours and after 3 mg lorazepam from the 2nd throughout the 8th hour ($P < 0 \cdot 05$–$0 \cdot 01$, Newman-Keuls test). Analysis of the inter-drug differences by means of the MANOVA showed significant F values in the 4th, 6th and 8th hours. A detailed analysis of the inter-drug differences by means of the Newman-Keuls test revealed that 3 mg lorazepam induced a significantly greater deterioration in attention than all the other substances in the 2nd through the 6th hour

was observed after 3 mg lorazepam ($P < 0 \cdot 05$–$0 \cdot 01$, Newman-Keuls test). 3 mg Lorazepam was thus also significantly different from all of the other substances in the 4th and 6th hours as well as from the other three active substances in the 8th hour (Fig. 5).

c. *Attention variability*
Attention variability, as measured by means of the differences between the extreme scores in the AD-test of Grünberger (1977), showed in the 3-way ANOVA significant ($P < 0 \cdot 01$) changes over time as well as significant inter-drug differences (Table 2). While there was a

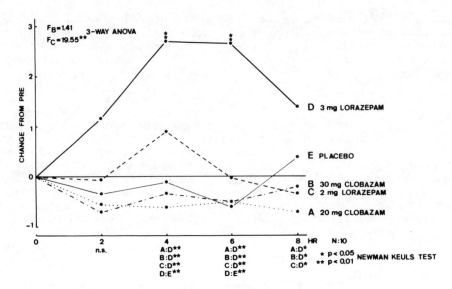

Figure 5. Changes in concentration (as evaluated by means of % errors in the AD-test) after clobazam, lorazepam and placebo (N:10). A significant increase of errors suggests a deterioration in concentration after 3 mg lorazepam, which is significantly different from the other substances.

Table 2

Time- and dose/treatment efficacy relations after clobazam, lorazepam and placebo (based on Friedman's rank ANOVA and the multiple Wilcoxon test of sign-free, placebo-corrected changes in all EEG variables; N:10)

Time-efficacy

Dose \ Time (h)	2	4	6	8	χ^2_{FR}	Multiple Wilcoxon
A 20 mg clobazam	33·5	42·5	42·5	41·5	2·14	n.s.
B 30 mg clobazam	42·5	36·5	44	37	1·63	n.s.
C 2 mg lorazepam	34	50	46	30	10·2	4:8*
D 3 mg lorazepam	31·5	62	43·5	33	10·41	2:4,* 4:8*
E placebo	41·5	38·5	37	43	0·84	n.s.

Dose/Treatment-efficacy

Time (h) \ Dose	A 20 mg clobazam	B 30 mg clobazam	C 2 mg lorazepam	D 3 mg lorazepam	E Placebo	χ^2_{FR}	Multiple Wilcoxon
2	36·5	46	52	63	42·5	10·19	A:D*
4	38·5	30·5	61	69·5	40·5	27·1	B:C,** A:D** B:D,** D:E*
6	33·5	44	54·5	67·5	40·5	17·6	A:D,** D:E*
8	43	46	44	66	44	16·82	n.s.

*P < 0.05, **P < 0.01.

trend towards a decrease in attention variability or only minimal changes after placebo, 20 and 30 mg clobazam as compared with baseline, an increase was seen after lorazepam, and significantly so in the 6th hour after 3 mg of this drug ($P < 0.05$). 3 mg Lorazepam was at that time also significantly inferior to placebo (Table 2) as well as to 20 mg clobazam ($P < 0.05-0.01$, Newman-Keuls test).

d. Tapping

Tapping demonstrated in the 3-way ANOVA significant inter-drug differences ($F_c = 14.6$, $P < 0.01$) (Fig. 6). While after 2 mg and especially after 3 mg lorazepam a decrease in motor speed was observed (significant in the 6th hour), no changes occurred after placebo and 30 mg clobazam, while after 20 mg clobazam improvement of motor speed was observed (Fig. 6). Inter-drug comparison by means of the Newman-Keuls test demonstrated that 20 and 30 mg clobazam were significantly superior to 2 and 3 mg lorazepam (Fig. 6). 3 mg Lorazepam were of course also significantly different from placebo in the 2nd hour.

e. Psychomotor activity

Psychomotor activity as determined by means of the FM test of Grünberger (1977) showed significant inter-drug differences in the 3-way ANNOVA ($F_c = 11.26$, $P < 0.01$). Both doses of lorazepam induced a deterioration of psychomotor activity, which reached the level of statistical significance in the 2nd, 4th and 6th hours after the higher doses ($P < 0.05-0.01$, Newman-Keuls test) as compared with pretreatment, while no changes or even a slight improvement was seen after placebo and the two clobazam doses. 3 mg Clobazam was significantly different from placebo (Table 2) as well as from clobazam (Table 3).

f. Reaction time

Reaction time as determined by means of the Viennese Reaktionsapparatus did not show any significant alterations over time in the single substances, nor were there any inter-drug differences ($P < 0.05$, Newman-Keuls test).

However, evaluation of errors in this test showed a marked inter-drug difference both in the 3-way ANOVA ($F_c = 13.97$, $P < 0.01$) as well as in the MANOVA. The latter exhibited significant F values in the 2nd, 4th and 8th hours (Fig. 7). This was due to the fact

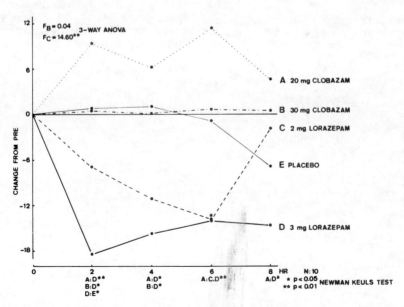

Figure 6. Changes in tapping after clobazam, lorazepam and placebo (N:10). Tapping improves after 20 mg clobazam but does not show any relevant changes after 30 mg clobazam and placebo and shows a slowing after 2 mg and especially after 3 mg lorazepam.

Table 3

Significant psychometric changes after cloba-
zam and lorazepam as compared with placebo
(N:10)

	Clobazam 20 mg	Clobazam 30 mg	Lorazepam 2 mg	Lorazepam 3 mg
Attention (AD test/total score)	ø	↓↓	↓↓	↓↓
Concentration (AD test/errors)	ø	ø	ø	↑↑
Attention/variability (AD test)	*	*	*	↑↑
Psychomotor activity	*	*	*	↓↓
Tapping	ø	ø	ø	↓
Reaction time	ø	ø	ø	ø
Reaction accuracy (errors)	ø	ø	↑↑	↑↑
Complex reaction	ø	ø	ø	ø
CFF	ø	ø	ø	↓↓
(PAULI test/total score)	ø	ø	ø	↓↓
(PAULI test/errors)	ø	ø	ø	ø
Mood (Bf-S)	ø	ø	↓↓	ø
Affectivity (semantic differential)	ø	ø	ø	ø
Skin conductance	ø	ø	↑	ø
Pupil size	↑	↑	↑↑	↑↑
Short-term memory (numerical)	ø	ø	ø	ø
Anterograde amnesia (verbal)	ø	↑	ø	↓
Retrograde amnesia (visual)	ø	ø	ø	ø

↓ = decrease $P < 0.05$ ↑ = increase $P < 0.05$
↓↓ = decrease $P < 0.01$ ↑↑ = increase $P < 0.01$
ø = no significant difference

that an increase in errors was observed after both lorazepam doses, while no changes or a decrease was observed after clobazam and placebo. Thus, based on the Newman-Keuls test 2 and 3 mg lorazepam were significantly different from placebo, as well as from clobazam.

g. *Complex reaction*

Complex reaction as determined by means of the Viennese Determinationsgerät of Schuhfried showed significant inter-drug differences in the 3-way ANOVA ($F_c = 10.54$, $P < 0.01$). MANOVA pointed out that the most significant differences were in the 6th and 8th hours. The latter was due to the fact that after 20 mg clobazam complex reaction improved, after 30 mg clobazam and placebo only minimal changes occurred, while after 2 mg and especially after 3 mg lorazepam (and significantly so in the 6th hour) a deterioration occurred. Thus, the latter dose was significantly inferior to 20 mg clobazam in the 4th hour throughout the 8th hour, in the 6th hour from both clobazam doses and in the 8th hour also from 2 mg lorazepam.

h. *Critical flicker frequency (CFF)*

Critical flicker frequency showed significant changes over time in the 3-way ANOVA ($F_c = 3.19$, $P < 0.05$). Analysis of each drug separately demonstrated only after 3 mg lorazepam in the 4th hour a significant decrease in CFF as compared with baseline (Fig. 9). Thus, 3 mg lorazepam significantly differed

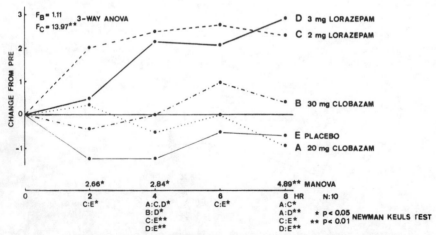

Figure 7. Changes in errors during the reaction time task after clobazam, lorazepam and placebo (N:10). In contrast to clobazam and placebo, lorazepam induces an increase of errors.

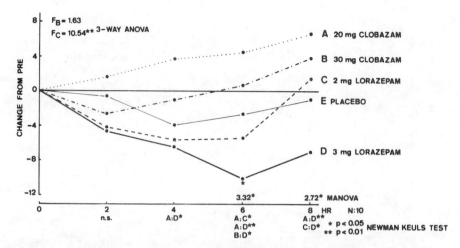

Figure 8. Changes in complex reaction as determined by the Viennese Determinationsgerät after clobazam, lorazepam and placebo (N:10). 20 mg clobazam tends to improve complex reaction; only minimal changes occur after 30 mg clobazam and placebo; while after lorazepam a dose-dependent deterioration may be observed.

from placebo, as well as 2 mg lorazepam and 30 mg clobazam at that time.

i. *Pauli test*

The total score (e.g. total sum of digit additions) in the Pauli test demonstrated in the 3-way ANOVA significant inter-drug differences ($F_c = 20.55$, $P < 0.01$). MANOVA showed that these differences were most pronounced in the 4th and 6th hours (Fig. 10). 3 mg Lorazepam produced a significant

deterioration of performance in the Pauli test, while this did not happen after the other substances. Thus, 3 mg lorazepam was also significantly different from all the other substances between the 2nd and 6th hours (except 2 mg lorazepam in the 4th hour). In the 8th hour the drug was significantly different from 30 mg clobazam (which actually showed an improvement in performance).

Errors in the Pauli test did not exhibit any significant differences between active drugs

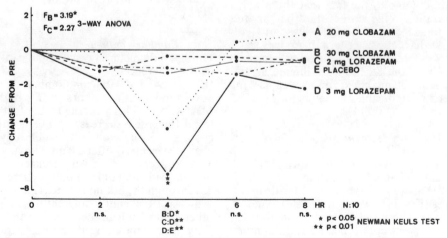

Figure 9. Changes in critical flicker frequency (descendent threshold) after clobazam, lorazepam and placebo (N:10). A significant decrease in CFF occurred only in the 4th hour after 3 mg lorazepam.

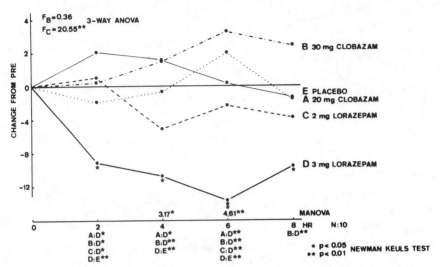

Figure 10. Changes in the Pauli test (total number of calculations) after clobazam, lorazepam and placebo (N:10). 3 mg lorazepam produced a significant deterioration of performance in the Pauli test.

and placebo based on the Newman-Keuls test. The only inter-drug difference was observed between 3 mg lorazepam and 20 mg clobazam.

j. *Well feeling (von Zerssen score)*
The von Zerssen score reflecting the subjectively experienced feeling of well-being demonstrated significant inter-drug differences in the 3-way ANOVA ($F_c = 8.09$, $P < 0.01$). This was largely due to the fact that there was a deterioration in the score in the 4th hour after 2 mg lorazepam ($P < 0.01$, Newman-Keuls test). At that time 2 mg lorazepam was significantly different from all the other substances, while in the 8th hour it differed significantly from 30 mg clobazam as well as 3 mg lorazepam (inducing a trend towards an improvement) (Fig. 11).

k. *Affectivity (semantic differential polarity profile)*
Affectivity showed in the 3-way ANOVA significant changes over time ($F_b = 5.81$, $P < 0.01$) as well as significant inter-drug differences ($F_c = 3.89$, $P < 0.01$ (Tables 2 and 3). Affectivity deteriorated over time in all treatment groups except in the 2nd and 8th hours after 30 mg clobazam and significantly so in the 4th and 6th hours after 2 mg lorazepam. At the latter hour this deterioration was

significantly more pronounced after 2 mg lorazepam than 20 mg clobazam.

l. *Skin conductance level (SCL)*
Skin conductance did not show any significant changes over time nor significant inter-drug differences in the 3-way ANOVA. Only in the 4th hour was the increase of the SCL after 2 mg lorazepam significantly more pronounced than after all the other substances (Table 2).

m. *Pupillary diameter*
Pupillary diameter showed significant inter-drug differences in the 3-way ANOVA ($F_c = 16.34$, $P < 0.01$), predominantly in the 4th and 6th hours ($P < 0.05$–0.01, MANOVA). This was due to the fact that a trend towards a decrease was seen after placebo and 30 mg clobazam, while only small changes occurred after 20 mg clobazam and 3 mg lorazepam; after 2 mg lorazepam a significant widening of the pupil occurred in the 4th through the 8th hour (Fig. 12). Thus, this drug was significantly different from all of the other compounds in the 6th hour and all but 3 mg lorazepam in the 4th hour. At that time there was also a significant difference between placebo and lorazepam. In the 8th hour placebo was significantly different (inducing a

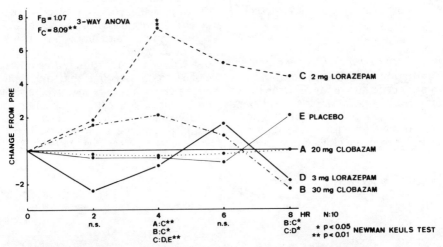

Figure 11. Changes in subjectively experienced well-being as evaluated by means of the von Zerssen score after clobazam, lorazepam and placebo (N:10). A deterioration occurs in the von Zerssen score, especially in the 4th hour after 2 mg lorazepam.

decrease in pupillary diameter) from all of the other substances.

n. *Short-term memory*
Short-term memory as evaluated by the numerical memory test (Grünberger, 1977) demonstrated in the 3-way ANOVA significant changes over time ($F_c = 4\cdot56$, $P < 0\cdot01$). Short-term memory declined over the record-

ing day after all 5 substances and significantly so in the 6th hour after 3 mg lorazepam. However, there were no inter-drug differences (Tables 2 and 3).

o. *Long-term memory/retrograde amnesia*
A card recognition test was presented before drug intake. The recall sessions at 4, 6 and 8 h did not show any significant differences

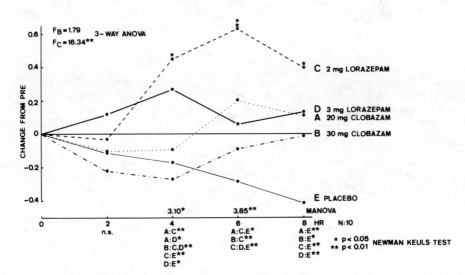

Figure 12. Changes in pupillary diameter after clobazam, lorazepam and placebo (N:12). A trend towards a decrease in pupillary diameter was seen after placebo, a significant increase occurred after 2 mg lorazepam.

between the active substances and placebo nor between the active substances themselves (Fig. 13).

p. *Longer-term memory/anterograde amnesia*
Word associations were presented to the subjects 2 h after drug intake (at the anticipated and confirmed time of peak blood levels). At the time of recall in the 4th, 6th and 8th hours lorazepam demonstrated a deterioration in this memory task, while clobazam showed an

psychotropic effects between the two active drugs and placebo as well as between two corresponding doses of the 1,4 and 1,5-benzodiazepine are summarized in Tables 2 and 3. The comparison of placebo versus drug showed significant differences after 20 mg clobazam in one variable only, and after 30 mg clobazam only in three variables (out of 18 variables), while after 2 mg and 3 mg lorazepam significant differences as compared to placebo were observed in five and ten variables, respectively (Table 2).

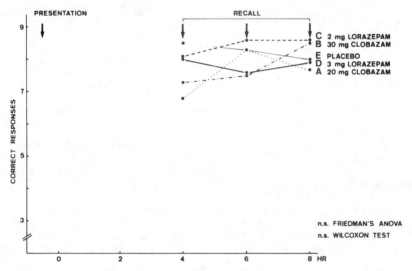

Figure 13. Mnestic changes regarding retrograde amnesia after clobazam, lorazepam and placebo (N:10). No significant differences can be observed between the five substances regarding retrograde amnesia.

improvement as compared with placebo. Inter-drug comparison by means of Friedman's ANOVA and multiple Wilcoxon test demonstrated in the 4th hour 3 mg lorazepam significantly inferior to placebo and 20 mg clobazam, in the 6th hour significantly inferior to placebo and 20 mg clobazam, while in the 8th hour it was statistically inferior to both clobazam doses (Fig. 14). At that time 30 mg clobazam was also significantly superior to placebo.

Dose treatment and time-efficacy relations based on psychometric changes

Pharmacodynamic differences in regard to

Table 3 demonstrates differences between two corresponding doses of clobazam and lorazepam. 2 mg Lorazepam differed significantly from 20 mg clobazam with respect to impairment of psychomotor and cognitive functions. The differences were seen in attention, reaction accuracy, tapping, complex reaction, pupillary diameter, skin conductance and mood alterations. 3 mg Lorazepam showed even more significant differences to the parallel dose of clobazam (30 mg) and led to significant impairment of psychomotor and cognitive functions (including attention, reaction accuracy, psychomotor activity, tapping, complex reaction, CFF, Pauli test) as compared with 30 mg clobazam. Anterograde amnesia was induced by 3 mg lorazepam in contrast to 30 mg clobazam. Pupil size

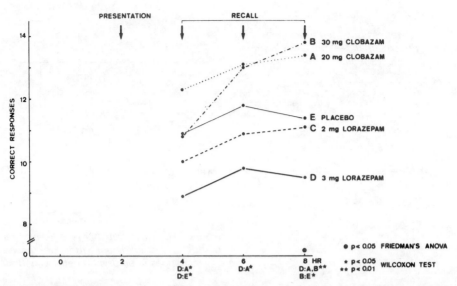

Figure 14. Mnestic changes regarding anterograde amnesia after clobazam, lorazepam and placebo (N:10). While lorazepam produced a dose-dependent increase in anterograde amnesia, improvement was seen after clobazam which reached the level of statistical significance as compared with placebo after 30 mg clobazam.

and mood changed significantly more with lorazepam than with 30 mg clobazam.

Dose/treatment efficacy calculations by means of the Friedman's rank ANOVA and multiple Wilcoxon test based on 16 psychometric variables (measured at all times) demonstrated in the 2nd throughout the 8th hours 3 mg lorazepam to be the most psychoactive substance followed by 2 mg lorazepam, 30 mg clobazam, placebo and 20 mg clobazam (Table 4). In the 2nd hour, 3 mg lorazepam differed significantly from 20 mg clobazam; in the 4th hour 3 mg lorazepam differed significantly from all the other substances; in the 6th hour 3 mg lorazepam was significantly different from placebo and 20 mg clobazam.

Figure 15 demonstrates a dose-efficacy relation based on discriminant function analyses of changes in all 16 psychometric variables at all time periods. As can be seen, the largest distance from placebo was observed after 3 mg lorazepam followed by 2 mg lorazepam and 30 mg clobazam, while 20 mg clobazam induced changes even in the opposite direction. Indeed, as one recalls alterations in single variables, there was a trend towards an improvement after low doses of clobazam in several measures, while deterioration occurred in the other substances. 3 mg Lorazepam differed overall significantly not only from placebo but also from 20 and 30 mg clobazam.

Time-efficacy calculations showed after clobazam no significant differences between the four recording periods, while after 2 and 3 mg clobazam the peak psychotropic effect was observed in the 4th hour (Table 4).

Tolerability and safety

Heart rate and blood pressure did not show any clinically relevant changes after five substances. From the statistical point of view there were significant inter-drug differences in heart rate ($F_c = 8.49$, $P < 0.01$), which were due to the fact that in the 2nd hour 3 mg lorazepam (inducing an increase in pulse rate by 6.5 beats/min) differed from all the other substances (inducing no changes). In the 6th hour similar findings were observed except that there were no significant differences as compared with placebo.

Systolic blood pressure demonstrated in the 2nd hour a significant inter-drug difference in the Newman-Keuls test between placebo (inducing an increase by 4.5 mm/Hg) as com-

Table 4

Significant differences between lorazepam- and clobazam-induced changes in psychometric variables

Variable	Cloba-zam vs. 20 mg	Loraze-pam 2 mg	Cloba-zam vs. 30 mg	Loraze-pam 3 mg
Attention (AD test/total score)		↓↓		↓↓
Concentration (AD test/errors)				↑↑
Attention/variability (AD test)				
Psychomotor activity				↓↓
Tapping		↓↓		↓
Reaction time				
Reaction accuracy (errors)		↑		↑
Complex reaction		↓		↓
CFF				↓
(PAULI test/total score)				↓↓
(PAULI test/errors)				
Mood (BF-S)		↓↓		↓
Affectivity (semantic differential)		↓		
Skin conductance		↑		
Pupil size		↑↑		↑↑
Short-term memory (numerical)				
Anterograde amnesia (verbal)				↓↓
Retrograde amnesia (visual)				

↓ = decrease $P < 0.05$ ↑ = $P < 0.05$
↓↓ = decrease $P < 0.01$ ↑↑ = increase $P < 0.01$

pared with 20 mg and 30 mg clobazam (inducing a decrease of 5 and 4 mm/Hg, respectively). Similarly, in *diastolic blood pressure*, placebo (inducing an increase by 7·5 mm/Hg) differed significantly from 20 mg clobazam (inducing an increase only by 1 mm/Hg), and in the 8th hour 2 mg lorazepam differed from placebo due to the fact that after 2 mg lorazepam blood pressure decreased slightly, while after placebo it slightly increased.

Side-effects were reported in one out of ten subjects after placebo, by four subjects each after 20 and 30 mg clobazam, as well as by five and six subjects after 2 and 3 mg lorazepam, respectively (Table 5). The main side-effect was drowsiness which was observed in one subject after placebo, in three subjects after 20 mg clobazam, in four subjects after

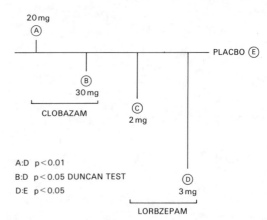

Figure 15. Dose/treatment efficacy relations based on discriminant function analysis of changes in all psychometric variables.

30 mg clobazam, in six subjects after 2 mg lorazepam and in seven subjects after 3 mg lorazepam. Corresponding to the memory test results, one subject complained about memory disturbances on the evening after intake of 3 mg lorazepam.

The *Romberg test* was performed to evaluate objectively and quantitatively drug-induced ataxia. Three measures were obtained—the standing time (with a maximal observation period of 2 min), gait speed and gait accuracy in walking a line of 10 m length.

Standing time (evaluated in seconds) demonstrated significant changes over time ($F_b = 4·46$, $P < 0·01$) as well as significant inter-drug differences ($F_c = 16·09$, $P < 0·01$). There was a dose-dependent decrease of standing time after both compounds but significantly so in the 2nd and 4th hours after 3 mg lorazepam ($P < 0·01$). At that time the highest dosage of lorazepam was also statistically significantly different from the other compounds. In the 6th hour 3 mg lorazepam were still significantly inferior to 2 mg lorazepam (Fig. 16).

Gait speed showed significant changes over time ($F_b = 5·1$) as well as significant inter-drug differences ($F_c = 12·4$, $P < 0·01$). There was a slight but significant increase in gait speed after placebo as well as after 30 mg clobazam (Table 6). On the other hand, a slowing of gait speed was observed after 3 mg lorazepam, so that this dosage differed from placebo at all times, and in addition in the 4th and 6th hours from 30 mg clobazam. In the

Table 5

Side effects after placebo, 20 mg and 30 mg clobazam and 2 and 3 mg lorazepam

Treatment group	Subject no.	Hour post R_x	Side effect	Severity
Placebo	9	2–4	Drowsiness	Light
20 mg Clobazam	7	2	Dizziness	Light
	8	1	Drowsiness	Light
	3	2	Drowsiness	Light
	6	2	Drowsiness	Moderate
		2	Dizziness	Light
30 mg Clobazam	6	0·5	Feeling of heaviness	Moderate
		0·5	Coordination problems	Moderate
		2	Drowsiness	Light
	7	2	Drowsiness	Light
	9	2	Drowsiness	Light
	10	2	Drowsiness	Light
2 mg Lorazepam	1	3	Sensation of coldness	Moderate
		3	Vertigo	Moderate
		4	Drowsiness	Moderate
		4	Vertigo	Moderate
		5	Drowsiness	Light
	3	6	Drowsiness	Moderate
	4	2	Drowsiness	Moderate
		2	Headaches	Moderate
		2	Vertigo	Moderate
		4	Drowsiness	Moderate
		4	Vertigo	Moderate
		6	Drowsiness	Moderate
		6	Vertigo	Moderate
	6	1	Drowsiness	Moderate
	6	1	Dizziness	Light
	7	4	Drowsiness	Severe
3 mg Lorazepam	1	2	Vertigo	Severe
		2	Drowsiness	Moderate
		6	Vertigo	Moderate
		6	Drowsiness	Moderate
	2	Test day evening	Memory disturbances	—
	4	0·5	Vertigo	Severe
		0·5	Sensation of coldness	Moderate
		0·5	Drowsiness	Severe
		4	Drowsiness	Moderate
		6	Drowsiness	Light
	6	2	Drowsiness	Light
	7	2	Drowsiness	Severe
	7	2	Drowsiness	Severe
		2	Dizziness	Moderate
		6	Euphoric feeling	Moderate

8th hour also 20 mg clobazam was significantly different from placebo.

Gait deviations measured in centimetres from the test line showed significant inter-drug differences ($F_c = 15·7$, $P < 0·01$), which was largely due to the fact that in the 2nd and 4th hours gait deviation increased markedly after 3 mg lorazepam (Table 6). Thus, this drug differed in the 4th hour from all of the other substances, in the 2nd hour from 20 mg clobazam, 2 mg lorazepam and placebo, while in the 6th hour it differed from placebo

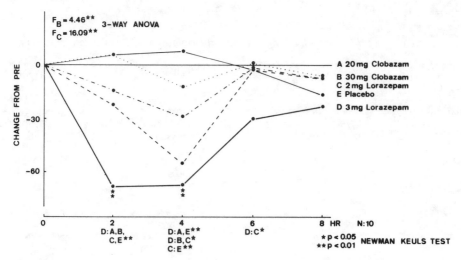

Figure 16. Changes in the Romberg test (standing time in seconds) after clobazam, lorazepam and placebo (N:10). 3 mg Lorazepam significantly shortened the standing time in the Romberg test.

Table 6

Changes in the Romberg test (gait speed in seconds) and deviations from the test
line (cm) after clobazam, lorazepam and placebo in ten normals

Gait speed (s)
$F_{time}=5.1$ $(P<0.01)$; $F_{drugs}=12.4$ $(P<0.01)$; 3-way ANOVA

Dose	Time (h) Baseline	2	4	6	8
A 20 mg Clobazam	8·4 (2·9)	0·5	−0·3	−0·6	−0·3
B 30 mg Clobazam	10·4 (3·2)	0	−1·8	−2·0	−2·5*
C 2 mg Lorazepam	10·1 (3·9)	−0·5	−1·3	−0·7	−1·7
D 3 mg Lorazepam	9·3 (2·4)	+0·9	+1·2	+0·5	−0·2
E Placebo	11·2 (6·4)	−1·5	−1·5	−2·4	−2·8*
		D:E**	D:E,B*	D:E,B*	E:A,D*

Gait speed (cm)
$F_{time}=2.5$ (n.s.); $F_{drugs}=5.7$ $(P<0.01)$; 3-way ANOVA

Dose	Time (h) Baseline	2	4	6	8
A 20 mg Clobazam	22·5 (12·7)	−6	0	−6	−1·5
B 30 mg Clobazam	21 (12·6)	12·5	−0·5	0	+3·0
C 2 mg Lorazepam	25·8 (27)	9·2	−4·3	−10·8	−8·8
D 3 mg Lorazepam	15 (10)	16·5*	16·5*	8·7	7·5
E Placebo	28·5 (17·4)	−6	3	−10·5	−1·5
		A:B,D**	D:A,B,E*	D:A*	n.s.
		B:C,E**	D:C**	D:C,E**	
		C:D**			
		D:E**			

*P<0.05; **P<0.01.
Newman Keuls

as well as 20 mg clobazam and 2 mg loraze-pam.

Discussion

Our double-blind, placebo-controlled trials demonstrated clear pharmacodynamic differences between two comparable doses of the 1,4-benzodiazepine lorazepam and the new 1,5-benzodiazepine clobazam based on neurophysiological, psychometric and tolerability/safety data.

Quantitative pharmaco-EEG investigations showed after both clobazam and lorazepam significant alterations in human brain function as compared with placebo, which were characterized by an increase of beta activity (especially in the middle fast frequency bands), decrease of alpha activity and acceleration of the centroid of the total activity. These changes have been described by us and other investigators as typical for anxiolytic drugs (Fink, 1969; Itil, 1974; Saletu, 1976; Saletu et al., 1981). However, differences were recorded in regard to slow delta activity: while there were no significant changes after clobazam, lorazepam produced a consistent and systematic increase of delta activity and a slowing of the centroid of the combined delta and theta activity indicating additional sedative/hypnotic properties. Dose/treatment efficacy calculations considering changes in all EEG variables demonstrated that 3 mg lorazepam produced the most encephalotropic effect followed by 2 mg lorazepam and 30 and 20 mg clobazam, while after placebo the least changes occurred. Time-efficacy calculations showed after both compounds the peak encephalotropic effect between the 2nd and 4th hours, which was in accordance with the blood level course.

Our psychometric investigations demonstrated further differential pharmacodynamic effects of the two drugs in regard to psychic functions: 20 and 30 mg clobazam induced only in one and three (out of 18) psychometric variables significant changes as compared with placebo, 2 and 3 mg lorazepam did so in five and ten variables, respectively. While after 20 mg clobazam only an increase in pupillary diameter was observed, 2 mg lorazepam induced a deterioration of attention, accuracy in a reaction task, mood and increased skin conductance and pupil size.

Even more marked were the differences between the two higher doses: while after 30 mg clobazam only a decrease in attention, an increase in pupil size and an improvement in mnestic performance occurred, 3 mg lorazepam produced a deterioration in attention, concentration, attention variability, psychomotor activity, tapping, accuracy in reaction, task performance and the Pauli test, decrease in critical flicker frequency, increase in pupil size as well as deterioration in verbal memory as compared with placebo. Significant differences, however, were also observed in the direct comparison between the two low doses and the two high doses of both benzodiazepines: 2 mg lorazepam produced a significantly more pronounced decrease in attention, tapping, reaction accuracy, complex reaction, mood and affectivity as well as a greater increase in skin conductance and pupillary size than 20 mg clobazam. Similarly, 3 mg lorazepam produced significantly greater deterioration in attention concentration, psychomotor, activity, tapping, reaction accuracy, complex reaction, performance in the Pauli test and mood, and furthermore a greater decrease in critical flicker frequency than 30 mg clobazam. The latter drug was also significantly superior to 3 mg lorazepam in regard to anterograde amnesia. Our findings confirmed earlier investigations indicating that, although the 1,5-benzodiazepine clobazam exhibits anxiolytic qualities like the 1,4-benzodiazepines (Hunt et al., 1974; Coste-Simonin and Krantz, 1975; Cottin et al., 1975; Martin, 1975), clobazam has no detrimental effects on psychomotor performance and on car driving behaviour (Berry et al., 1974; Borland and Nicholson, 1974; Hindmarch et al., 1977; Hindmarch and Gudgeon, 1980).

Our present psychometric findings corroberate our neurophysiological results suggesting that the 1,5-benzodiazepine clobazam exerts less sedative effects and impairs less vigilance than the 1,4-benzodiazepine lorazepam if one compares doses used in daily prescriptions. This does not of course exclude the possibility that exceedingly high doses would not induce some sedation, nor does it say that this is a typical difference between all 1,5- and 1,4-benzodiazepines, as clinical experience with the former is still limited to clobazam. On the other hand, the class of 1,4-benzodiazepines includes both substances with pronounced (as for instance flunitrazepam, brotizolam, flurazepam) and only light sedative effects (as for instance prazepam) (Saletu *et al.*, 1981, 1983). Moreover, as can be repeatedly shown, the encephalotropic and psychotropic effects of these drugs are very much dependent both on the dosage and the baseline arousal. While high doses of anxiolytic sedatives like brotizolam, lopirazepam, etc. produce a deterioration of performance in normal volunteers, low doses induce improvement while medium doses fall in between (Saletu and Grünberger, 1979; Grunberger *et al.*, 1978). The baseline CNS arousal plays a further important role: for instance, 10 mg of the same compound lopirazepam in both a normal and an anxiety population produced an "anxiolytic" pharmaco-EEG profile, but only the normals exhibited an augmentation of delta and theta activity indicating sedation (Saletu *et al.*, 1979). This was also pointed out by Hindmarch (1979) who investigated the effects of an acute dose of 20 mg clobazam on complex psychomotor behaviour with respect to anxiety of the individual subjects and found a U-shaped relationship. Subjects with high anxiety demonstrated poor performance; when the anxiety is reduced by a drug they move towards the bell of the curve with the performance improving accordingly. Normal subjects on the other hand receiving anxiety-reducing drugs are expected to show a performance impairment, as Malpas *et al.* (1974) postulated, because they would move to the lower (impairment) part of the curve.

A further interesting difference between the 1,5-benzodiazepine clobazam and the 1,4-benzodiazepine lorazepam was in regard to mnestic functioning: while the short-term memory, but also the long-term memory in regard to retrograde amnesia, remained unchanged by both drugs, long-term memory in regard to anterograde amnesia exhibited a deterioration after lorazepam and an improvement after clobazam. This confirms not only previous studies showing that clobazam does not impair memory functions in animals (Hock and Kruse, 1982; Giurgea, in press), but also investigations in man by Siegfried *et al.* (1981) and Paes De Sousa *et al.* (1981). Specifically, Siegfried *et al.* (1981) described almost identical results: while short-term memory and retrograde amnesia were not influenced by 1,4- and 1,5-benzodiazepines, anterograde amnesia was only observed with 1,4-benzodiazepines. Various representatives of the latter class have shown amnestic effects (mostly in anaesthesiological studies): flunitrazepam (Bixler *et al.*, 1979; George and Dundee, 1977; Heermann, 1979; Pacquet *et al.*, 1978; Tolksdorf *et al.*, 1979), nitrazepam (Liljequist and Mattila, 1979), oxazepam and methyloxazepam (Liljequist *et al.*, 1979), midazolam (Dundee and Wilson, 1980), temazepam (Liljequist and Mattila, 1979), nordiazepam (Liljequist *et al.*, 1979) and triazolam (Poitras, 1980; Roth *et al.*, 1980). Diazepam seems to induce more rapid but shorter and less severe amnestic effects than lorazepam (Dundee *et al.*, 1979; Galloon *et al.*, 1977; George and Dundee, 1977; Studd and Eltringham, 1980).

The amnestic effects of benzodiazepines are dependent on factors like dose (Pandit *et al.*, 1976), time of drug application and retrieval (Roth *et al.*, 1980), learning material (e.g. verbal or numerical) (Jones *et al.*, 1979) and method of presentation and reproduction (e.g. memory impairment with free recall but not with recognition procedure) (Clarke *et al.*, 1980). furthermore, the amnestic effects of benzodiazepines are most pronounced after acute doses, but significant memory impairment still has been reported after three weeks of benzodiazepine administration (Ghoneim *et al.*, 1981).

The mechanism of amnestic action of 1,4-benzodiazepines may be due to an impairment of the process of consolidation of the learning material (Clark *et al.*, 1979; Ghoneim and Mewaldt, 1975). This process is supposed to be a selective transfer of the memory material from a short-lasting labile state immediately after information input (electrophysiological state, short-term memory) to the relatively stable engram (biochemical state, long-term memory) (Sinz, 1979). The amnestic action of benzodiazepines seems to be different from that of other drugs: e.g. physostigmine counteracted the anterograde amnesia of scopolamine, but failed to do the same in anterograde amnesia induced by diazepam (Ghoneim and Mewaldt, 1977).

The question arises whether or not bad mnestic performance is the consequence of sedation. While we could on the one hand show that subjects with good mnestic performance show a better vigilance as determined by the computer-analysed EEG, both at the time of the acquisition and the time of the recall (Saletu *et al.*, 1982), McKay and Dundee (1980), Roth *et al.* (1980) and Siegfried *et al.* (1981) are of the opinion that mnestic and sedative effects of benzodiazepines are independent. Giurgea (personal communication) observed recently that the differences between 1,4- and 1,5-benzodiazepines in regard to amnesia remained evident even when doses were titrated to such an extent that the sedation was matched.

Finally, our blood level and pulse rate data demonstrate that both 1,4- and 1,5-benzodiazepines did not effect the cardiovascular system in a significant way. Evaluation of spontaneously reported side-effects suggested a better tolerability after the 1,5-benzodiazepine, which could be shown also by the Romberg test including standing time, gait speed and gait deviations from a test line. Our pharmacodynamic data suggests that the 1,5-benzodiazepine clobazam should be utilized as a daytime tranquilizer, while the 1,4-benzodiazepine lorazepam should be prescribed as a night-time tranquilizer.

Summary

In a double-blind, placebo-controlled study the pharmacodynamic effects of two therapeutically equivalent doses of the 1,4-benzodiazepine lorazepam and the 1,5-benzodiazepine clobazam were investigated utilizing quantitative EEG and psychometric analyses. Ten normal volunteers received randomized (latin square), and at weekly intervals, single oral doses of placebo, 20 mg and 30 mg clobazam as well as 2 mg and 3 mg lorazepam. Blood level samplings, EEG recordings, psychometric tests, evaluation of pulse, blood pressure, side-effects and the Romberg test were carried out at 0, 2, 4, 6 and 8 h postdrug. Computer-assisted spectral-analysis of the EEG demonstrated after both compounds an anxiolytic profile characterized by an increase of beta activity, decrease of alpha activity and an acceleration of the centroid of the total activity. However, in contrast to clobazam, lorazepam induced an additional augmentation of delta activity and a slowing of the centroid of the combined delta and theta activities indicating sedative/hypnotic properties. Dose/treatment efficacy calculations revealed 3 mg lorazepam as the most CNS effective compound followed by 2 mg lorazepam, 30 mg and 20 mg clobazam, while after placebo the least changes were observed. Time-efficacy calculations showed the peak CNS effect after both compounds in the 2nd and 4th hours which paralleled the blood level course. Psychometric investigations demonstrated that after 20 and 30 mg clobazam significant changes as compared with placebo occurred in only one and three variables respectively (out of 18), while after 2 mg and 3 mg lorazepam significant alterations occurred in five and ten variables, respectively. Inter-drug comparison showed after lorazepam (and specifically after 3 mg) a significantly more pronounced decrease in attention, concentration, psychomotor activity, tapping, reaction accuracy, complex reaction, performance in the Pauli test, mood and critical flicker frequency than after the corresponding doses of clobazam. No inter-drug differences were observed in short-term or long-term memory regarding retrograde amnesia. However, anterograde amnesia deteriorated dose-dependently after lorazepam, while it improved after clobazam as compared with placebo. Pulse and blood pressure did not show any clinically relevant changes after both compounds. Clobazam was superior to lorazepam in regard to side-effects and performance in the Romberg test. Our findings point to the employment of clobazam as a daytime tranquilizer, and lorazepam as a night-time tranquilizer.

References

Berry, P. A., Burtles, R., Grubb, D. J. and Hoare, M. V. (1974). An evaluation of the effects of clobazam on human motor coordination, mental acuity and mood. *British Journal of Clinical Pharmacology* **1**, 346.

Bixler, E. O., Scharf, M. B. and soldatos, C. R. (1979). Effects of hypnotic drugs on memory. *Life Science* **25**, 1379–1388.

Borland, R. G. and Nicholson, A. N. (1974). Immediate effects on human performance of a 1,5-benzodiazepine (clobazam) compared with the 1,4-benzodiazepines, chlordiazepoxide, hydrochloride and diazepam. *British Journal of Clinical Pharmacology* **2**, 215–221.

Braestrup, C. and Squires, R. (1977). Brain specific benzodiazepine receptors in rats characterized by high affinity ^{3}H-diazepam binding. *Proceedings of the National Academy of Science USA* **74**, 3805–3809.

Clark, E. O., Glanzer, M. and Turndorf, H. (1979). The pattern of memory loss resulting from intravenously administered diazepam. *Archives of Neurology* **36**, 296.

Clarke, P. R. F., Bennet, N. R. and Thornton, J. A. (1980). Gone but not forgotten: Benzodiazepine-induced amnesia. *British Journal of Anesthesia* **52**, 231p.

Coste-Simonin, A. and Krantz, D. (1975). *Etude clinique d'un nouvel anxiolytique en cardiologie: le clobazam. Gazette Méd. de France* **82**, 4460–4464.

Cottin, M., Dachary, J. M., Marie, C., Pagott, R., Ramant, J. and Sales, M. (1975). Etude d'un nouvel anxiolytique, le clobazam, dans l'anxiété résiduelle des psychotiques. *J. Pharmac. Clin.* **2**, 81–87.

Dundee, J. W. and Wilson, D. B. (1980). Amnesic action of midozolam. *Anaesthesia* **35**, 459–465.

Dundee, J. W., McGowan, W. A. W., Lilburn, A. C. and Hegarty, J. E. (1979). Comparison of the actions of diazepam and lorazepam. *British Journal of Anaesthesia* **51**, 439–443.

Fink, M. (1969). EEG and human psychopharmacology. *A. Rev. Pharmac.* **9**, 241–258.

Galloon, N.S., Gale, G.D. and Lancee, W.J. (1977). Comparison of lorazepam and diazepam as premedicants. *British Journal of Anaesthesia* **49**, 1265–1268.

George, K. A. and Dundee, J. W. (1977). Relative amnesic actions of diazepam, flunitrazepam and lorazepam in man. *British Journal of Clinical Pharmacology* **4**, 45–50.

Ghoneim, M. M. and Mewaldt, S. P. (1975). Effects of diazepam and scopolamine on storage, retrieval and organisational processes in memory. *Psychopharmacology* **44**, 257–262.

Ghoneim, M. M. and Mewaldt, S. P. (1977) Studies on human memory: the interactions of diazepam, scopolamine and physostigmine. *Psychopharmacology* **52**, 1–6.

Ghoneim, M. M., Mewaldt, S. P., Berie, J. L. and Hinrichs, J. V. (1981). Memory and performance effects of single and 3-week administration of diazepam. *Psychopharmacology* **73**, 147–151.

Giurgea, C. (1978). Benzodiazepines (BDZ); mecanismes d'action et effets secondaires. BCNBP, Annual Forum (Brussels), 1–10.

Greenblatt, D. J. and Shader, R. (1978). Pharmacotherapy of anxiety with benzodiazepines and beta-adrenergic blockers. In "Psychopharmacology" (Edited by Lipton, M. A., DiMascio, A. and Killam, F.), pp. 1381–1390. Raven Press, New York.

Grünberger, J. (1977). "Psychodiagnostik des Alkoholkranken. Methodischer Beitrag zur Bestimmung der Organizität in der Psychiatrie." Maudrich, Wien.

Grünberger, J. and Saletu, B. (1980). Determination of pharmacodynamics of psychotropic drugs by psychometric analysis. In *Progress of Neuro-Psychopharmacology* **4**, 469–489.

Grünberger, J., Saletu, B., Linzmayer, L., Kalk, A. and Berner, P. (1978). Pharmacodynamic investigations with WE 941, a new triazolodiazepine by means of psychometric analyses. *Currect Therapeutic Research* **24**, 427–440.

Hajdu, P., Uihlein, M. and Damm, D. (1980). Quantitative determination of clobazam in serum and urine by gas chromatography, thin layer chromatography and fluorometry. *Journal of Clinical Chemistry and Clinical Biochemistry* **18**, 209–214.

Heermann, J. (1979). Flunitrazepam mit anterograder Amnesie und Bluthochdrucksenkung vor der Lokalanästhesie ohne Intubation bei 3000 HNO—Operationen. *Laryngologie, Rhinologie, Otologie. Ihre Grenzgebiete* **58**, 162–168.

Hindmarch, I. (1979). Some aspects of the effects of clobazam on human psychomotor performance. *British Journal of Clinical Pharmacology* **7**, 77S–82S.

Hindmarch, I. and Gudgeon, A. C. (1980). The effects of clobazam and lorazepam on aspects of psychomotor performance on car handling ability. *British Journal of Clinical Pharmacology* **10**, 145–150.

Hindmarch, I., Hanks, G. W. and Hewett, A. J. (1977). Clobazam, a 1,5-benzodiazepine, and car-driving ability. *British Journal of Clinical Pharmacology* **4**, 573–578.

Hock, F. J. and Kruse, H. J. (1982). Differential effects of psychotropic drugs on ECS—induces amnesia in a passive avoidance task. Anxiolytic drugs: Diazepam versus clobazam. *IRCS Medical Science* 10, 221–222.

Hsieh, M. T. (1982). The involvement of monoaminergic and GABA ergic systems in locomotor inhibition produced by clobazam and diazepam in rats. *Int. J. Clin. Pharmac. Ther. Toxicol.* 20/5, 227–235.

Hunt, B. J., George, A. J. and Ridges, A. P. (1974). Preliminary studies in humans on clobazam (HR 376)—a new anti-anxiety agent. *British Journal of Clinical Pharmacology* 1, 174–175.

Itil, T. M. (1974) Quantitative pharmaco-electroencephalographie. In "Psychotropic Drugs and the Human EEG" (T. M. Itil, ed.), Vol. 8, pp. 43–75. Karger, Basel.

Jones, D. M., Jones, M. E. L., Lewis, M. J. and Spriggs, L. B. (1979). Drugs and human memory: Effects of low doses of nitrazepam and hyoscine on retention. *British Journal of Clinical Pharmacology* 7, 479–483.

Liljequist, R. and Mattila, M. J. (1979). Acute effects of temazepam and nitrazepam on psychomotor skills and memory. *Acta Pharmacologica and Toxicologica* 44, 364–369.

Liljequist, R., Palva, E. and Linnoila, M. (1979). Effects on learning and memory of 2 weekstreatment with chlordiazepoxide lactam, N-desmethyldiazepam, oxazepam and methyloxazepam, alone or in combination with alcohol. *International Pharmacopsychiatry,* 14, 190–195.

Malpas, A., Legg, N. J. and Scott, D. F. (1974). Effects of hypnotics on anxious patients. *British Journal of Psychiatry* 124, 482–484.

Martin, J. C. (1975). Essai contrôlé d'un nouveau tranquillisant (le clobazam) chez des alcooliques chroniques en phase de sevrage. *J. Pharmac. Clin.* 1, 21–27.

McKay, A. C. and Dundee, J. W. (1980). Effect of oral benzodiazepines on memory. *British Journal of Anaesthesia* 52, 1247–1257.

Mohler, H. and Okada, T. (1977). Benzodiazepine receptor: Demonstration in the central nervous system. *Science* 198, 849–851.

Osgood, C. E., Suci, G. J. and Tannenbaum, P. H. (1957). "The Measurement of Meaning." Urbana.

Paes de Sousa, M., Figuiera, M. L., Loureiro, F. and Hindmarch, J. (1981). Lorazepam and clobazam in anxious elderly patients. In "Clobazam" (I. Hindmarch and P. D. Stonier, eds), Royal Society of Medicine International Congress and Symposium Series No. 43, pp. 119–123. Royal Society of Medicine, London.

Pandit, S. K., Heisterkamp, D. V. and Cohen, P. J. (1976). Further studies of the anti-recall effect of lorazepam. *Anaesthesiology* 45, 496–500.

Paquet, C., Gaillard, J. M. and Tissot, R. (1978). Flunitrazepam et mémoire. *Acta Psychiatrica Belgica* 78, 374–378.

Poitras, R. (1980). A propos d'épisodes d'amnesies anterogrades associés a l-utilisation du triazolam. *Union Médicale du Canada* 109, 427.

Roth, T., Hartse, K. M., Saab, P. G., Piccione, P. M. and Kramer, M. (1980). The effects of flurazepam, lorazepam and triazolam on sleep and memory. *Psychopharmacology* 70, 231–237.

Saletu, B. (1976). "Psychopharmaka, Gehirntätegkeit und Schlaf." Karger, Basel.

Saletu, B. and Grünberger, J. (1979). Evaluation of pharmacodynamic properties of psychotropic drugs: Quantitative EEG, psychometric and blood level investigations in normals and patients. *Pharmacopsychiatria* 12, 45–58.

Saletu, B., Saletu, M., Grünberger, J. and Mader, R. (1979). Drawing inferences about the therapeutic efficacy of drugs in patients from their CNS effect in normals: Comparative quantitative pharmaco-EEG and clinical investigations. In "Neuro-Psychopharmacology" (B. Saletu, P. Berner and L. Hollister, eds), pp. 393–407. Pergamon Press, Oxford.

Saletu, B., Grünberger, J., Linzmayer, L. and Flener, R. (1981). Anxiolytics and beta blockers: Evaluation of pharmacodynamics by quantitative EEG, psychometric and physiological variables. *Agressologie* 22, 5–16.

Saletu, B., Grünberger, J., Linzmayer, L. and Pietschmann, H. (1982). Neurophysiological aspects of aging, dementia and its pharmacotherapy. In "WPA Regional Symposium Kyoto" (H. Ohashi, K. Nakayama, M. Saito and B. Saletu, eds), pp. 272–281. The Japanese Society of Psychiatry and Neurology, Tokyo.

Saletu, B., Grünberger, J., Linzmayer, L. and Sieghart, W. (in press). Zur zentralen Wirkung hoher Benzodiazepindosen: Quantitative Pharmako-EEG und psychometrische Studien mit Prazepam. In "Proceedings des 2. Kongresses der Deutschen Gesellschaft für Biologische Psychiatrie, Dusseldorf, 23–25. September, 1982."

Schacht, U. and Baecker, G. (1982). Effects of clobazam in benzodiazepine-receptor binding assays. *Drug Development Research* (Suppl.) **1**, 83–93.

Siegfried, K., Koeppen, D., Taeuber, K., Malerczyk, V. and Sittig, W. (1981). A double-blind comparison of the acute effects of clobazam and lorazepam on memory and psychomotor functions. In "Clobazam" (I. Hindmarch and P. D. Stonier, eds), Royal Society of Medicine International Congress and Symposium Series No. 43, pp. 13–21. Royal Society of Medicine, London.

Sinz, R. (1979). "Neurobiologie und Gedächtnis." Fischer and Gustav, Stuttgart. ISBN: 3-437-00287-2.

Stöhr, H., Grünberger, J., Linzmayer, L., Saletu, B. and Thoma, H. (1982). Der Einsatz des Mikrocomputers in der klinischen Psychodiagnostik. *Wissenschaftliche Berichte zur BMT Jahrestagung 1982*, pp. 30–33. Osterreichische, deutsche und schweizer Gesellschaft für biomedizinische Technik, Graz 1982.

Studd, C. and Eltringham, R. J. (1980). Lorazepam as night sedation and premedication; a comparison with diazepam. *Anaesthesia* **35**, 60–64.

Subhan, Z. (1981). A dose-range comparison of clobazam and diazepam: II. Effects on memory. In "Clobazam" (I. Hindmarch and P. D. Stonier, eds), Royal Society of Medicine International Congress and Symposium Series No. 43, pp. 7–12. Royal Society of Medicine, London.

Thompson, P. J. and Trimble, M. R. (1981). Clobazam and cognitive functions: effects in healthy volunteers. In "Clobazam" (I. Hindmarch and P. D. Stonier, eds), Royal Society of Medicine International Congress and Symposium Series No. 43, pp. 33–38. Royal Society of Medicine, London.

Tolksdorf, W., Berlin, J., Bethke, U., Striebel, J. P., Westphal, K. T. and Lutz, H. (1979). Rohypnol (Flunitrazepam) als Sedativum bei Leitungsanästhesien unter besonderer Berücksichtigung der amnestischen Wirkung. *Prakt. Anaesth.* **14**, 59–66.

Wilson, J. E. (1973). Oral premedication with lorazepam (Ativan): A comparison with heptabarbitone (Medonin) and Diazepam (Valium). *British Journal of Anaesthesia* **45**, 738–744.

Wittenborn, J. R., Flaherty, C. F., McGough, W. E. and Nash, R. J. (1979). Psychomotor changes during initial day of benzodiazepine medication. *British Journal of Clinical Pharmacology* **7**, 69–76.

Zerssen, V. D., Koeller, D. M. and Rey, E. R. (1970). Die Befindlichkeitsskala (B-S)—ein einfaches Instrument zur Objektivierung von Befindlichkeitsstörungen, insbesondere im Rahmen von Längsschnittuntersuchungen. *Arzneimittelforschung* **20**, 915–918.

Clobazam, Personality, Stress and Performance

A. C. PARROTT

Institute of Naval Medicine, Alverstoke, Gosport, Hampshire, UK*

Introduction

Clobazam is a 1,5-benzodiazepine derivative with anxiolytic effects (Hanks, 1979; Koeppen, 1981); a property also demonstrated by meprobamate, alcohol, barbiturates and 1,4-benzodiazepine derivatives (Gray, 1982). Drug-induced reduction of anxiety should not however be considered as a phenomenon which occurs under all circumstances of drug administration. Anxiety reduction depends upon the internal condition of the individual at the time of drug action—such as the characteristic propensity of the personality to experience anxiety; and upon the external conditions at the time of drug action—such as the conditions of external stress or threat. Studies investigating the influences of the above factors will be presented in two sections; first, studies not involving clobazam, and secondly a more comprehensive review of studies involving clobazam.

Studies Not Involving Clobazam

Janke *et al.* (1979) in a lengthy review of studies in this area, suggested that the emotionality of the personality was an important modifier of response to drugs. Emotionality was described as:

"A broad personality area ... called anxiety by Cattell and neuroticism by Eysenck"

Levels of emotionality were assessed on questionnaires such as the Taylor manifest anxiety scale, Eysenck personality inventory neuroticism scale, Middlesex Hospital Questionnaire, Scheir and Cattell anxiety questionnaire, and Speilberger state/trait anxiety scales. Janke *et al.* (1979) concluded:

"In the literature regarding emotional changes after the administration of tranquilizing and sedating drugs (e.g. meprobamate, bromazepam, diazepam, chlordiazepoxide, oxazepam, promazine, fluphenazine) in neurotic and non-neurotic subjects ... one might conclude that people with low neuroticism scores usually tend to respond to depressant drugs with paradoxical increase of self-reported emotional tension. People with high neuroticism scores tend to react with a reduction of symptoms connected with emotional tension."

Performance changes under anxiolytic drugs were also shown to be influenced by personality factors. For instance, Janke (1964) showed that emotionally labile (high anxiety) subjects improved their finger dexterity performance under meprobamate, while emotionally stable (low anxiety) subjects showed no difference between meprobamate and placebo. Performance changes are, however, frequently quite complex. Di Mascio and Barrett (1965) demonstrated improved tapping speed with high anxiety subjects following 30 mg oxazepam, while tapping speeds with low anxiety subjects were unchanged. However, co-ordination test and steadiness test performance levels were not changed in either group, although subjective self-reports demonstrated reduced anxiety levels in the high anxiety subjects and increased anxiety levels in the low anxiety subjects. Barnett *et al.* (1981) demonstrated a significant interaction between drug conditions (5 mg diazepam or placebo) and Speilberger state anxiety levels, in errors on a running memory test. Low anxiety subjects demonstrated increased errors under diazepam, while high anxiety subjects demonstrated decreased error rates under diazepam. Several further studies have demonstrated significant differential effects:

---

* *Former address:* The work reviewed was undertaken while the author held a temporary lectureship in the Department of Psychology, University of Leeds, Leeds LS2 9JT, UK

Richter and Hobi (1975) with bromazepam; Idestrom and Schalling (1970) with amylobarbital; Boucsein (1976) with diazepam. However, these differential effects have not been produced with consistency. They sometimes occur with certain drug conditions or dose levels, but not others; for instance, Barrett and Di Mascio (1966) reported them with lower doses of diazepam (7·5 mg) and chlordiazepoxide (15 mg), but not with higher doses (15 mg diazepam and 30 mg chlordiazepoxide). Furthermore, some studies have used several dependent variables (multiple performance assessments, and more than one "feeling state" scale), and differential effects have been found with one or two of the dependent variables, but not with the other variables (Janke et al., 1979, pp. 30–43). As Janke et al. (1979) concluded:

"The correlation between drug response and neuroticism is not constant."

In conclusion, there is a consistent tendency for the emotionality of the personality to affect responses to drugs with anxiolytic actions (benzodiazepines, barbiturates, meprobamate). High anxiety subjects frequently respond to anxiolytic drugs with a reduction in their levels of anxiety, and performance is sometimes improved. Low anxiety subjects sometimes respond to these same drug conditions with paradoxical increases in levels of anxiety, and performance levels are sometimes impaired. Although these changes have been frequently reported, they are not particularly robust. This is probably because the emotionality of the personality is only one of several important factors which may influence the nature of a drug response. Other important factors include age, extraversion, test sensitivity, test practice and learning, maturation, and time of testing following drug administration.

Some studies into the effects of anxiolytic drugs have investigated the influence of task stressors. Various experimental procedures have been utilized with the aim of modifying the level of externally provoked stress. The procedures have incorporated the following factors: loud noise, viewing distressing films, threat of electric shock and being tested in front of a group of peers. The main problem with these procedures is that the perception of an environmental event as "stressing" is a highly individual response. It is, therefore, very difficult to generate an experimental situation with a reliable and consistent

environmental stressor. Janke et al. (1979) reviewed studies into the effects of stressors upon anxiolytic drug action. With reference to studies using loud noise (80–95 dB) they concluded that objective performance measures showed little effect, but subjective self-reports of anxiety feelings and emotional stability were frequently affected. Under loud noise, emotionally labile subjects demonstrated reduced emotional tension, or no change in tension. Under the control condition of low environmental stress (low noise volume), feeling states sometimes demonstrated general deactivation, and either no change in emotional tension, or paradoxical increases in emotional tension. For instance, Janke and Stoll (1965) reported a significant interaction between the noise level at testing, and the effects of oxazepam upon emotionally labile subjects. Semantic differential reports of emotional stability were significantly improved under the high noise condition, but were unchanged under low noise. Boucscein (1974) used the "threat of electric shock" to induce anxiety; 20 mg chlordiazepoxide led to reduced levels of anxiety under the "threat of shock" condition, but paradoxical increases in emotional lability were found in the "no threat of shock" condition. Janke et al. (1979) reviewed a number of similar studies to the above, but concluded that most studies had failed to demonstrate reduced levels of anxiety under drug influence, in situations specifically designed to generate stress. However, some studies not covered in the Janke review have produced positive findings. McNair (1975) reported reduced levels of anxiety in the period of anticipation and waiting before public speaking, following diazepam; subjective self-ratings and electrodermal responsiveness were the dependent variables. Molander (1982) investigated electrodermal responses during aversive classical conditioning. Anticipatory aversive responses to the stimuli were reduced by 10 mg diazepam, as were the numbers of conditioned and unconditioned aversive responses. Kohnen and Lienert (1980) induced three levels of social stress: high, being filmed on video; medium, tested in front of a group of four spectators; and low, tested individually. Subjects were tested on a memory task following either cloxazolam or placebo. There was a significant interaction between the level of stress at testing and drug response. Under low stress, performance following placebo was better than performance following cloxazolam. Under high stress, performance following cloxazolam was better than performance following placebo.

In conclusion, some investigations have generated different anxiety provoking situations, where differential drug responses have been evident. Under conditions of high environmental stress (loud noise, being filmed, performing in front of a group, prior to aversive stimulation) anxiolytic drug assessments were frequently better than placebo assessments. In contrast, under conditions of low environmental stress, anxiolytic drug assessments tended to be worse than placebo assessments.

Studies Involving Clobazam

Parrott and Hindmarch (1975a,b) investigated the arousal performance relationship by testing choice reaction time performance under CNS stimulant drugs (dexamphetamine, pemoline, dimethylxanthine, methylphenidate), CNS depressant drugs (amylobarbitone, chlorpromazine), clobazam and placebo. Performance was assessed under two conditions of environmental stress: high stress, when stimulus light onset was accompanied by a raucous high volume (98 dB) tone; and low stress, when stimulus light onset was accompanied by an equivalent low volume (68 dB) tone. Yerkes-Dodson inverted-U functions between arousal (CFF thresholds) and performance (response speeds and errors) were empirically generated (Fig. 1). Under the high stress condition, all eight drug conditions fitted the inverted-U curves. Under the low stress condition, seven of the eight drug conditions fitted the inverted-U curves, the exception being clobazam. Clobazam performance levels were lower than would be expected on the basis of arousal level on the empirically generated curves (Fig. 1). Clobazam performance was, therefore, unimpaired under high stress, but impaired under low stress. This was demonstrated with both dependent variables tested: response speeds and response errors.

In a second study, Parrott and Hindmarch (1977) investigated the effects of three benzodiazepines (20 mg clobazam, 5 mg nitrazepam, 15 mg flurazepam) upon performance in the reaction time task used previously. Under low stress, performance speeds were significantly slower with all three benzodiaze-

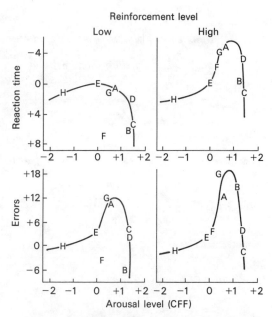

Figure 1. *Changes in performance on a reaction time task, under different levels of arousal, as indicated by critical flicker fusion (CFF) threshold changes. Two levels of external stress or reinforcement were present, low and high. All scores represent pre-drug, post-drug administration difference scores (after Parrott and Hindmarch 1975b). A, 20 mg methylphenidate; B, 400 mg dimethylxanthine; C, 40 mg pemoline; D, 10 mg dexamphetamine; E, placebo; F, 20 mg clobazam; G, 100 mg amylobarbitone; H, 50 mg chlorpromazine.*

pines compared to placebo. Under high stress, performance speeds were significantly impaired following nitrazepam, but were not impaired following flurazepam or clobazam (Table 1). The differential effect of high and low environmental stress was, therefore, demonstrated with 20 mg clobazam and 15 mg flurazepam, but not 5 mg nitrazepam. Performance levels demonstrated near zero correlations with EPI neuroticism scores, with placebo and nitrazepam, but were generally significant with flurazepam and clobazam. Under clobazam and flurazepam, performance changes were comparatively better with the high neuroticism subjects, and comparatively worse with the low neuroticism subjects (Table 1). This was found with clobazam for low noise performance, high noise performance, and low/high noise perfor-

Table 1

Comparative effects of acute single doses of three benzodiazepine derivatives upon choice reaction times under two conditions of task stress. All data represents pre-drug, post-drug administration difference scores, $1\frac{1}{2}$ h following drug administration (after Parrott and Hindmarch, 1977)

		Drug condition		
Response time differences (s)		Nitrazepam/ placebo	Flurazepam/ placebo	Clobazam/ placebo
Low stress		−0·09**	−0·08*	−0·07*
High stress		−0·08*	−0·03	−0·02
	Placebo	5 mg Nitrazepam	15 mg Flurazepam	20 mg Clobazam
Correlations between low/ high stress performance differences, and EPI neuroticism scores	$r=0·15$	$r=0·09$	$r=0·76*$	$r=0·63*$

$** P<0·01; * P<0·05.$

mance differences (i.e. high neuroticism subjects showed a greater differential stress effect). It was found with flurazepam for high noise performance and low/high noise performance differences, but under low noise the correlation value was negative (i.e. the high neuroticism subjects under flurazepam produced comparatively worse performance under low stress).

In a third study, Parrott and Hindmarch (1978) compared the effects of two dose levels of clobazam (10 and 20 mg) upon performance in the same choice reaction time task. Performance changes under high stress were better following clobazam than placebo, while under low stress, performance changes were comparatively worse following clobazam than placebo. This differential effect was statistically significant with 10 mg clobazam, but not 20 mg clobazam (Table 2). Performance values were correlated with EPI neuroticism scores, and MHQ anxiety subscale scores (Table 2). Under placebo, performance/neuroticism correlations were near zero or slightly negative. Under 20 mg clobazam, performance/neuroticism correlations were non-significantly positive. Under 10 mg clobazam an interesting pattern of changes was found. Under low stress, the performance/neuroticism correlation was significantly negative: the high neuroticism subjects' performance was worse than the low neuroticism subjects' performance. Under high stress the performance/neuroticism cor-

relations were positive, and the low/high stress difference correlations were also positive: the high neuroticism subjects performed comparatively better under high stress conditions under clobazam.

A theoretical explanation for the complex findings described above was proposed by Parrott and Hindmarch (1978). This explanation is paraphrased below.

"The differential changes in response speed according to task stress conditions are interpreted as depending upon clobazam's anxiolytic properties. By reducing state anxiety it is hypothesized that the overall drive or motivation to respond quickly is lowered. In the low stress (low noise) condition, speeds were therefore reduced, but in the high stress (high noise) condition, where incentives for responding quickly are intrinsic to the task, response speeds were as fast as they would be normally. This explanation relates performance changes to the extent of anxiolytic activity, and leads to the prediction that the more anxious subjects should show the greatest differential stress effect. This has been generally shown. Following 10 mg clobazam and 15 mg flurazepam, trait anxiety and response speed at low stress correlated inversely, while trait anxiety and response speed at high stress correlated positively. The more anxious subjects produced the greatest performance decrements at low

Table 2

Effects of two dose levels of clobazam upon choice reaction times under two conditions of task stress. All data represents pre-drug, post-drug administration difference scores, $1\frac{1}{2}$ h following drug administration (after Parrott and Hindmarch, 1978)

		Drug condition	
Response Time Differences (s)		10 mg Clobazam /placebo	20 mg Clobazam /placebo
Low Stress		−0·06*	−0·06
High stress		+0·05	−0·03
Low/high stress difference		+0·11*	+0·03

Correlations between response time performance changes and EPI neuroticism and MHQ anxiety scale scores		Placebo	10 mg Clobazam	20 mg Clobazam
Low stress	MHQ anxiety	0·21	−0·62	0·31
	EPI neuroticism	0·01	−0·84**	0·57
High stress	MHQ anxiety	−0·38	0·62	0·41
	EPI neuroticism	−0·05	0·32	0·46
Low/high stress	MHQ anxiety	0·05	0·70*	0·29
	EPI neuroticism	−0·47	0·64	0·62

** $P<0·01$; * $P<0·05$.

stress, and the greatest performance increments at high stress. With 20 mg clobazam, subjects with high anxiety and neuroticism scores produced comparatively better performance changes than subjects with low levels of anxiety, at both stress levels, but a similar relationship between anxiety level and performance was found. Differences in response speed between the low and high stress conditions correlated positively with neuroticism scores. Subjects with higher anxiety or neuroticism profiles, therefore, performed comparatively better under the high stress condition."

Parrott and Munton (1981) attempted to investigate the effect of different environmental stress conditions upon performance in cognitive information processing tasks, using two volumes (68 dB, 98 dB) of white background noise provided through earphones. Various dose levels of clobazam (10, 20, 30, 40, and 60 mg), diazepam (5, 10, 15, 20, and 30 mg), and placebo were investigated. Critical Flicker Fusion values were not affected by the noise conditions, suggesting that cortical arousal was not significantly affected by the noise. Speeds on the concept identification task were non-significantly slower under the low noise ($P<10$, two-tailed), while speeds were also slower on the other task investigated—the serial subtraction of numbers. However, there were no drug/noise interaction effects, and no tendencies towards such effects were apparent. In retrospect, the use of continuous background noise as a potential "stressor" in this study seems to have been unsuccessful. There are various possible reasons for this. First, continuous noise may be less effective than intermittant noise as a stressor (Broadbent, 1971). Secondly, cognitive (pigeon-holing) tasks such as concept identification and number subtraction, may be less affected by noise than tasks with a larger perceptual (stimulus filtering) component (Broadbent, 1971). Thirdly, in the previous studies (Parrott and Hindmarch, 1975a,b, 1977, 1978), noise conditions were linked directly to stimulus occurrence, whereas in Parrott and Munton (1981), noise was uninformative in relation to task requirements.

Clyde (1981) compared low doses of clobazam (10 mg, 20 mg), nitrazepam (2·5 mg, 5 mg), and placebo, for their effects upon choice reaction time, card sorting, serial subtraction of numbers, and self-reported levels of anxiety and drowsiness, in low and high trait-anxiety subgroups. Significant interactions between drug condition and trait-anxiety subgroup were found with clobazam (10 mg and 20 mg); high trait-anxiety subjects demonstrated reduced state-anxiety following clobazam, while low trait-anxiety subjects demonstrated no change in state-anxiety. Similarly, high trait-anxiety subjects demonstrated increased relaxation under clobazam, while low trait-anxiety subjects demonstrated unchanged levels of relaxation. On simple reaction time there were no drug/trait-anxiety interactions, while on eight choice reaction time, all drug conditions led to significant performance impairments, but they were mainly due to the low trait-anxiety subjects. With the serial subtraction of threes, significant drug/trait-anxiety interactions were found with clobazam (10 mg and 20 mg); performance was comparatively improved in high trait-anxiety subjects, and comparatively impaired in low trait-anxiety subjects. However, no significant interactions were found with the serial subtraction of 7s, or 17s. Clyde (1981) concluded:

> "Trait-anxiety level modifies responses to clobazam and nitrazepam in mood and performance areas. The reduction in anxiety seen in high anxious individuals, is replaced by sedation and slight increases in anxiety in the low anxiety group."

Berry et al. (1974) compared acute single doses of 10 mg clobazam, 10 mg diazepam, and placebo. Pursuit rotor performance was significantly impaired by both clobazam and diazepam. Braking reaction time on a driving simulator was significantly impaired by diazepam, but not clobazam. One possible interpretation for these findings is that the pursuit rotor represents a boring low stress task, whereas braking on a driving simulator represents an interesting high stress task. It could, therefore, be suggested that clobazam impaired performance on the low stress task (pursuit rotor), but not on the high stress task (braking reaction time). It should be noted that 10 mg diazepam did not produce this "differential" effect.

Biehl (1979) demonstrated that high neuroticism subjects were significantly more "ready to brake" following 20 mg clobazam than placebo. In contrast, following 10 mg diazepam, these subjects were significantly less "ready to brake" than after placebo or clobazam. It should be noted that in this study, mood states for "activity" and "depression"

were significantly lower under diazepam than clobazam ($P < 0.01$), with intermediate placebo values.

Leygonie et al. (1975) investigated sleep and performance in "normal" and "anxious" subjects, stratified on the basis of the Rorschach test. The performance tests demonstrated marked learning effects; performance changes under 20 mg clobazam were, therefore, compared to scores "predicted" on the basis of placebo pre-drug and post-drug values. Statistical comparisons were not consistently reported but, in general, pre-drug performance scores for the anxious subjects were lower than those for the normals, while following clobazam, performance scores were similar for the two subject groups.

Hindmarch (1979) demonstrated a significant U-shaped relationship between choice reaction time performance changes and EPI neuroticism scores. Following 20 mg clobazam, subjects with medium neuroticism scores (N scale: 10–16) demonstrated improved performance, while subjects with low and high neuroticism scores demonstrated unchanged or slightly impaired performance (Hindmarch, 1979, p. 80).

Parrott (1982a) combined the critical flicker fusion (CFF) values from several studies involving single acute single doses of 20 mg clobazam and placebo. Subjects with high anxiety (MHQ anxiety subscale score: 7+), generally demonstrated comparatively better CFF values following clobazam. Subjects with lower anxiety scores (MHQ anxiety subscale score: 6−) demonstrated either little change in CFF values, or slight CFF decrements (Parrott, 1982a, Fig. 6). Following this, Parrott (1982b) undertook a comprehensive analysis of the effects of clobazam upon CFF thresholds, combining data from 15 previous studies. No significant interactions between drug condition and anxiety subgroup were found, however.

Parrott and Davies (1983) utilized the experimental social stress procedures described by Kohnen and Lienert (1980). Subjects were tested while being filmed on video (high stress), or while not being filmed (low stress), following 20 mg clobazam or placebo. Under high stress, clobazam performance was comparatively better than placebo performance, whereas under low stress clobazam was worse than placebo. This general tendency was present with each of the five performance assessments (choice reaction total times, recognition times, critical flicker fusion, serial subtraction of 3s and 17s), although none were significant (Table 3).

Parrott and Kentridge (1982) used Kelly's repertory grid technique to assess self-perceptions of anxiety feelings. The repertory grid technique (Kelly, 1955) allows each person to describe their own feelings and personal constructs. Constructs specifically relating to anxiety were elicited in lengthy individual interviews (lasting 60–120 min). Anxiety constructs were translated into ten-point linear self-rating scales, and scores on these scales were obtained following 20 mg clobazam and placebo.

The high trait-anxiety group demonstrated reduced anxiety feelings under clobazam, while the low trait-anxiety group demonstrated increased anxiety feelings under clobazam: the drug/trait-anxiety interaction was significant ($P < 0.01$; Table 4). Findings from individual subjects were also statistically analysed. Eight of the ten high trait-anxiety subjects demonstrated reduced anxiety (three significantly, five non-significantly); nine of the ten low trait-anxiety subjects demonstrated increased anxiety (eight significantly, one non-significantly).

Discussion

This review has demonstrated that the emotionality of the personality, and the level of task-related stress, can have important influences upon responses to clobazam. In general, psychological assessments with high trait-anxiety subjects were comparatively improved by clobazam, while psychological assessments with low trait-anxiety subjects were comparatively impaired by clobazam. This general pattern was found both with subjective self-assessments of feeling states, and with objective measures of performance. Under conditions of high environmental stress, performance was comparatively improved by clobazam; while under low stress, performance was comparatively impaired by clobazam. Although fewer investigations in this area have been carried out using other specific drug conditions, similar conclusions can be proposed for the actions of other anxiolytic drugs such as the 1,4-benzodiazepine derivatives and meprobamate. It should be emphasized that although these above findings have been reported from many studies, in many cases they have not been demonstrated.

Most theoretical explanations for these phenomena have been described using models based upon activation theory: Janke *et al.* (1979), Clyde (1981), and Debus (1981). The following explanation is paraphrased from Janke *et al.* (1979):

"Many interactions can be explained by activation theory concepts. Particularly important is the inverted relationship between arousal, on the one hand, and performance or hedonic tone of emotions

Table 3

Effects of clobazam upon five performance assessments, under two conditions of stress. All data was collected 1½ h following drug administration (after Parrott and Davies, 1983)

Performance assessment	20 mg Clobazam			Placebo			Clobazam/ placebo drug stress difference
	High stress	Low stress	Stress difference	High stress	Low stress	Stress difference	
Choice reaction time— recognition (s)	0·32	0·31	+0·01	0·35	0·29	+0·06	−0·05
Choice reaction time— total (s)	0·53	0·54	−0·01	0·62	0·51	+0·11	−0·12
Serial subtraction of threes (s)	2·53	2·78	−0·25	2·48	2·52	−0·04	−0·21
Serial subtraction of seventeens (s)	7·27	8·16	−0·89	8·11	7·20	+0·91	−1·80
Critical Flicker Fusion (Hz)	32·50	31·30	+1·20	30·20	33·10	−2·90	+4·10

Table 4

Personal constructs of anxiety, using Kelly's repertory grid technique, following clobazam in low and high trait-anxiety subjects (after Parrott and Kentridge, 1982)

Group mean scores (Lower scores indicate lower anxiety feeling states)	Drug condition	
Trait-anxiety subgroup	Placebo	20 mg Clobazam
Low trait-anxiety	81	90
High trait-anxiety	106	102
Analysis of Variance	F-value	Significance
Trait-anxiety (low/high)	8·11	$P < 0·01$
Drug condition (clobazam/ placebo)	1·18	
Trait-anxiety × drug (interaction)	7·83	$P < 0·01$

on the other hand. ... Under normal experimental conditions, normal subjects are assumed to be slightly below the optimum level of activation. A depressant drug will reduce the performance, which is usually accompanied by negative feelings ... however ... when subjects are in a state of heightened activation (i.e. past the peak of the inverted-U function) then it is possible to obtain no change or even improvement in performance after administration of drugs."

These changes are illustrated in Fig. 2, which is based upon a figure presented by Debus (1981). The effects of environmental stressors can also be explained by this model, since they will lead to increased levels of drive or arousal (i.e. will push the pre-drug levels to the right, in Fig. 2). The greatest drug benefits will, therefore, be obtained with high trait-anxiety subjects tested under high stress conditions. The greatest drug decrements will occur with low trait-anxiety subjects tested under low stress conditions.

Clyde (1981) similarly used the Yerkes-Dodson inverted-U curve in her explanation of different drug responses between high and low trait-anxiety subjects. She stated:

"The effects on performance are concomitant with the changes that would be predicted from the Yerkes-Dodson law. ... High anxiety subjects are assumed to be overaroused ... a decrease in anxiety in

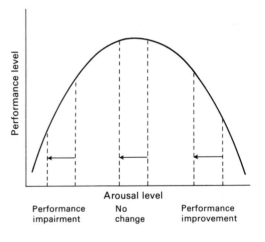

Figure 2. The inverted-U model of the relationship between arousal (drive) level and performance (after Debus, 1981). (Note: the arrow represents a reduction in arousal with drug.)

this group reduces arousal, and performance therefore improves. ... In the low anxiety group, reduced arousal causes sedation and impaired performance."

Clyde emphasized that low doses produced slight activation level changes, and moved performance levels close to the peak of the inverted-U. Larger doses reduced activation levels past the peak of the inverted-U and performance levels deteriorated.

Parrott and Hindmarch (1975a,b) also utilized the inverted-U curve, but importantly did not assume a change in arousal level (or activation) with the anxiolytic agent. It was explicitly stated that arousal levels were not changed:

"Clobazam was indistinguishable from placebo in changing subjective estimates of alertness and arousal. On the other hand placebo did not affect anxiety ($F = 0.18$, NS) whereas clobazam significantly reduced self-reported anxiety ($F = 2.32$, $P < 0.05$)."

Critical flicker fusion thresholds were also unchanged by clobazam. They suggested that the performance reductions found under low stress reflected a reduced motivation to respond, performance was therefore less than would have been otherwise expected at *that* level of arousal. Under high stress, the motivation to respond quickly was provided by the stress conditions of the task, and performance was "at the level predicted by the inverted-U curve for that particular arousal level".

The Parrott and Hindmarch (1975b) explanation was based essentially upon changes in the motivation/anxiety to respond, and did not assume changes in arousal/activation level with drugs. The Janke *et al.* (1979) and Clyde (1981) explanations were based upon drug-induced changes in arousal/activation level.

There are, however, several problems with the explanations based upon arousal changes. These are briefly listed below.

1. The model can be applied only to depressant drugs. An anxiolytic drug which does not reduce arousal/alertness cannot be explained by the model.

2. The model sometimes describes a positive correlation between arousal and anxiety. For instance, with high trait-anxiety subjects on drug, a decrease in anxiety reduces arousal (Clyde, 1981). However an inverse correlation between arousal and anxiety is also sometimes described, as when low trait-anxiety subjects demonstrate reduced alertness on drug, but "paradoxical" increases in anxiety. The inverted-U function, therefore, relates to alertness/arousal, but not consistently to anxiety. No function describing anxiety

change is present in the model, other than it will always tend towards a central mean value, following any change in arousal!

3. The inverted-U model is basically a unidimensional arousal model, yet current theories of arousal are multidimensional. Debus (1981) has stated: "The relationship between drive and performance is already complicated even with the assumptions of a single drive concept. Most authors today however accept a multiple drive concept."

4. Debus (1981) has elegantly expanded the inverted-U model to take account of many further factors of importance (such as task complexity, multiple drives, and other personality dimensions). However, the increased number of interrelated factors, added to the inherent ambiguity of the inverted-U model (any performance changes can be explained with the right assumptions), make the model very complex and difficult to test.

In conclusion, the inverted-U model is essentially an arousal model, and therefore adequate only as a basis for explanations of sedative or alerting drugs. It is not an adequate model for anxiolytic drugs. A model for drug effects is required which is based not upon arousal/activation theory, but upon anxiety theory. In the next section, Gray's (1981, 1982) neurophysiological model of anxiety is briefly described, and drug effects are discussed in relation to it.

Anxiolytic Drug Action, Related to Gray's Neurophysiological Model of Anxiety

Gray (1981a, 1981b) postulated a behavioural inhibition system (BIS), where activity in the BIS "constitutes anxiety". Gray (1981b) stated:

"On this view ... anxiety in animals consists of a central state elicited by threats of punishment, frustration or failure, novelty or uncertainty."

The suggested neuroanatomical site for the behavioural inhibition system is the septo-hippocampal system. Furthermore:

"Anti-anxiety drugs act on the septo-hippocampal system to produce those changes which are critical for their anti-anxiety effects (as distinct from, say, the sedative or anticonvulsant effects they may also produce)."

The BIS acts as a stimulus comparator system, to check actual input with expected events, and becomes activated into a control mode when mismatch occurs. This leads to increased checking of stimulus events, increased overall behavioural inhibition of previous ongoing motor actions, increased arousability, and increased (narrowed?) attention (Fig. 3).

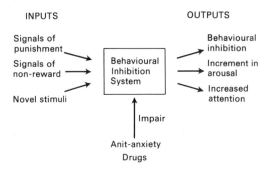

INPUTS   OUTPUTS

Signals of   Behavioural
punishment   inhibition

Signals of   Behavioural   Increment in
non-reward   Inhibition   arousal
                System
                                Increased
Novel stimuli   attention

                Impair

                Anit-anxiety
                Drugs

Figure 3. The Behavioural Inhibition System (BIS) of Gray's neurophysiological model of anxiety (after Gray, 1981).

Gray's model is based almost entirely upon animal experimental data, but Gray (1981b) has stated that an extension of the model to human anxiety is conceptually simple.

". . . the greater the reactivity of the B.I.S., the more susceptible the individual is to anxiety ... although in practice there remains much to be done to spell out and test the predictions."

Some interpretations of human psychopharmacological findings presented in this paper, are now discussed, using Gray's neurophysiological model.

According to the model, high trait-anxiety subjects will demonstrate greater BIS reactivity; they will therefore demonstrate increased stimulus checking, identify a wide range of stimuli as stressing/threatening, and will tend to check and inhibit their patterns of motor actions. High trait-anxiety subjects given anxiolytic drugs will demonstrate reduced BIS reactivity. Under low stress conditions, there will be a reduced tendency for

the stimuli to be labelled as threatening or important; thus high trait-anxiety subjects under a low stress condition may demonstrate reduced levels of performance, although the reduced levels of "motor inhibition" may counter this, and lead to unchanged performance. Under a high stress condition, the high stress stimulus will still be correctly identified as important, and performance will not be impaired. Performance improvements may occur, since the reduced levels of general motor inhibition may lead to less inhibited and generally faster motor performance. Resources may also be allocated more efficiently to the central performance task of importance.

With low trait-anxiety subjects, under normal conditions, the BIS is operating efficiently, and only important stimuli are responded to. The administration of an anxiolytic drug will, however, impair the BIS. Stimuli which were previously adequately processed by the BIS will no longer be appropriately analysed following drug administration. Under low stress conditions performance levels will be reduced because of the general interference with systems which were previously operating adequately. Under high stress conditions, the high stress stimuli will still alert the BIS system and motor actions relevant to the high stress stimulus will occur, although they may be slightly impaired. Except under conditions of high stress, low trait-anxiety subjects may experience a loss of control over stimulus events, and this may cause the paradoxical increase in anxiety reported by some low trait-anxiety subjects.

In order to further investigate these suggested relationships, Parrott and Kentridge (1982) suggested that it was important to assess the feeling states of high and low trait-anxiety subjects under drug in more detail. In particular, the following are suggested as important: feelings of control over events; self-perceptions of performance abilities; changed patterns of motor control; sensory reception mechanisms; and attribution of stress/threat/importance to particular environmental stimuli. Kelly's repertory grid technique is considered to be a particularly useful tool for such an investigation. For future research in this area, and in order to investigate the implications of Gray's model, it is seen as most important to be able to accurately identify the attributions given to events by the individual.

Summary

The effects of the 1,5-benzodiazepine derivative clobazam in human psychopharmacological studies were reviewed. In many studies, high trait-anxiety subjects demonstrated reduced feelings of anxiety under clobazam compared to placebo, whereas low trait-anxiety subjects demonstrated paradoxical increases in feelings of anxiety under clobazam. Under conditions of high environmental stress, clobazam performance tended to be better than placebo; in contrast, under conditions of low stress, clobazam performance tended to be worse than placebo performance. Similar differential effects have also been reported with other anxiolytic agents such as meprobamate and some 1,4-benzodiazepines. Several explanations for these effects have been proposed on the basis of the Yerkes-Dodson inverted-U function relating arousal and performance. These explanations were critically reviewed and it was concluded that anxiolytic drug effects would be best explained using anxiety theory, rather than arousal/activation theory. Gray's neurophysiological model of anxiety is briefly presented, and the differential personality and stress effects discussed on the basis of Gray's model.

References

Barnett, D. B., Taylor-Davies, A. and Desai, N. (1981). Differential effect of diazepam on short term memory in subjects with high or low level anxiety. *British Journal of Clinical Pharmacology* **11**, 411–412.

Barrett, J. E. and Di Mascio, A. (1966). Comparative effects on anxiety of the minor tranquilisers in high and low anxious student volunteers. *Diseases of the Nervous System* **27**, 483–486.

Berry, P. A., Burtles, R., Grubb, D. J. and Hoare, M. (1974). An evaluation of the effects of clobazam on human motor co-ordination, mental activity and mood. *British Journal of Clinical Pharmacology* **1**, 346.

Biehl, B. (1979). Studies of clobazam and car driving. *British Journal of Clinical Pharmacology* (Suppl.) **7**, 85–90.

Boucsein, W. (1974). Die wirkung von chlordiazepoxyd unter angstbedingungen im psychophysiologischen experiment. *Arzneimittel-Forsch.* **24**, 1112–1114.

Boucsein, W. (1976). Experimental psychologie untersuchung zur wirkung von tranquilizern (diasepam und einer prüfsubstanz) unter berucksichtigung von personlichkeitsmerk-malen. *Arzneimittel-Forsch.* **26**, 28–31.

Broadbent, D. E. (1971). "Decision and Stress." Academic Press, London.

Clyde, C. A. (1981). The influence of personality on response to low doses of benzodiazepines. *Royal Society of Medicine International Symposium Series* **43**, 75–86.

Di Mascio, A. and Barrett, J. (1965). Comparative effects of oxazepam in high and low anxious student volunteers. *Psychosomatics* **6**, 298–302.

Debus, G. (1981). Models of the connection between sedation, relaxation and performance. *Royal Society of Medicine International Symposium Series* **43**, 43–49.

Gray, J. A. (1981a) Anxiety as a paradigm case of emotion. *British Medical Bulletin* **37**, 193–197.

Gray, J. A. (1981b). "The Neuropsychology of Anxiety: An Enquiry into the Functions of the Septo-hippocampal System." Oxford University Press, Oxford.

Hanks, G. W. (1979). Clobazam: pharmacological and therapeutic profile. *British Journal of Clinical Pharmacology* **7**, 151S–155S.

Hindmarch, I. (1979). Some aspects of the effects of clobazam on human psychomotor performance. *British Journal of Clinical Pharmacology* **7** (Suppl. 1), 77S.

Idestrom, C. M. and Schalling, D. (1970). Objective effects of dextroamphetamine and amobarbital and their relations to psychaesthetic personality traits. *Psychopharmacology* **17**, 339.

Janke, W. (1964). "Experimentelle Untersuchungen zur abhangigkeit der Wirkung psycho-

troper Substanzen von personlichkeitsmerkmalen." Akademische Verlagsge-
sellschaft, Frankfurt.
Janke, W. and Stoll, K. D. (1965). Untersuchungen zur wirkung eines tranquilizers auf
emotional labile personen. *Arzneimittel-Forsch.* **15**, 366–374.
Janke, W., Debus, G. and Longo, N. (1979). Differential psychopharmacology of tranquiliz-
ing and sedative drugs. In "Differential Psychopharmacology of Anxiolytics
and Sedatives. Modern Problems of Pharmacopsychiatry" (J. R. Boissier,
ed.), Vol. 14, pp. 13–98. Karger, Basel.
Kelly, G. A. (1955). "The Psychology of Personal Constructs," Vols 1 and 2. Norton, New
York.
Koeppen, D. (1981). Clinical experience with clobazam 1968–1981. *Royal Society of Medicine
International Symposium Series* **43**, 193–198.
Kohnen, R. and Lienert, G. A. (1980). Defining tranquilizers operationally by non-additive
effect in experimental stress situations. *Psychopharmacology* **68**, 291–294.
Leygonie, F., Rethore, A., Yuceyatak, F. and Yuceyatak, A. (1975). A new anxiolytic drug,
clobazam; effects on sleep and performance levels on waking. *Gazette
médicale de france* **82**, 1303–1310.
McNair, D. M. (1975). Sensitivity of two mood state factors to anxiety and antidepressant
drugs. In "Neuropharmacology" (J. R. Boissier, ed.), vol. 9, CINP Conference 1974, Amsterdam and New York.
Molander, L. (1982). Effect of melperone, chlorpromazine, haloperidol and diazepam on
experimental anxiety in normal subjects. *Psychopharmacology* **77**, 109–113.
Parrott, A. C. (1982a). Critical Flicker Fusion Thresholds and their relationship to other
measures of alertness. *Pharmacopsychiatia* **15** (Suppl.), 39–43.
Parrott, A. C. (1982b) The effects of clobazam upon critical flicker fusion thresholds: a review.
Drug Development Research **1** (Suppl.), 57–66.
Parrott, A. C. and Davies, S. (1983). Effects of a 1,5-benzodiazepine derivative upon
performance in an experimental stress situation. *Psychopharmacology* **79**,
367–369.
Parrott, A. C. and Hindmarch, I. (1975a). Arousal and performance—the ubiquitous
inverted-U relationship. *IRCS Medical Science* **3**, 176.
Parrott, A. C. and Hindmarch, I. (1975b). Clobazam, a 1,5-benzodiazepine derivative: effects
on anxiety, arousal and performance compared with those of CNS stimu-
lants, sedatives and tranquilizers. *IRCS Medical Science* **3**, 177.
Parrott, A. C. and Hindmarch, I. (1977). Comparative effects of three benzodiazepine
derivatives—clobazam, nitrazepam, and flurazepam, upon psychomotor
performance under different reinforcement conditions. *IRCS Medical Science* **5**, 166.
Parrott, A. C. and Hindmarch, I. (1978). Clobazam, a 1,5-benzodiazepine derivative: effects
upon human psychomotor performance under different levels of task reinforcement. *Archives internationales de Pharmacodynamie et de Therapie* **232**,
261.
Parrott, A. C. and Kentridge, R. (1982). Personal constructs of anxiety under the 1,5-
benzodiazepine derivative clobazam, related to trait-anxiety levels of the
personality. *Psychopharmacology* **78**, 353–357.
Parrott, A. C. and Munton, A. (1981). Comparative effects of clobazam and diazepam on
psychological performance under different levels of background noise. *Royal
Society of Medicine International Symposium Series* **43**, 51–57.
Richter, R. and Hobi, V. (1975). Die personlichkeitsspezifische. Wirkung eines Tranquilizers.
Arzneim.-Forsch. **25**, 26–28.

The Effects of Combining Clobazam with Nomifensine on Psychomotor Performance in Healthy Subjects: A Brief Review

P. D. STONIER

Medical Department, Hoechst UK Ltd., Salisbury Road, Hounslow, Middlesex, UK

and I. HINDMARCH

Human Psychopharmacology Research Unit, University of Leeds, Leeds, UK

Introduction

Clobazam is a 1,5-benzodiazepine which has been shown to be an effective anxiolytic in comparison with placebo and standard, 1,4-benzodiazepines (Brogden *et al.*, 1980). At the anxiolytic dosage of 20–30 mg per day it has minimal sedative activity and does not impair psychomotor performance (Hindmarch, 1979; Borland and Nicholson, 1974). In particular clobazam has been shown not to impair laboratory assessments of skills related to car driving (Hindmarch, 1979) or actual car handling ability (Hindmarch *et al.*, 1977).

Nomifensine is an antidepressant with a novel chemical structure and pharmacological profile (Hanks, 1977). In extensive clinical studies it has been shown to be an effective antidepressant in comparison with placebo and to have equal efficacy to the tricyclic antidepressants, whilst being relatively free from troublesome side-effects (Brogden *et al.*, 1979). In particular, it has minimal anticholinergic activity and is free from sedative effects (Hanks, 1977). Studies with nomifensine on psychomotor performance (Hindmarch and Parrott, 1977) and simulated aspects of car driving ability (Hindmarch, 1977) have shown the drug to be relatively free from disruptive effects.

HOE 8476 is a fixed ratio combination (10:3) of nomifensine 25 mg and clobazam 7·5 mg. The monosubstances have been shown not to have pharmacokinetic interactions (Rupp *et al.*, 1979). A series of experiments was designed to compare the effects of HOE 8476 on sleep, mood and psychomotor performance including car handling ability, with those of its monosubstances (clobazam and nomifensine) placebo and an internal control (verum) of a combination of amitriptyline and chlordiazepoxide. The effects of giving HOE 8476 at different dose levels and at different times of day were also investigated.

The four studies summarized here, when viewed together, are an illustration of the human pharmacodynamics of HOE 8476 in comparison to the monosubstances and the verum. These experiments also indicate the dose regimens to be used in the clinical situation. The first three experiments have been published in full (Hindmarch *et al.*, 1980; Parrott *et al.*, 1982; Stonier *et al.*, 1982) and the fourth will be published in full elsewhere.

Methods

The experiments reported were carried out at the Human Psychopharmacology Research Unit, University of Leeds, using groups of 10–16 healthy female volunteer car-drivers. The volunteers were not taking any concurrent medication, other than the contraceptive pill; the use of alcohol was discouraged throughout the study and not permitted during pretreatment days or on the study days. Each gave informed verbal consent to participate.

The individual designs are summarized for each experiment. The medication, presented in matching capsules, was given for 48 h prior to testing in three experiments whilst the fourth was an acute dose study.

Table 1 shows the medication schedules for active drugs. Matching placebos were used as a treatment group and to balance treatment regimens to ensure blindness.

Assessments

Subjects were familiarized with the assessment procedures and allowed to practise on all measures prior to the start of the study. The following summarizes all assessment measures employed, although not all were used in each study. All have been described in full elsewhere.

Middlesex Hospital Questionnaire (MHQ) (Crown and Crisp, 1970). All subjects completed the MHQ before entry into the study; this was to screen out any subjects with abnormal anxiety ratings.

Leeds Sleep Evaluation Questionnaire (LSEQ) (Hindmarch, 1975; Parrott and Hindmarch, 1978). The effects of treatments on subjective sleep factors, namely getting to sleep (GTS), quality of sleep (QOS), awaking from sleep (AFS), and behaviour following waking (BFW) were assessed on the LSEQ, which consists of a series of 10 cm visual analogue scales. The LSEQ was completed on the morning of the test day following pre-dosing.

Linear Analogue Rating Scales (LARS) (Hindmarch, 1980). These consist of a series of 10 cm visual analogue scales relating to mood and subjective feeling states (e.g. alertness, anxiety, tension, depression, etc.) which in normal volunteers are thought to represent responses to general sedative properties of medications.

Critical Flicker Fusion Threshold (CFFT) (Hindmarch, 1980) was used as an objective index of CNS arousal and measured using the Leeds Psychomotor Tester. The mean threshold was determined in a set of four light-emitting diodes in foveal fixation at one metre from six presentations according to the psychophysical method of limits.

Choice Reaction Time (CRT) (Hindmarch and Parrott, 1978) was used as an index of sensori-motor performance, the mean latency of response for 25 stimulus presentations being the assessment measure recorded on the Leeds Psychomotor Tester.

Serial Subtraction of Numbers (SSN) (Parrott and Munton, 1981) assessed mental arithmetic ability at three levels of difficulty, namely the mean time taken to make 20 sequential subtractions of threes, sevens or seventeens from a five figure number.

Car driving performance was scored on a ten-point scale by independent marshals of an advanced Driver Training Centre on a set of tests similar to those used in other studies (Betts *et al.*, 1972; Hindmarch, 1976; Hindmarch *et al.*, 1977; Hindmarch and Gudgeon, 1980). Five aspects of car handling were assessed—namely reversing, parking, width estimation, brake reaction time, and slalom driving. Each test was repeated twice and the mean score taken as the assessment measure.

Brake reaction time was measured using an onboard computer mounted in a car and attached to the brake system of the vehicle. Accurate measures of brake response latency to an "emergency stop signal" on the bonnet of the car were made while the car was being driven along the private roads of a disused airfield.

Table 1

	Experiment 1	Experiment 2	Experiment 3	Experiment 4
HOE 8476 (nomifensine 25 mg/ clobazam 7·5 mg)	1 cap t.d.s.	1 cap t.d.s. 2 caps t.d.s. 3 caps nocte	2 caps b.d.	4 caps mane
Nomifensine 25 mg	1 cap t.d.s.	—	2 caps b.d.	4 caps mane
Clobazam 7·5 mg	—	—	2 caps b.d.	4 caps mane
Amitriptyline 25 mg/ chlordiazepoxide 10 mg	1 cap t.d.s.	1 cap t.d.s.	—	2 caps mane

Card sorting was used as a measure of psychomotor performance comprising a conceptual and a motor element; three levels of difficulty were assessed, namely colours, suits and numbers. The time taken for correct sorting was recorded.

Peg board. A standard peg board was used to assess motor coordination and the times taken for rivet and washer assembly, as well as the dismantling of the rivet/washer unit, were recorded.

Concept Identification Test (COITEST). A COITEST (Parrott and Munton, 1981) was used to measure the speed of processing cognitive information.

The results were analysed using a one-way ANOVAR for drug effects and a two-way ANOVAR for drug and period effects. A post-hoc pairwise comparison of means in discriminant tests was derived from Duncan's New Multiple Range Tests, or 95% confidence limits or Dunnet tests.

Experiment 1

The effect of sub-acute doses of HOE 8476 (25/7·5 mg t.d.s.), AMI/CHLOR (25/10 mg t.d.s.), nomifensine (25 mg t.d.s.) and placebo on car driving and related psychometric and performance measures.

Subjects and methods

Sixteen consenting female volunteers, mean age 32 years, were admitted to the study. Each subject acted as her own control and received all treatments in a double-blind design in accordance with four self-conjugate standard squares to balance order effects. Testing took place at weekly intervals and was preceded by a period of 48 h drug administration. A further single dose of medication was administered on the morning of the test day. Medication consisted of HOE 8476 (nomifensine 25 mg, clobazam 7·5 mg), one capsule t.d.s.; AMI/CHLOR (amitriptyline 25 mg, chlordiazepoxide 10 mg), one capsule t.d.s.; nomifensine 25 mg t.d.s. or matching placebo, one capsule t.d.s.

Assessments as described earlier consisted of Critical Flicker Fusion Thresholds (CFFT), Choice Reaction Time (CRT), Mental Arithmetic by Serial Subtraction of threes,

sevens and seventeens (SSN), Concept Identification Test (COITEST), short-term memory by nonsense trigrams, subjective mood states by 100 mm line visual analogue scales (LARS), and the Leeds Sleep Evaluation Questionnaire (LSEQ). Car driving ability was scored by marshals of the Tockwith Driver Training Centre on four aspects of car handling. Side-effects were rated by two judges.

Results

Summary results are displayed in Table 2. Significant differences with respect to placebo are given for two-tailed values and derived from paired *t*-tests. Non-significant test measures are also listed.

Discussion

AMI/CHLOR showed positive sedative and impairing activity across a broad range of the tests of alertness and psychomotor performance. On the subjective assessments it improved depression and tension as measured by visual analogue scales but impaired alertness in keeping with its generally sedative profile. This was further demonstrated on the Leeds Sleep Evaluation Questionnaire.

In contrast both HOE 8476 and low-dose nomifensine showed alerting properties by increasing Critical Flicker Fusion Threshold and nomifensine also significantly improved Choice Reaction Time in contrast to AMI/CHLOR.

The car-driving tests failed to demonstrate statistically significant differences between active drugs and placebo. However, AMI/CHLOR produced a strong trend towards impairment and the detailed results showed a close concordance between drug effects on overall car driving performance and tests of psychomotor activity (Hindmarch *et al.*, 1980).

In this experiment the fixed ratio combination of amitriptyline and chlordiazepoxide produced results consistent with the known central sedative properties of the preparation and, through its use as a positive control established the sensitivity of the majority of measures to drug-induced changes. Nomifensine, as in previous studies, is shown to possess mentally alerting properties manifest as an increase in both subjective and objective

Table 2

Experiment 1: changes v. placebo

	AMI/CHLOR (25/10 mg t.d.s.)	HOE 8476 (25/7·5 mg t.d.s.)	Nomifensine (25 mg t.d.s.)
CFFT	↓	↑	↑
CRT (movement)	↓	—	↑
Driving	(↓)	—	—
SSN (errors)	↓	—	—
COITEST (easy)	↓	—	—
LARS—Depression	↑	—	—
LARS—tension	↑	—	—
LARS—alertness	↓	—	—
LSEQ—GTS	↑	—	—
—QOS	↑	—	—
—AFS	↓	—	—
—BFW	↓	—	—
Side-effects	↓[a]	—	—

Significant differences (paired *t*-tests) $P<0·05$; ( ) $=P<0·1$.
↓ = impairment, ↑ = improvement.
n.s.: CRT (recognition); SSN (time); COITEST (hard) (errors); memory; LARS (anxiety).
[a]Wilcoxon matched-pairs signed ranks test.
GTS = ease of getting to sleep; QOS = perceived quality of sleep; AFS = impairment of the ease of waking; BFW = integrity of early morning behaviour.

measures of arousal. HOE 8476 is generally free from any significant effect on car driving and laboratory assessment of psychomotor performance. The objective measure of arousal, CFF threshold, is significantly increased by HOE 8476 in accord with the findings for the two component drugs, nomifensine and clobazam.

Experiment 2

The effects of three dose regimens of HOE 8476 on mood, sleep and psychomotor performance relating to car-driving.

Subjects and methods

Ten consenting female volunteers, mean age 32 years, were selected for the study. Each subject acted as her own control and received all treatments in turn with the order allocated according to a randomized balanced-block design. Testing took place at weekly intervals preceded by a 48 h period of drug administration, leaving a four-day washout period between treatments. A further single dose of medication (or placebo) was administered on the morning of the test day 1 h prior to testing. Following the morning session subjects were given a light lunch, followed by a further dose of medication (or placebo) 1 h prior to the afternoon test session, during which many of the tests were repeated. Medication consisted of HOE 8476 (nomifensine 25 mg, clobazam 7·5 mg) one capsule t.d.s., two capsules t.d.s., three capsules in a single dose at night; AMI/CHLOR (amitriptyline 25 mg, chlordiazepoxide 10 mg) one capsule t.d.s.; placebo one capsule t.d.s.

Assessments as described earlier consisted of a battery of psychometric and psychomotor performance tasks and subjective evaluation of sleep variables, mood states and side-effects. Car-driving performance was scored on a ten-point scale by marshals of the Tockwith Driver Training Centre. Five aspects of car driving were assessed—namely, reversing, parking, width estimation, brake reaction time, and slalom driving. Each test was repeated twice and the mean score taken as the assessment measure.

Results

Summary results are displayed in Table 3. The results were analysed using analysis of

Table 3

Experiment 2: changes v. placebo

	AMI/CHLOR (25/10 mg t.d.s.)	HOE 8476 (25/7·5 mg t.d.s.)	HOE 8476 (50/15 mg t.d.s.)	HOE 8476 (75/22·5 mg nocte)
CFFT	↓ (a.m.) (p.m.)	—	—	—
SSN—7s	↓ (p.m.)	—	—	—
—17s	↓ (a.m.)	—	—	—
Card sorting[a]				
—suits	↓	—	↓	—
—numbers	↓	—	↓	—
LARS[a]—mood	↓	—	—	—
LSEQ—GTS	↑	—	—	—
—QOS	↑	↑	↑	↑
—AFS	(↓)	—	—	—
—BFW	(↓)	—	—	—

Significant differences $P < 0.05$; ( ) $= P < 0.1$.
↓ = impairment, ↑ = improvement.
n.s.: CRT, SSN (3s), COITEST, peg board, driving, card sorting (colours).
[a]Morning test only.

variance, and factors for drug and period of administration were included. Pairwise comparisons of treatment means were made using the Duncan New Multiple Range Test.

Discussion

As in experiment 1, AMI/CHLOR impaired CFFT and Serial Subtraction of Numbers, although the broad range of impairment was not as marked as in experiment 1. No test impairment was seen with the low dose regimen of HOE 8476 given as a single dose at night or in divided dose. However, there was an impairment of serial subtraction of numbers at the higher repeated dose. AMI/CHLOR impaired mood states (LARS) and demonstrated sedative activity on the LSEQ, whilst all dose regimens of HOE 8476 showed effects on sleep by improvement of the subjective assessment of the quality of sleep. This property is not accompanied, however, by a significant hangover the next morning, as is seen with AMI/CHLOR.

As in experiment 1 the battery of car-driving tests did not show statistically significant drug effects but a dose- and time-dependent trend was apparent as shown in Fig. 1. Here there was an increased tendency to impaired performance in the afternoon with AMI/CHLOR and the high dose of HOE 8476, compared with either the low dose of HOE 8476 or the single night-time dose, with the latter showing an improvement in the afternoon compared with the morning assessment. In this dosage group there was of course no midday dosing of active substance.

As in experiment 1, this study demonstrates important differences between AMI/CHLOR and HOE 8476. The sedative activity of AMI/CHLOR is shown on virtually all the sensitive subjective and objective measures of behaviour, whilst, in contrast, there is a relative lack of sedation attributed to HOE 8476. Nevertheless, the effects of HOE 8476 on the card sorting task and on the quality of sleep factor of the LSEQ indicate its powerful psychotropic properties, although this activity is present in a different form from that characterizing AMI/CHLOR, as it is not accompanied by sedation and drowsiness.

Experiment 3

The effect of higher sub-acute twice daily doses of HOE 8476 50/15 mg, nomifensine 50 mg, clobazam 15 mg, and placebo on psychometric and psychomotor performance measures, mood states and sleep.

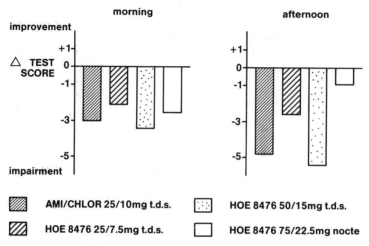

Figure 1. Experiment 2: car-driving tests.

Subjects and methods

Twelve female volunteers participated (mean age 34·3 years). Each subject acted as her own control and received all treatments in a double-blind Latin square design. Each treatment was given twice a day for two consecutive days and once more on the morning of the third day. Testing took place at weekly intervals and a four-day washout period separated each treatment regimen. On the test day laboratory assessments commenced 30 min after the final medication. A second battery of tests was given in the afternoon after a light lunch. Medication consisted of HOE 8476 (nomifensine 50 mg, clobazam 15 mg), nomifensine 50 mg, clobazam 15 mg, and placebo, with each dose being given in the morning and at night. A battery of assessment measures from those described earlier was administered.

Results

Summary results are displayed in Table 4. The assessment measures were analysed by two-way analysis of variance for drug effects, time of testing effects, and drug/time interactions. Placebo values were compared with those for each drug condition by Dunnet's t-test.

Discussion

In experiment 3 few assessment measures showed significant drug effects, and those

Table 4

Experiment 3: changes v. placebo

	HOE 8476 (50/15 mg b.d.)	Nomifensine (50 mg b.d.)	Clobazam (15 mg b.d.)
CRT	—	—	↓
COITEST (hard)	—	–.–	↓
LARS—anxiety	↑	—	(↑)
LSEQ–GTS	—	—	↑

Significant differences $P < 0·05$; ( ) = $P < 0·1$.
↓ = impairment, ↑ = improvement—both morning session only.
n.s. CFFT (memory); DSST, SSN, LARS (depression, alertness, clumsiness); LSEQ (QOS, AFS, BFW)

differences that could be demonstrated from placebo were in the morning session. Clobazam impaired choice reaction time and COI-TEST (hard). It also showed significant effects on the LSEQ (getting to sleep). Both HOE 8476 and clobazam improved LARS ratings of anxiety. Neither HOE 8476 nor nomifensine impaired objective tests of performance.

In this experiment, therapeutic daily doses of nomifensine and clobazam were used, and indications from clinical trials suggested that HOE 8476 50/15 mg b.d. was a suitable therapeutic dose in treatment of mixed anxiety depression. The results show that HOE 8476 does not impair performance on ány measure compared with one of its components, clobazam, which at the dose regimen used here impairs both choice reaction time and difficult concept identification, which suggests that the inclusion of nomifensine in this fixed-dose combination in some way attenuates the effects of clobazam. Nevertheless, the combination shows positive anxiolytic activity as assessed by the visual analogue rating scale in normal volunteers, which is in contrast to nomifensine. Some of the properties of HOE 8476 and its components in active doses were further evaluated in experiment 4, together with an active dose of AMI/CHLOR.

Experiment 4

An acute dose comparison of single morning doses of HOE 8476 (100/30 mg), nomifensine (100 mg), clobazam (30 mg), AMI/CHLOR (50/20 mg), and placebo on psychometric and psychomotor performance tasks.

Subjects and methods

Ten healthy female volunteers (mean age 32 years) entered this double-blind five-way crossover study in which treatment order was determined by two 5×5 Latin squares. Each subject acted as her own control and received all treatments. Testing took place at weekly intervals 2 h after administration of medication or placebo. Medication consisted of HOE 8476 (nomifensine 100 mg, clobazam 30 mg), nomifensine 100 mg, clobazam 30 mg, AMI/CHLOR (amitriptyline 50 mg, chlordiazepoxide 20 mg), and placebo. AMI/CHLOR was administered at half the equivalent dose of HOE 8476 due to the limits of single-dose tolerability.

All subjects were assessed on cognitive and performance measures 2 h following administration of treatment. The assessment measures were CFFT, CRT, Visual Analogue Scale for Sedation (LARS), two simulated car-tracking tasks (A and B), a memory scanning test (MST), a real car-driving assessment, and a side-effects check list.

Results

The summary results are displayed in Table 5. The assessment measures were analysed by two-way analysis of variance for drug effects. Placebo values were compared with those for each drug condition by paired t-tests.

Table 5

Experiment 4: changes v. placebo

	AMI/CHLOR (50/20 mg)	HOE 8476 (100/30 mg)	Nomifensine (100 mg)	Clobazam (30 mg)
CFFT	↓	—	—	↓
CRT	↓	↓	—	↓
Tracking A	—	↓	—	—
Tracking B	↓	—	—	—
Memory	↓	↓	↑	—
Sedation	↓	↓	—	↓

Significant differences $P < 0.05$.
↓ = impairment, ↑ = improvement.
n.s.: driving tests.

Discussion

Table 5 shows that with high acute doses AMI/CHLOR, HOE 8476, and clobazam impair performance on a range of tests, albeit selectively. Both AMI/CHLOR and clobazam reduce CFFT. This is not unexpected for clobazam at an acute dose of 30 mg 2 h after administration. The addition of nomifensine in HOE 8476 appears to alleviate this activity. AMI/CHLOR, HOE 8476, and clobazam all slow total reaction time. Nomifensine speeds CRT but not significantly. In the simulated car-tracking tasks, HOE 8476 impairs performance only in task A although AMI/CHLOR and clobazam but not nomifensine tend in that direction. In task B, AMI/CHLOR greatly impairs performance, although HOE 8476 tends in that direction whilst nomifensine and clobazam tend to improve performance although not significantly. The results of these tasks indicate that the activity of HOE 8476 is not an additive one of the two monosubstances. This is again indicated in the memory task which is impaired by AMI/CHLOR and HOE 8476 but not by clobazam alone, whilst nomifensine alone "improves" memory (Fig. 2).

In the driving tests, whilst the overall results show no significant drug effects, AMI/CHLOR and clobazam show trends towards impairment, whilst nomifensine and HOE 8476 tend towards improved performance, again indicating that the activity of HOE 8476 is not a simple additive effect of the monosubstances. The VAS assessment of sedation shows significant positive effects of all treatment conditions apart from nomifensine.

General Discussion and Conclusions

This series of experiments evaluated the effects of a fixed-combination of nomifensine (25 mg) with clobazam (7.5 mg) in a battery of objective and subjective tests of psychomotor and cognitive performance, car handling ability, mood states, and sleep. The activity of various doses of HOE 8476 were compared with the monosubstances and an active control group in double-blind, placebo-controlled studies.

For the purposes of this brief review it is possible to draw some conclusions regarding the psychopharmacological effects of HOE 8476 based on the results of these experiments, on the known properties of the monosubstances and on the comparison with placebo effects and the effects of the verum, a combination of amitriptyline and chlordiazepoxide, chosen as a positive internal control because of its known sedative and impairing properties.

The combination of amitriptyline and chlordiazepoxide was confirmed in these experiments to have a wide ranging sedative effect and to impair performance on tests of central nervous system arousal, reaction

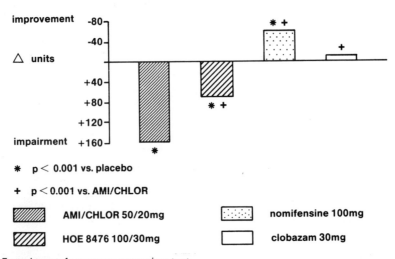

* p < 0.001 vs. placebo

+ p < 0.001 vs. AMI/CHLOR

| //// | AMI/CHLOR 50/20mg | :::: | nomifensine 100mg |
| //// | HOE 8476 100/30mg | | clobazam 30mg |

Figure 2. Experiment 4: memory scanning test.

time, memory, and skilled behaviours. In subjective tests its action is to improve depression and tension ratings and to impair alertness. The effects on all three of these scales as measured in normal healthy volunteers probably reflects an overall sedative action with consequent effects on scales of mood and feeling states. This sedative action is clearly reflected in the sleep variable of the Leeds Sleep Evaluation Questionnaire with improvement in sleep onset and quality at the expense of an impairment in ease of waking and subsequent behaviour.

In contrast, HOE 8476 shows dose-differential activity, with relatively little performance impairment at daily doses of nomifensine 75 mg/clobazam 22·5 mg, whether given as a single dose at night or in divided doses. Little impairment is produced by nomifensine 100 mg/clobazam 30 mg given in a twice daily divided dose (50 mg/15 mg b.d.). However, at higher divided doses of nomifensine 50 mg/ clobazam 15 mg three times daily, or nomifensine 100 mg/clobazam 30 mg as a single dose in the morning, some selective performance impairment is seen. Comparison of this performance impairment between the combination and its monosubstances suggests that this is not in all respects due to a simple additive effect of nomifensine and clobazam (see especially experiment 4) and that HOE 8476 has specific psychotropic activity. This needs further evaluation and confirmation.

In conclusion, the psychoactive profile of HOE 8476 suggests it to be a non-alerting, non-sedating, non-impairing antidepressant/ benzodiazepine combination at therapeutic doses. Sedative properties and selective impairment of performance emerge with higher acute single morning and total daily doses.

Summary

Four studies in healthy volunteers to investigate the psychopharmacological effects of a fixed combination (HOE 8476) of nomifensine (25 mg) and clobazam (7·5 mg) are reviewed.

A battery of tests of CNS arousal, reaction time, skilled behaviour including car handling, memory and subjective ratings of mood states and sleep variables were made in double-blind, placebo-controlled studies of HOE 8476 at various doses, the monosubstances and a positive internal control, amitriptyline/chlordiazepoxide.

HOE 8476 at doses of 25/7·5 mg t.d.s., 50/ 15 mg b.d., and 75/22·5 mg nocte produced relatively little performance impairment. At higher doses of 100/30 mg mane and 50/ 15 mg t.d.s. HOE 8476, some selective impairment of performance occurred, although this was not a simple additive effect of the monosubstances.

The psychoactive profile of HOE 8476 suggests it to be a non-alerting, non-sedating, non-impairing antidepressant/benzodiazepine combination at known therapeutic doses, with sedative properties and selective impairment of performance emerging at higher acute single and total daily doses.

References

Betts, T. A., Clayton, A. B. and Mackay, G. M. (1972). Effect of four commonly used tranquilisers on low-speed driving performance tests. *British Medical Journal* 4, 580–584.

Borland, R. G. and Nicholson, A. N. (1974). Immediate effects on human performance of a 1,5-benzodiazepine (clobazam) compared with the 1,4-benzodiazepines, chlordiazepoxide, hydrochloride and diazepam. *British Journal of Clinical Pharmacology* 2, 215–221.

Brogden, R. N., Heel, R. C., Speight, T. M. and Avery, G. S. (1979). Nomifensine: A review of its pharmacological properties and therapeutic efficacy in depressive illness. *Drugs* 18, 1–24.

Brogden, R. N., Heel, R. C., Speight, T. M. and Avery, G. S. (1979). Clobazam: A review of its pharmacological properties and therapeutic use in anxiety. *Drugs* 20, 161–178.

Crown, S. and Crisp, A. H. (1970). "Manual of the Middlesex Hospital Questionnaire". Psychological Test Publication, Barnstaple.

Hanks, G. W. (1977). A profile of nomifensine. *British Journal of Clinical Pharmacology* 4 (Suppl. 2), 2435–2488.

Hindmarch, I. (1975). A 1,4-benzodiazepine, temazepam (K3917): its effect on some psychological parameters of sleep and behaviour. *Arzneimittel-Forschung, Drug Research* **25**, 1836–1839.

Hindmarch, I. (1976). The effects of sub-chronic administration of an anti-histamine, clemastine on tests of car driving ability and psychomotor performance. *Current Medical Research and Opinion* **4**(3), 197–206.

Hindmarch, I. (1977). Laboratory investigation of effect of acute doses of nomifensine on a simulated aspect of night-time car driving performance. *British Journal of Clinical Pharmacology,* **4** (Suppl. 2), 175S–178S.

Hindmarch, I. (1979). Some aspects of the effects of clobazam on human psychomotor performance. *British Journal of Clinical Pharmacology* **7**, 77S–82S.

Hindmarch, I. (1980). Psychomotor function and psychoactive drugs. *British Journal of Clinical Pharmacology* **10**, 189–209.

Hindmarch, I. and Gudgeon, A. C. (1980). The effect of clobazam and lorazepam on aspects of psychomotor performance and car handling. *British Journal of Clinical Pharmacology* **10**, 145–150.

Hindmarch, I. and Parrott, A. C. (1977). Repeated dose comparison of nomifensine, imipranine and placebo on subjective assessments of sleep and objective measures of psychomotor performance. *British Journal of Clinical Pharmacology* **4** (Suppl. 2), 1675–1745.

Hindmarch, I. and Parrott, A. C. (1978). The effect of a sub-chronic administration of three dose levels of a 1,5-benzodiazepine derivative, clobazam, on subjective assessments of sleep and aspects of psychomotor performance the morning following night time medication. *Arzneimittel Forschung, Drug Research* **28**, 2169–2172.

Hindmarch, I. and Parrott, A. C. (1979). The effect of repeated nocturnal doses of clobazam, dipotassium chlorazepate and placebo on subjective ratings of sleep and early morning behaviour and objective measures of arousal, psychomotor performance and anxiety. *British Journal of Clinical Pharmacology* **8**, 325–329.

Hindmarch, I., Hanks, G. W. and Hewett, A. (1977). Clobazam, a 1,5-benzodiazepine, and car-driving ability. *British Journal of Clinical Pharmacology* **4**, 573–578.

Hindmarch, I., Parrott, A. C. and Stonier, P. D. (1982). The effects of nomifensine and HOE 8476 on car-driving and related psychomotor performance. *Royal Society of Medicine International Congress and Symposium Series* **25**, 47–54.

Parrott, A. C. and Hindmarch, I. (1978). Factor analysis of a sleep evaluation questionnaire. *Psychological Medicine* **8**, 325.

Parrott, A. C. and Munton, A. (1981). Comparative effects of clobazam and diazepam on psychological performance under different levels of background noise. *Royal Society of Medicine International Congress and Symposium* **43**, 51–58.

Parrott, A. C., Hindmarch, I. and Stonier, P. D. (1982). Nomifensine, clobazam and HOE 8476: Effect on aspects of psychomotor performance and cognitive ability. *European Journal of Clinical Pharmacology* **23**, 309–313.

Rupp, W. *et al.* (1979). Pharmacokinetics of single and multiple doses of clobazam in humans. *British Journal of Clinical Pharmacology* **7** (Suppl. 1), 51S–58S.

Stonier, P. D., Parrott, A. C. and Hindmarch, I. (1982). Clobazam in combination with nomifensine (HOE 8476): Effects on mood, sleep and psychomotor performance relating to car-driving ability. *Drug Development and Research,* Suppl. 1, 47–56.

Anxiety in Depression. Short Report.

A. GJERRIS

Rigshospitalet, Copenhagen, Denmark

In neurotic states anxiety is the crucial symptom, but also in depression anxiety constitutes a central feature (Bech *et al.*, 1975).

Looking at the Hamilton Depression Scale items, "psychic anxiety" appeared to carry as much weight as "depressed mood", "guilt" and "retardation", and on this basis "psychic anxiety" has been included in the Bech-Rafaelsen Melancholia Scale (BRMES), a modification of the Hamilton Depression Scale (Bech *et al.*, 1979; Bech and Rafaelsen, 1980). Furthermore, a drug trial quantifying the antidepressant effect of imipramine showed that "anxiety" was influenced to the same degree as "depressed mood", "guilt" and "retardation" (Bech *et al.*, 1981).

In more atypical forms of depression "anxiety" is often even more pronounced, and it has been claimed that particularly these types of depression benefit from treatment with monoamine oxidase inhibitors (Quitkin *et al.*, 1979).

How then do we measure depressive features in anxiety states and how do we measure anxiety features in depressive states? Hamilton (1959, 1969) developed an anxiety scale (HAS) to be used in neurotic anxiety, and this scale has also been applied by various researchers to assess anxiety in depressive states (McEnvoy *et al.*, 1980; Tyrer *et al.*, 1980). The 1969 version is now included in the National Institute of Mental Health Standard Assessment Battery (Guy, 1976).

In general, the usefulness and value of a rating scale depends upon several properties: reliability (inter-rater agreement), homogeneity (internal consistency), and transfer-ability (applicability).

With this background we found it important to evaluate the inter-rater reliability and homogeneity of the HAS when applied to patients diagnosed with depressive disorders (Bech *et al.*, 1978; Rafaelsen *et al.*, 1981; Gjerris *et al.*, 1983). We also correlated the total HAS score, i.e. a quantitation of anxiety to the total BRMES score, i.e. a quantitation of depression.

Twenty-two patients with depressive symptomatology were divided into 13 with endogenous depression (= melancholia) and nine with non-endogenous depression, using the 8th edition of the WHO International Classification of Diseases (IDC-8).

The inter-rater reliability was found statistically significant for both the HAS and the BRMES. On the other hand, the test for homogeneity comparing each item with the total score of the remaining items (using mean values for the participating raters), showed statistical significance for only seven of the 14 items on the HAS, whereas nine of 11 items on the BRMES had statistically significant correlation values.

The seven items of statistical significance on HAS were "anxious mood", "tension", "fear", "insomnia", "general somatic symptoms (sensory)", "cardiovascular symptoms", and "behaviour at interview", whereas the following items showed insignificant levels of correlation: "intellectual retardation", "depressed mood", "general somatic symptoms (muscular)", "respiratory symptoms", "autonomic symptoms", "gastrointestinal symptoms", and "genito-urinary symptoms".

A statistically positive correlation was found between the scale scores of the two rating systems (Spearman correlation coefficient r_S being 0.53, $P \leq 0.05$). When classifying the patients according to the ICD-8, this correlation seemed to be due to the group of endogenous depressions ($r_s = 0.73$, $P \leq 0.01$).

As we have felt the need for a more stringent set of research diagnostic criteria, the Multi-Axial Classification of Affective Disorders (MULTI-CLAD) was developed (Shapiro *et al.*, 1976), and when these criteria were applied, no significant intercorrelations of the HAS and the BRMES could be demonstrated within the subtypes of depression.

These findings are in accordance with Watts (1966), who obtained a positive correlation between severity of depression and anxiety. Crisp (1978) described that patients diagnosed with depressions reported very high levels of anxiety, whereas patients diagnosed as having anxiety disorders reported only moderate degrees of depressive symptoms. On the other hand, the difference in intercorrelation of HAS and BRMES between sub-types of depression was not confirmed when patients were classified according to MULTI-CLAD. This discrepancy between the diagnostic systems might be due to the small number of patients within the various classification categories of MULTI-CLAD.

In conclusion the present study has shown:

1. that the inter-observer reliability of the Hamilton Anxiety Scale in patients with depressive disorders is adequate, corresponding with the inter-observer reliability found by Hamilton (Roberts and Hamilton, 1958) in patients with anxiety neurosis;

2. that the homogeneity of the HAS compared with the homogeneity of the BRMES when applied on a group of depressed patients is unsatisfactory, but that the group of intercorrelated HAS-items correspond largely to the Hamilton factor of psychic anxiety (Hamilton 1969) and

3. that a positive correlation between the HAS-score and the BRMES-score can be demonstrated for the total group of depressed patients.

Hence, the summed score of HAS on patients with depressive disorders is not transferable to patients with anxiety neurosis. However, we have to consider that the present study is based upon our HAS item definitions making comparison to previous HAS studies difficult.

References

Bech, P. and Rafaelsen, O. J. (1980). The use of rating scales exemplified by a comparison of the Hamilton and the Bech-Rafaelsen Melancholia Scale. *Acta Psychiatr. Scand.* **62** (Suppl. 285), 128–132.

Bech, P., Gram, L. F., Dein, E., Jacobsen, O., Vitger, J. and Bolwig, T. G. (1975). Quantitative rating of depressive states. *Acta Psychiatr. Scand.* **51**, 161–170.

Bech, P., Allerup, R. and Rosenberg, R. (1978). The Marke-Nyman Temperament Scale: evaluation of transferability using the Rasch item analysis. *Acta Psychiatr. Scand.* **57**, 49–58.

Bech, P., Bolwig, T. G., Kramp, P. and Rafaelsen, O. J. (1979). The Bech-Rafaelsen Mania Scale and the Hamilton Depression Scale: evaluation of homogeneity and inter-observer reliability. *Acta Psychiatr. Scand.* **59**, 420–430.

Bech, P., Allerup, P., Gram, L. F. *et al.* (1981). The Hamilton Depression Scale: evaluation of objectivity using logistic models. *Acta Psychiatr. Scand.* **63**, 290–299.

Crisp, A. H. (1980). A biological factor operative with depression. *Br. J. Clin. Pract.* (Suppl. 7), 47–50.

Gjerris, A., Bech, P., Bøjholm, S., Bolwig, T. G., Kramp, P., Clemmesen, L., Andersen, J., Jensen, E. and Rafaelsen, O. J. (1983). The Hamilton Anxiety Scale. Evaluation of homogeneity and inter-observer reliability in patients with depressive disorders. *J. Affective Disord.* **5**, 163–170.

Guy, W. (1976). "ECDEU Assessment Manual." National Institute of Mental Health, Maryland.

Hamilton, M. (1959). The assessment of anxiety states by rating. *Br. J. Med. Psychol.* **32**, 50–55.

Hamilton, M. (1969). Diagnosis and rating of anxiety. In *Br. J. Psychiatry*, special publication, No. 3, 76–79.

McEnvoy, J. P., Sheridan, W. F., Stewart, W. R. C., Thomas, A. B., Wilson, W. H., Guy, W. and Schaffer, J. D. (1980). Viloxazine in the treatment of depressive neurosis: a controlled clinical study with doxepin. *Br. J. Psychiatry* **137**, 440–443.

Quitkin, F., Rifkin, A. and Klein, D. F. (1979). Monoamine oxidase inhibitors. A review of antidepressant effectiveness. *Arch. Gen. Psychiatry* **36**, 749–759.

Rafaelsen, O. J., Gjerris, A., Bolwig, T. G., Kramp, P., Bøjholm, S., Andersen, J. and Bech, P. (1981). Hamilton Anxiety Scale—evaluation of homogeneity and inter-observer reliability in patients with depressive disorders. In "Symposium on Psychopathology of Anxiety and its Management." Cairo.

Roberts, M. J. and Hamilton, M. (1958). Treatment of anxiety states: the effects of suggestion on the symptoms of anxiety states. *J. Ment. Sci.* **104**, 1052–1055.

Shapiro, R. W., Bock, E., Rafaelsen, O. J., Ryder, L. P. and Svejgaard, A. (1976). Histocompatibility antigens and manic-depressive disorders. *Arch. Gen. Psychiatr.* **33**, 823–825.

Tyrer, P., Gardner, M., Lambourn, J. and Whitford, M. (1980). Clinical and pharmakinetic factors affecting response to phenelzine. *Br. J. Psychiatry* **136**, 359–365.

Watts, C. A. H. (1966). "Depressive Disorders—In the Community." John Wright & Sons, Bristol.

The Effectiveness of Repeated Nocturnal Doses of Clobazam and Dipotassium Clorazepate on Clinical Measures of Anxiety, Patient Ratings of Mood and Sleep and Objective Assessments of CNS Activity

M. GRINGRAS and G. BEAUMONT

The Surgery, Priorslegh, London Road, Poynton, Cheshire, UK

Introduction

Nocturnal treatment with antianxiety agents with long pharmacological activity, has advantages in allowing unwanted side-effects to dissipate during sleep and in providing a residual antianxiety activity the day following medication (Nicholson *et al.*, 1976). Sedation and drowsiness are common side-effects of benzodiazepine derivatives used as antianxiety agents (Wittels and Stonier, 1981) and, while these are unwanted in ambulatory patients' operating machinery or driving motor vehicles, they are useful concomitants of nocturnal administration in assisting the induction of sleep.

However, it has been shown that drugs which improve sleep have a tendency to produce a "hangover" of detrimental effects the morning following medication (Bixler *et al.*, 1972) and this has been shown for a variety of 1,4-benzodiazepine derivatives (Hindmarch, 1984a).

Dipotassium clorazepate, a precursor of *N*-desmethyldiazepam, is used clinically for the treatment of anxiety on a nocturnal regimen because, like clobazam, it has pharmacological properties suggesting a long duration of antianxiety activity. Clobazam, a 1,5-benzodiazepine derivative has been shown to be effective in the clinical treatment of anxiety (Koeppen, 1981) and anxiolytic activity has been detected in the afternoon of the day following nocturnal doses of 30 mg clobazam (Hindmarch and Parrott, 1978). Clinical studies in general practice patients with anxiety (Hill *et al.*, 1981) have shown nocturnal doses of both 20 and 40 mg of clobazam are effective as day-time antianxiety agents without producing any untoward sedation.

This study compares the effects of clobazam and dipotassium clorazepate on subjective ratings of sleep, early morning behaviour and anxiety and objective assessments of CNS activity following repeated nocturnal doses in anxious patients.

Patients and Methods

Patients were selected from general practice. Anxiety was their major presenting symptom and included chronic free-floating anxiety, phobic anxiety states, acute anxiety states due to environmental or other stress, and combinations of these. Patients of either sex aged 15–70 years with a clinical diagnosis of anxiety and suitable for general practice management were admitted to the study. Exclusion criteria were pregnancy or suspected pregnancy, patients with known renal or hepatic disease, alcoholics, patients with psychotic illness, patients in whom underlying depression was suspected or patients who must continue with other CNS-active drugs including hypnotics.

The study was designed as a double-blind three parallel group comparison for two weeks with a preceding week placebo wash-out period and a placebo withdrawal period of two weeks. The treatment groups were clobazam 20 mg, clobazam 30 mg and clorazepate 15 mg. Placebo and active treatments were presented in identical capsules, patients being "blind" to the whole treatment regimen and clinicians "blind" to the active treatment conditions.

Ninety patients, 30 per group, were to be entered into the study from three general practice groups. Those satisfying the inclusion criteria were admitted to the study and had a practice session on the psychomotor testing equipment. Initially patients were assessed by the clinician on a four-point clinical global rating scale, and completed the

Middlesex Hospital Questionnaire (MHQ) and line analogue scales of symptoms. At the first visit patients were assessed clinically and given placebo tablets for one week and then were assessed again and randomly allocated to one of the three treatment groups. Patients were required to take the medication nightly 30 min before retiring to bed. Clinical and psychological assessments were again made after one and two weeks active treatment and following one and two weeks withdrawal, while receiving placebo.

Assessments at each visit were as follows:

(1) Clinical Global Rating (CGR) was made by the physician on a four-point rating scale.
(2) Line Analogue Symptom Rating Scales (LARS) were completed by the patients to measure the subjective symptoms of anxiety (Hill *et al.*, 1981).
(3) The Leeds Sleep Evaluation Questionnaire (LSEQ) (Hindmarch, 1975, 1984b) was used to assess the patients' ability to get to sleep, the perceived quality of sleep, the ease of waking and the integrity of behaviour on waking.
(4) Side-effects, adverse life events, drop-outs due to concurrent illness, change in medication, and compliance checks were recorded as and when they occurred.
(5) Critical Flicker Fusion Threshold (CFFT) was measured on the Leeds Psychomotor Tester (Hindmarch and Parrot, 1978) for four light-emitting diodes in foveal fixation at 1 m, using the psychophysical method of limits for three ascending and three descending scales (Woodworth and Schlosberg, 1958).

The MHQ was repeated at the end of the active treatment period. The assessments and treatments schedules are summarized in Table 1.

Results

Complete data was obtained from 35 patients—ten in the clobazam 20 mg group, 14 in the clobazam 30 mg group and 11 in the clorazepate group. Analyses of variance for repeated measures were performed on the data and post hoc comparisons of treatment means made using 95% confidence limits. On analysis of the pre-test, LARS, for symptoms of anxiousness, tiredness, feeling happy,

drowsiness, dizziness, energy, and sadness, the group allocated to clobazam 30 mg were found to be less severely anxious and this was confirmed by the CGR scores made by the clinicians which showed the patients in this treatment group to be significantly less anxious than those in the other two groups. Scores in the 30 mg clobazam group on CFFT were also significantly higher, indicating less anxiety, than those in the two other treatment groups. It was felt that not sufficient data was available to use covariant analyses of variance to take account of pre-test differences in baselines and it was decided to drop the 30 mg clobazam condition from the present analysis.

Line Analogue Symptom Rating Scales (LARS)

Figure 1 shows the patients' response week by week on a 10 cm VAS for "anxiousness". Both groups have similar pre-test levels but, after one week's medication with clobazam, there is a dramatic decrease in anxiety symptoms which is statistically significant both from the pre-test level and when compared with the clorazepate group, which had a smaller decrease in anxiety. After two weeks clorazepate had an equivalent anxiolytic effect which was significantly different from baseline. In the first post-active treatment week there is very little difference between the two groups, but a divergence in scores shows up very obviously during the second placebo week where patients on clobazam are still significantly improved, whilst patients on clorazepate are reporting an increase in their "anxiousness". The response to the question "More or less happy than usual?" is shown in Fig. 2. Both active treatment groups have similar baseline scores, but the clobazam group shows a more rapid response which persists two weeks after treatment, whilst the clorazepate group again deteriorates during the placebo follow-up period.

Figure 3 shows the ratings of relaxation from the LARS and it can be seen that after one week of medication with clobazam and after two weeks of medication with clorazepate there are significant drug related improvements in relaxation. Those patients treated with clobazam sustain their improvement in contrast to the cessation of effect on withdrawal of clorazepate.

Figures 4, 5 and 6 show a similar pattern of

Table 1

Assessments and treatment schedule

	Week					
	0	1	2	3	4	5
Middlesex Hospital Questionnaire (MHQ)		×			×	
Clinical Global Rating (CGR)		×	×	×	×	×
Line Analogue Symptom Rating Scale (LAR)		×	×	×	×	×
Leeds Sleep Evaluation Questionnaire (LSEQ)			×	×	×	×
Critical Flicker Fusion Threshold (CFFT)		×	×	×	×	×
Treatment dispensed	P	D	D	P	P	—

P, Placebo; D, clobazam 20 mg, 30 mg, clorazepate, 15 mg.
Week 1 is pre-test baseline following one-week placebo.

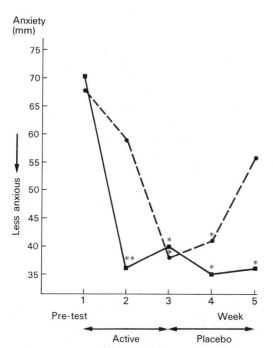

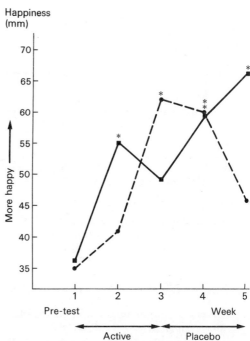

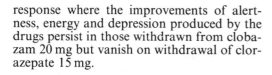

Figure 1. Line Analogue Scale for anxiety. *, different from pre-test (P <0·05); +, different from clorazepate (P <0·05). ■——■, clobazam 20 mg; ●--●, clorazepate 15 mg.

Figure 2. Line Analogue Scale for happiness. *, different from pre-test (P <0·05). ■——■, clobazam 20 mg; ●--●, clorazepate 15 mg.

response where the improvements of alertness, energy and depression produced by the drugs persist in those withdrawn from clobazam 20 mg but vanish on withdrawal of clorazepate 15 mg.

Clinical Global Rating (CGR)

CGRs scored by the physicians (Fig. 7)

showed that both drugs improved overall ratings of the severity of anxiety, which persisted on withdrawal of medication in spite of a recorded worsening of the CGRs.

The Leeds Sleep Evaluation Questionnaire (LSEQ)

Analysis of the Leeds Sleep Evaluation Questionnaire on the four variables of getting

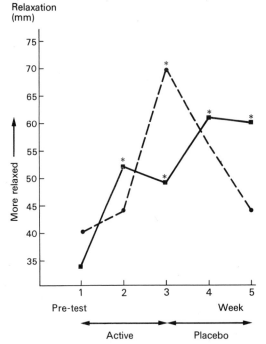

Figure 3. Line Analogue Scale for relaxation. *, different from pre-test (5% level); +, different from cloraxepate (5% level). ■——■, clobazam 20 mg; ●——●, clorazepate 15 mg.

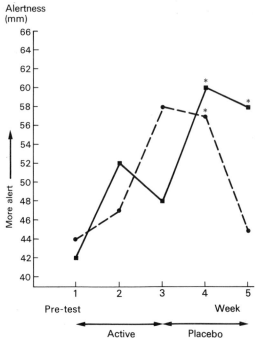

Figure 4. Line Analogue Scale for alertness. *, different from pre-test ($P < 0.05$). ■——■, clobazam 20 mg; ●——●, clorazepate 15 mg.

to sleep, quality of sleep, awaking from sleep, and behaviour following waking, showed no significant difference between the two treatment groups.

Critical Flicker Fusion Threshold (CFFT)

The clobazam 20 mg group and the clorazepate 15 mg group had similar pre-test CFFT levels, but after both one week and two weeks of treatment there was a significant improvement shown in the clobazam 20 mg group which was maintained during the two weeks placebo follow-up (Fig. 8).

Middlesex Hospital Questionnaire (MHQ)

The MHQ analysed into its six constituent factors showed no significant difference between the two treatment groups, as can be seen from the results in Table 2.

Side-effects

There were no significant reports of side-

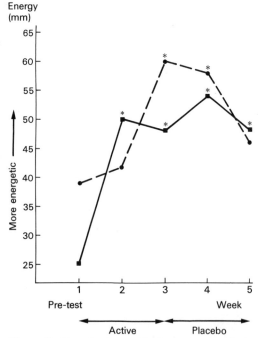

Figure 5. Line Analogue Scale for energy. *, different from pre-test ($P < 0.05$). ■——■, clobazam 20 mg; ●——●, clorazepate 15 mg.

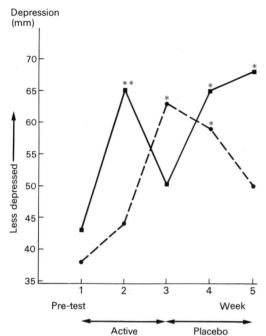

Figure 6. Line Analogue Scale for depression. *, different from pre-test (P <0·05); +, different from clorazepate (P <0·05). ■——■, clobazam 20 mg; ●--●, clorazepate 15 mg.

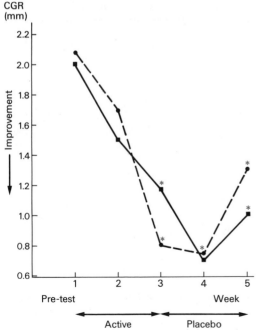

Figure 7. Clinical Global Rating (CGR). *, different from pre-test (P <0·05). ■——■, clobazam 20 mg; ●--●, clorazepate 15 mg.

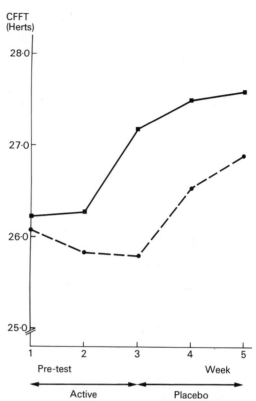

Figure 8. Critical Flicker Fusion Threshold (CFFT). *, different from pre-test (P <0·05); ⊙, pre-test level of clobazam 30 mg group. ■——■, clobazam 20 mg; ●--●, clorazepate 15 mg.

effects associated with either of the active treatments and no noticeable life events or problems with compliance reported.

Discussion

It was planned to admit 90 patients to the study from three general practice centres, and six months after the start of the project, in mid-1981, one centre had completed its quota. The other two centres failed to provide any patients for the study and the recruitment of further centres did not significantly improve the patient numbers. The reason for the poor recruitment (a final complement of 35 patients) was identified as a rapidly changing attitude to benzodiazepine prescribing and clinical trial participation amongst both general practitioners and patients.

The results from patients' blind ratings of drug efficacy (LARS) shows that clobazam

Table 2

Middlesex Hospital Questionnaire

	MHQ Score						
	A	P	O	S	D	H	
Clobazam 20 mg	10·0	4·8[a]	9·5	7·8	6·3	4·3	Pre-test
(n = 10)	10·0	5·0	9·8	6·3	6·5	3·9	Post-test
Clorazepate 15 mg	11·0	6·4	7·5	8·8	6·3	3·6	Pre-test
(n = 12)	10·6	6·5	8·1	7·4	5·7	3·3	Post-test

[a]Significant difference clobazam/clorazepate, $P < 0.05$.
A, Anxiety; O, obsession; D, depression; P, phobia; S, somatic; H, hysteria.

20 mg achieved a more rapid antianxiety effect than clorazepate 15 mg, although both drugs were rated as effective antianxiety agents at some point during active medication. On withdrawal of active medication there was a noticeable rebound, i.e. return of the symptoms of anxiety, in the patients' ratings following clorazepate but not clobazam.

CFF thresholds reflect the LARS results quite closely. Such a concordance of objective (CFF) and subjective (LARS) measures suggest that the clinical effects observed by the patients have, as their basis, some intrinsic property of the drug. Indeed the striking difference between clobazam and clorazepate in the speed of onset of patient rated antianxiety activity and upon withdrawal, might be a further reflection of basic differences between 1,4-benzodiazepines (clorazepate) and the 1,5-benzodiazepine (clobazam). The deterioration of patient ratings of "relaxation" following cessation of treatment with clorazepate could well pose problems in withdrawing patients from sub-chronic and chronic treatments with the drug. The maintained "relaxation" on withdrawal of clobazam suggests that patients experience fewer difficulties on withdrawal of active treatment.

The persistent improvement in CFF scores during and upon cessation of treatment with clobazam concurs closely with the work of Hill *et al.* (1981) and Ponciano *et al.* (1981). These authors reported a significant increase in CFF following repeated doses of clobazam in anxious patients. Krugman (1947), Goldstone (1955), Bühler (1955), and Jones (1958) established a definite correlation between anxiety levels and CFF. Anxious patients have, in general, a lower CFF than age- and sex-matched "normals". In terms of this present study a clear augmentation of CFF levels is found following treatment with clobazam 20 mg and this is commensurate with improvement in patient ratings. Both CFF improvements, lower anxiety and LARS ratings of antianxiety activity, persist after treatment with clobazam. Clorazepate does not rapidly reduce LARS ratings and on cessation of treatment there is a worsening of LARS and CFF measures.

There are many situations in clinical practice where short sub-chronic courses of antianxiety treatment are required. Clobazam has shown itself to be superior to clorazepate as the latter drug is slower to exert an anxiolytic effect and has more problems associated with its withdrawal upon cessation of treatment.

Summary

A double-blind comparative study in anxious patients in general practice compared clobazam 20 mg and clorazepate 15 mg given at night for three weeks. Both drugs significantly improve anxiety ratings after one week's treatment, with clobazam having a significantly greater effect when compared with clorazepate.

Assessments in a two-week withdrawal period following active treatment indicate that the effects of clobazam are maintained during this period whilst those patients who had been treated with clorazepate showed evidence of deterioration. Possible reasons for this are discussed.

Acknowledgements

The authors are grateful to the following general practitioners for contributing patients to this study: Drs H. Williams, D. John, W. E. Helliwell, J. Caisley, P. Franks, K. Shearer, and A. G. E. Smith.

References

Bixler, E. O., Scharf, M. B. and Kales, A. (1972). "NATO symposium on drugs, sleep and performance." Aviemore, Scotland (mimeo).
Bühler, R. A. (1955). Flicker fusion threshold and anxiety level. *Psychological Abstracts* **39**, 701.
Goldstone, S. (1955). Critical flicker fusion measurement and anxiety level. *Journal of Experimental Psychology* **49**, 200.
Hill, A. J., Hindmarch, I. and Walsh, R. D. (1981). Tolerability of nocturnal doses of clobazam in anxious patients in general practice. *Royal Society of Medicine International Congress and Symposium Series* **43**, 133–140.
Hindmarch, I. (1975). A 1,4-benzodiazepine, temozepan (K3917). Its effects of some psychological parameters of sleep and behaviour. *Arzneimittel-Forschung* **25**, 1836–1839.
Hindmarch, I. (1984a). "Drugs and Psychiatry", Vol. II, 217–229. Elsevier, Amsterdam.
Hindmarch, I. (1984b). "Biological psychiatry: Recent studies", pp. 228–239. Hibbey, London.
Hindmarch, I. and Parrott, A. C. (1978). The effect of a sub-chronic administration of three doses levels of a 1,5-benzodiazepine derivative, clobazam, on subjective assessments of sleep and aspects of psychomotor performance the morning following night time medication. *Arzneimitel-Forschung* **28**, 2169–2172.
Jones, O. (1958). Relationship between visual and auditory discrimination and anxiety level. *Journal of General Psychology* **59**, 111.
Koeppen, D. (1981). Clinical Experience with clobazam 1968–81. *Royal Society of Medicine International Congress and Symposium Series* **43**, 193–198.
Krugman, H. (1947). Flicker fusion frequency as a function of anxiety reaction: An exploratory study. *Psychomatic Medicine* **4**, 269.
Nicholson, A. N., Stone, B. M., Clarke, C. H. and Ferres, H. M. (1976). Effects of N-desmethyldiazepam and a precursor potassium clorazepate on sleep in man. *British Journal of Clinical Pharmacology* **3**, 429–438.
Parrott, A. C. and Hindmarch, I. (1978). Clobazam—A 1,5-benzodiazepine derivative: Effect upon human psychomotor performance under different levels of task reinforcement. *Archives Internationales de Pharmacodynamie et de Thérapie* **232**, 261–268.
Ponciano, E., Relvas, J., Mendes, F., Lameiras, A., Vazserra, A. and Hindmarch, I. (1981). Clinical effects and sedative activity of bromazepam and clobazam in the treatment of anxious out-patients. *Royal Society of Medicine International Congress and Symposium Series* **43**, 125–131.
Wittels, P. Y. and Stonier, P. D. (1981). The effects of benzodiazepines on psychomotor performance in patients. *Royal Society of Medicine International Congress and Symposium Series* **43**, 111–118.
Woodworth, R. S. and Schlosberg, H. (1958). *Experimental Psychology*. Methuen, London.

Differential Effects of Three Benzodiazepines in the Treatment of Neurotic Patients

C. DISAYAVANISH, S. MAHATNIRUNKUL and P. DISAYAVANISH

Department of Psychiatry, Faculty of Medicine, Chiang Mai University, Chiang Mai, Thailand

Introduction

For more than two decades, benzodiazepines have been amongst the most widely prescribed anti-anxiety drugs in clinical practice. Their record of safety and efficacy in treating anxiety and its related symptoms is remarkable. 1,4-Benzodiazepines are a class of centrally active compounds which possess sedative-hypnotic, anti-anxiety, anti-convulsant and muscle-relaxant properties to varying degrees (Hollister, 1978; Richter, 1981). The best known of these compounds are chlordiazepoxide, diazepam, clorazepate, lorazepam and oxazepam.

Diazepam is one of the most popularly used 1,4-benzodiazepines. The major metabolic pathway of diazepam in humans involves N-demethylation, yielding its pharmacologically active metabolite, N-desmethyldiazepam. The plasma half-life of diazepam shows two phases when the drug is given intravenously—a rapid, distributive phase and a second, slower phase. The latter has varied between 26 and 53 h with different subjects. Peak plasma levels at a steady-state showed a two-fold variation both for diazepam and its major plasma metabolite—N-desmethyldiazepam (Berlin *et al.*, 1972). Steady-state conditions are reached for diazepam at the end of one week, with a half-life of 54 h, and for N-desmethyldiazepam at the beginning of the second week, with a half-life for the metabolite of 92 h (Hillestad *et al.*, 1974).

Lorazepam, a conventional 1,4-benzodiazepine, is considered to be one of the most highly potent anti-anxiety agents. It is biotransformed by direct conjugation to glucuronic acid, yielding a water-soluble glucuronide metabolite which is excreted in the urine (Greenblatt *et al.*, 1976). Active metabolic products are not produced. The elimination half-life of lorazepam is shorter than that of diazepam, ranging from 10 to 20 h in most individuals (Shader and Greenblatt, 1981).

Clobazam is the first 1,5-benzodiazepine and thus differs structurally from all previous 1,4-benzodiazepines used in the treatment of anxiety. This drug is metabolized in the body by demethylation and hydroxylation, yielding norclobazam or N-desmethyl-clobazam as the principal active metabolite.

Clobazam has a half-life of 18 h and is thus long-acting. Moreover, it also has an active metabolite, whose half-life is even longer, i.e. 50 h (Fielding and Hoffmann, 1979).

Both laboratory and clinical research have shown that clobazam possesses pronounced anxiolytic activity without the disruption of psychomotor performance normally found following the administration of anxiety-reducing 1,4-benzodiazepines (Hindmarch, 1979; Wittenborn *et al.*, 1979). Some studies suggested that diazepam might exert detrimental effects on learning and memory capabilities at therapeutic doses (Subhan, 1981). Another study was performed to investigate the effects of clobazam and lorazepam on memory functions in relation to their effects on psychomotor performance, vigilance, and mood state. Anterograde amnesia after lorazepam was significantly stronger than after both clobazam and placebo. It was suggested that the anterograde amnestic effects of benzodiazines were related to their detrimental effects on other functions such as vigilance and psychomotor performance (Siegfried *et al.*, 1981).

The objective of this study is to investigate the possible differences among the three benzodiazepines (i.e. diazepam, clobazam and lorazepam) both in the treatment of anxiety and in the withdrawal effects following discontinuation of medication.

Methods

Patients

The study was carried out in the Department of Psychiatry, Faculty of Medicine, Chiang Mai University, Chiang Mai, Thailand. A total of 60 inpatients were admitted to the study; of these, 50 completed the six-week period of this study. All patients (27 male, 23 female) were aged between 11 and 60 years with a mean of 31·25 years (Table 1), and were diagnosed as suffering primarily from anxiety with various clinical manifestation. Anxiety neurosis was the most frequent diagnosis (40%), followed by hypochondriacal neurosis (16%). The diagnostic groups are given in Table 2.

Materials and Design

The study lasted six weeks. On entry to the study all patients received a week's treatment with placebo, three times daily, to wash out the residual effects of previously administered psychoactive drugs. The baseline assessments were made after one week. Patients were allocated to one of three types of tablets using a randomized set of letter codes: A, B and C.

Table 1

Age and sex of patients

Age range	No. of patients
11–20	10
21–30	14
31–40	13
41–50	10
51–60	3
	$N = 50$
	(27 males, 23 females)

    Group A received 5 mg diazepam t.i.d. for a four-week period. Group B and Group C received 10 mg clobazam t.i.d. and 1 mg lorazepam t.i.d. respectively for a similar length of time. After one month of drug treatment all patients received placebo three times daily for one week. Placebo and active treatments

Table 2

Diagnosis in patients

Diagnosis	Group		
	A	B	C
Anxiety neurosis	7	6	7
Hypochondriacal neurosis	2	3	3
Phobic neurosis	—	—	1
Obsessive-compulsive neurosis	1	1	—
Hysterical neurosis	2	2	1
Depressive neurosis	2	2	1
Adjustment reaction	1	—	—
Neurotic alcoholism	—	1	1
Psychophysiologic disorders	2	3	1
Total	17	18	15

were presented in identical matching tablets. After the code was revealed, it appeared that Group A's 17 patients were given diazepam, Group B's 18 patients were given clobazam and Group C's 15 patients received lorazepam.

    The physicians were unaware as to which treatment condition the patients had been allocated until the code was broken at the end of the study. Assessments for all measures were made by individual physicians at the initial interview with the patient, after a one-week treatment with placebo, after two weeks of treatment with either diazepam, clobazam, or lorazepam, after four weeks of drug treatment, and following a one-week wash out with placebo.

Assessments

All patients were assessed on the Hoechst Anxiety Rating Scale which was completed by the physician and scores computed for psychic, somatic and overall levels of anxiety. In this rating scale, 11 items were scored from 1 (not present) to 5 (very severe).

Results

During the six-week period of the study, ten patients dropped out of the trial as they left the hospital before the schedule and did not return for follow-up. The mean scores at each assessment session regarding the effects of three drugs, obtained on the anxiety rating scale, is presented in Table 3.

Analyses of variance (McCall, 1970) were used to test the significance of the changes produced by the drug treatment and to assess possible differences among diazepam, clobazam and lorazepam. Where significant effects ($P < 0.05$) were found by the analysis of variance a Duncan's new multiple range test (Edwards, 1970) was employed as a post-hoc procedure to compare the drug treatment.

The comparisons among the average total scores of Group A, Group B and Group C are given in Fig. 1. None of the analyses of variance among drug differences proved significant ($P < 0.05$) after two and four weeks of treatment. However, there was a significant differential effect ($P < 0.05$) found on the withdrawal period.

Figure 2 shows the mean psychic anxiety scores of Group A, Group B and Group C. The analyses of variance revealed similar results as presented in Fig. 1. The difference in the efficacy of the three drugs in reducing the psychic anxiety symptoms was not statistically significant ($P < 0.05$) after two and four weeks of treatment but, however, it became significant ($P < 0.05$) one week following the cessation of medication.

The analyses of variance showed no significant differential effect of the three drugs in reducing the somatic anxiety symptoms on any of the assessment measures (Fig. 3).

The differences among the mean psychic anxiety scores of three drugs were assessed by means of a Duncan's new multiple range test after the final week on placebo. The analysis showed that the patients treated with diaze-pam and lorazepam developed the recurrence of the symptom of anxiety during the placebo withdrawal period (Table 4).

Some side-effects were observed in 11 patients: in five patients (29·41%) as a result of diazepam, in two (11·11%) after clobazam and in four (26·67%) after lorazepam. The side-effects are listed in Table 5. Three patients who were treated with diazepam developed rather severe ataxia and lethargy after one week of treatment and the dose had to be reduced to 2 mg t.i.d. The incidence of side-effects on clobazam (four complaints) was significantly low as compared to diaze-pam (13 complaints) and lorazepam (nine complaints).

Discussion

It is obvious from this study that there is no significant difference discernible between dia-zepam, clobazam and lorazepam in the treatment of anxiety. Physicians were unable to discriminate among the three drugs in terms of efficacy during the four-week treatment period. The statistical computations also confirm that there is no way of differentiating the effects of one drug from another on anxiety rating scales.

On withdrawal of medication, reduction of anxiety was maintained in the clobazam group with no significant change in the mean total and mean psychic anxiety scores, whereas in the diazepam and lorazepam groups there was a notable worsening of anxiety in both mean scores. The recurrence

Table 3

Effects of three drugs on the Anxiety Rating Scale (average scores at each assessment session)

Anxiety Rating Scale	Drug	Pretest	Placebo	Acter two weeks on drug	After four weeks on drug	After one week on placebo
Psychic	A Diazepam	15·00	14·29	10·35	8·35	11·59
	B Clobazam	15·72	15·16	11·55	8·77	8·94
	C Lorazepam	14·60	14·00	9·60	8·73	12·33
Somatic	A Diazepam	9·76	9·23	7·53	6·59	6·59
	B Clobazam	10·67	10·22	8·22	7·05	6·89
	C Lorazepam	9·40	9·00	7·47	6·73	7·40
Total	A Diazepam	24·76	23·52	17·88	14·94	18·17
	B Clobazam	26·38	25·38	19·77	15·83	15·83
	C Lorazepam	24·00	23·00	17·06	15·46	19·73

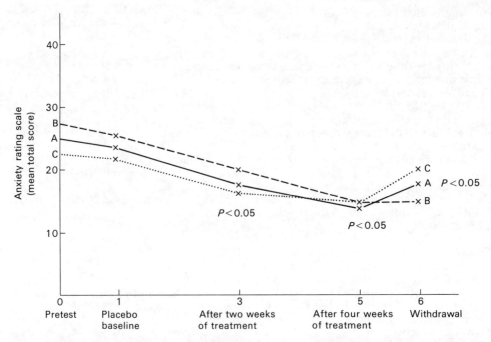

Figure 1. Comparison between the average scores on Anxiety Rating Scale. A=15 mg diazepam per day (n=17); B=30 mg clobazam per day (n=18); C=3 mg lorazepam per day (n=15).

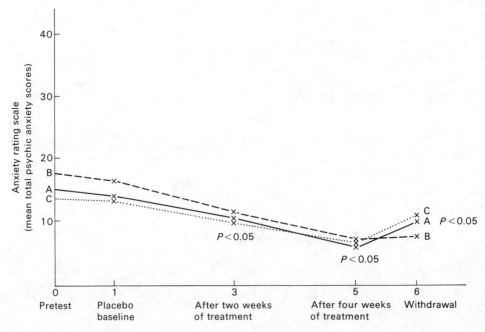

Figure 2. Comparison between the mean psychic anxiety scores. A=15 mg diazepam per day (n=17); B=30 mg clobazam per day (n=18); C=3 mg lorazepam per day (n=15).

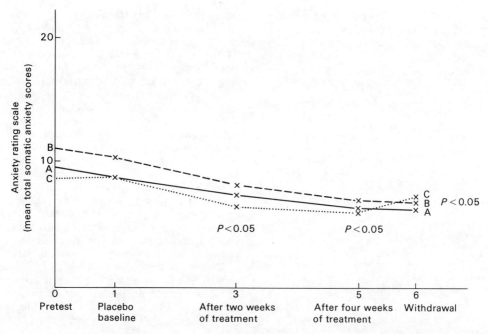

Figure 3. Comparison between the mean somatic anxiety scores. A=15 mg diazepam per day (n=17); B=30 mg clobazam per day (n=18); C=3 mg lorazepam per day (n=15).

of anxiety on the total psychic anxiety scores following discontinuation of treatment with diazepam and lorazepam was significantly different from clobazam ($P<0.05$).

De Figueiredo *et al.* (1981) studied 60 anxious patients who received either lorazepam or clobazam for four weeks, preceded and followed by a one-week placebo treatment. Both drugs were equally effective in changing the rating of anxiety. Statistically significant differences between the two drugs were observed after the final week on placebo. In the patients treated with lorazepam the psychic anxiety scores worsened and began to return to their pre-drug levels. This reoccurrence of the symptoms of anxiety was not noticed in the patients treated with clobazam.

Doongaji *et al.* (1979) analysed the data on 40 patients and found that the differences between clobazam and diazepam failed to reach statistical significance either on the total scores of the Hamilton Anxiety Scale or the psychic anxiety and somatic anxiety clusters of this scale. At the end of the post-drug

Table 4

Differences between means of three groups (withdrawal period)

Duncan's New Multiple Range Test		
Group	A	B	C
Mean	11·59	8·94	12·33

Least significant range $= 1.65$ ($n_A = 17$, $n_B = 18$)
$= 1.81$ ($n_C = 15$, $n_A = 17$)
$= 1.74$ ($n_C = 15$, $n_B = 18$)

D–C $= 2.65 > 1.65$ Significance ($P<0.05$)
L–D $= 0.74 < 1.81$ Non-significance ($P<0.05$)
L–C $= 3.39 > 1.74$ Significance ($P<0.05$)
∴Diazepam and lorazepam develop the recurrence of the symptoms of anxiety

D = diazepam, C = clobazam, L = lorazepam

placebo period, the clobazam series maintained greater anxiolytic efficacy compared with the diazepam series.

Although our results indicate that diazepam, clobazam, and lorazepam have equipotent anti-anxiety activity, they do display significant differences on the anxiety rating scale following discontinuation of active treatment. Clobazam is an anxiolytic agent with a long pharmacological activity, due probably to its principal active metabolite N-desmethylclobazam. On the other hand, lora-

Table 5

Side-effects

	Treatment Groups		
	Diazepam (n = 17)	Clobazam (n = 18)	Lorazepam (n = 15)
Number reporting side-effects	5 (29·41%)	2 (11·11%)	4 (26·67%)
Side-effects reported			
Drowsiness	4	2	4
Dry mouth	2	1	2
Lethargy	4	1	2
Ataxia	3	0	1
Total side-effects reported*	13	4	9

*The numbers refer to complaints, not patients. The total number of complaints exceeds the number of patients because of multiple side-effects in some patients.

zepam is much shorter in the duration of its action and has no active metabolites. Clobazam with its active metabolite has an elimination half-life of between 18 and 72 h (Rupp et al., 1979), while lorazepam has an elimination half-life of between 9 and 22 h (Greenblatt et al., 1977).

Thus it can be postulated that the difference observed between clobazam and lorazepam in this study and the others is due to the dissimilarity of their elimination half-lives. The lorazepam group would be experiencing the withdrawal of active compound after one week on placebo, whereas the clobazam group would still have residual active metabolite to provide anxiolytic effect.

Since the elimination half-life of diazepam is 20 and 70 h (Mandelli et al., 1978) when diazepam therapy at usual therapeutic dose is abruptly terminated, the drug is by no means rapidly eliminated from the body. Clinically important amounts of diazepam and desmethyldiazepam may persist in the blood and in the body for days and even weeks after the termination of treatment. However, objective withdrawal syndromes associated with diazepam therapy do occur, but they are probably not common. After abrupt discontinuation, occasional patients show symptoms which are suggestive of withdrawal. Some report insomnia or waking from sleep with sweating and nightmares. Other patients show a clinical picture consistent with the classical sedative-hypnotic withdrawal syndrome long associated with barbiturates, though occurring somewhat later (Shader and Greenblatt, 1981; Seppälä et al., 1976; Berry et al., 1974; Borland and Nicholson, 1974).

Several studies have commented on the sedative-hypnotic activity of diazepam and lorazepam and the relative lack of unwanted effect of sedation attributable to clobazam. Such sedative-hypnotic activity might be perceived by the patient as an habitual concomitant of drug administration. When diazepam or lorazepam is abruptly terminated, subjective awareness of drug activity and support will rapidly disappear giving rise to the patient's feeling of insecurity and anxiety.

On the contrary, the relative lack of sedative effect associated with the administration of clobazam and the presence of its anxiolytic metabolite with a rather long half-life, will make the transition from drug to placebo states less noticeable to the patient.

The side-effects of three drugs consisted chiefly of drowsiness, dryness of the mouth, lethargy and ataxia and all of them appeared at the beginning of therapy. However, the unusually low incidence of side-effects on clobazam was impressive.

Since the sudden withdrawal of benzodiazepines may cause the relapse of anxiety, Goldstein (1982) suggests physicians should discontinue both short- and long-acting benzodiazepines gradually, especially when given for longer than four months and even if doses were in the therapeutic range. A reasonable schedule to follow would be to reduce the dose by 10 to 25% each week, depending on the dose and length of time that the patient has taken the medication.

Summary

This randomized double-blind study consisted of 60 patients with neurotic disorders. Each patient received either 15 mg diazepam, 30 mg clobazam or 3 mg lorazepam daily for four weeks. This period was preceded and followed by a one-week placebo treatment to wash out the residual effects of previously administered psychoactive drugs and to monitor withdrawal effects, respectively. All three drugs were equally effective in changing the ratings of anxiety obtained on the Hoechst anxiety rating scale ($P < 0.05$).

After the final week on placebo, the significant differences among the three drugs were observed. In the patients treated with loraze-

pam and diazepam the psychic anxiety scores worsened and began to return to their pre-drug levels. The recurrence of the symptoms of anxiety was not noticed in the patients treated with clobazam.

References

Berlin, A., Siwers, B., Agurell, S., Hiort, A., Sjoquist, F. and Strom, S. (1972). Determinations of bioavailability of diazepam in various formulations from steady-state plasma concentration data. *Clinical Pharmacology and Therapeutics* **13**, 733–744.

Berry, P. A., Burtles, R., Grubb, D. J. and Hoare, M. V. (1974). An evaluation of the effects of clobazam on human motor coordination, mental activity and mood. *British Journal of Clinical Pharmacology* **1**, 346.

Borland, R. G. and Nicholson, A. N. (1974). Immediate effects on human performance of a 1,5-benzodiazepine derivative (clobazam) compared with the 1,4-benzodiazepines chlordiazepoxide hydrochloride and diazepam. *British Journal of Clinical Pharmacology* **2**, 215–221.

De Figueiredo, R., Franchini, A., Martinho, A. and Hindmarch, I. (1981). Differences in the effect of two benzodiazepines in the treatment of anxious outpatients. *International Pharmacopsychiatry* **16**, 57–65.

Doongaji, D. R., Sheth, A., Apṭe, J. S., Lakdawala, P. D., Khare, C. B. and Thatte, S. S. (1979). Clobazam versus diazepam: A double-blind study in anxiety neurosis. *British Journal of Clinical Pharmacology* **7**, 119s.

Edwards, A. L. (1970). "Experimental Design in Psychological Research." Holt, Rinehart and Winston, London.

Fielding, S. and Hoffmann, I. (1979). Pharmacology of anti-anxiety drugs with special reference to clobazam. *British Journal of Clinical Pharmacology* **7**, 7s–15s.

Goldstein, B. J. (1982). The risk of abuse/dependence: A perspective. In "Benzodiazepines in the 80s: Era of Change." Proceedings from a Symosium. Biomedical Information Corporation, New York.

Greenblatt, D. J., Schillings, R. T., Kyriakopoulos, A. A., Sader, R. I., Sisenwine, S. F., Knowles, J. A. and Ruelius, H. W. (1976). Clinical pharmacokinetics of lorazepam. I. Absorption and disposition of oral ^{14}C-lorazepam. *Clinical Pharmacology and Therapeutics* **20**, 329–341.

Greenblatt, D. J., Joyce, T. H., Comer, W. H., Knowles, J. A., Shader, R. I., Kyriakopoulos, A. A., MacLaughlin, D. S. and Ruelius, H. W. (1977). Clinical pharmacokinetics of lorazepam. II. Intramuscular injection. *Clinical Pharmacology and Therapeutics* **21**, 222–230.

Hillestad, L., Hansen, T. and Melsom, H. (1974). Diazepam metabolism in normal man. II. Serum concentration and clinical effect after oral administration and accumulation. *Clinical Pharmacology and Therapeutics* **16**, 485–489.

Hindmarch, I. (1979). Some aspects of the effects of clobazam on human psychomotor performance. *British Journal of Clinical Pharmacology* **7**, 77s–82s.

Hollister, L. E. (1978). Antianxiety drugs. In "Clinical Pharmacology of Psychotherapeutic Drugs", pp. 12–49. Churchill Livingstone, Edinburgh and New York.

McCall, R. B. (1970). "Fundamental Statistics for Psychology." Harcourt Brace and World, New York.

Mandelli, M., Togoni, G. and Garattini, S. (1978). Clinical pharmacokinetics of diazepam. *Clinical Pharmacokinetics* **3**, 72–91.

Richter, J. J. (1981). Current theories about the mechanisms of benzodiazepines and neuroleptic drugs. *Anesthesiology* **54**, 66–72.

Rupp, W., Badian, M., Christ, D., Hajdu, R. D., Kulkarni, R. D., Taeuber, K., Uihlein, M., Bender, R. and Vanderbeke, O. (1979). Pharmacokinetics of single and multiple doses of clobazam in humans. *British Journal of Clinical Pharmacology* **7**, 51–57.

Seppälä, T., Kortilla, K., Häkkinen, S. and Linnoila, M. (1976). Residual effects and skills related to driving after a single oral administration of diazepam, medazepam or lorazepam. *British Journal of Clinical Pharmacology* **3**, 831–841.

Shader, R. I. and Greenblatt, D. J. (1981). The use of benzodiazepines in clinical practice. *British Journal of Clinical Pharmacology* **11**, 5s–9s.

Siegfried, K., Koeppen, D., Taeuber, K., Badian, M., Malerczyk, V. and Sittig, W. (1981). A double-blind comparison of the acute effects of clobazam and lorazepam on memory and psychomotor functions. *Royal Society of Medicine International Symposium Series* **43**, 13–21.

Subhan, Z. (1981). A dose-range comparison of clobazam and diazepam. II. Effect on memory. *Royal Society of Medicine International Symposium Series* **43**, 175–179.

Wittenborn, J. R., Flaherty, J. R., McGough, W. E. and Nash, R. J. (1979). Psychomotor changes during initial day of benzodiazepine medication. *British Journal of Clinical Pharmacology* **7**, 69s–76s.

A Comparison of Clobazam and Diazepam in Anxious Patients

C. HARRISON, I. HINDMARCH, C. A. CLYDE

*Human Psychopharmacology Research Unit, Department of Psychology,
University of Leeds, Leeds, UK*

and G. M. WELHAM

The Shaftesbury Health Centre, Harehills Lane, Leeds, UK

PART A

Introduction

Studies using normal volunteer subjects suggest that clobazam, the first 1,5-benzodiazepine, has less sedative properties than standard 1,4-benzodiazepines such as diazepam, while possessing equivalent anxiolytic activity. Diazepam has been shown to impair adaptive tracking (Borland and Nicholson, 1974), reaction time (Borland and Nicholson, 1974; Hindmarch, 1979) and critical flicker fusion (Hindmarch, 1979), in contrast to clobazam, which had no effect on these performance measures. Comparisons of clobazam with two other benzodiazepines, lorazepam and chlordiazepoxide, strengthen this distinction with lorazepam causing an impairment of memory, reaction time and critical flicker fusion (Siegfried *et al.*, 1981) and chlordiazepoxide adversely affecting both reaction time and flicker fusion thresholds (Hindmarch, 1979). Clobazam may even be associated with an enhancement of performance rather than the detriment generally found after benzodiazepines, since Wittenborn *et al.* (1979) reported improved balancing skills after clobazam compared to both diazepam and placebo and Steiner-Chaskel and Lader (1981) noted improved performance after clobazam on a wide range of tests, again relative to diazepam and placebo.

The above results, however, emanate wholly from investigations with volunteer subjects, usually after single acute doses of the medications and, as such, cannot simply be assumed to apply to anxious patient populations. The clinical significance of this apparently greater separation of anxiolytic and sedative properties with clobazam as compared to other benzodiazepines needs to be thoroughly assessed, since obviously an anxiolytic with less accompanying sedation would have important advantages especially for patients who drive or who are engaged in any other skilled performance. The present study was undertaken to assess the clinical response to three weeks treatment with either clobazam or diazepam and to compare the effects of the two drugs on measures of self-rated mood, sleep and psychomotor performance.

Patients and Methods

Patients diagnosed by their general practitioner as having anxiety as their major presenting symptom were referred to the trial. The clinical definition of anxiety included chronic free-floating anxiety, phobic anxiety states, acute anxiety due to environmental or other stress, or any combination of these. For inclusion in the trial patients had to be aged between 16 and 65, without a history of renal or hepatic disorder, have no suspected alcoholism, underlying depression or psychotic illness, have no possibility of pregnancy and not be receiving concurrent psychoactive medication. Patients had also to be suitable for general practice management and give their informed consent prior to the trial.

Sixty-three patients fulfilled these criteria and were admitted to the trial. Forty-seven of these initial entrants completed the whole study period, with the remaining 16 excluded mainly due to failure to attend.

Treatments

Patients were randomly assigned to treatment with either clobazam 10 mg t.d.s. or diazepam 5 mg t.d.s. Both active treatments and placebo were identically packaged in pale blue capsules which patients were instructed to take thrice daily.

Design

This was a double-blind parallel two-group comparison. Each patient acted as his/her own control and received one week of treatment with placebo, followed by three weeks of active treatment, then a final week on placebo. Assessments by the clinician and psychologist took place at weekly intervals over the six-week trial period.

Assessments

All patients were assessed on clinical rating scales, subjective self-completed question-naires and psychomotor performance in accordance with the schedule shown in Table 1. The baseline for comparison of drug effects was taken as week 2 to allow for full familiarization with the assessment techniques.

The overall severity of anxiety was rated by the physician on the four-point clinical global rating scale (CGR) on four occasions—on admission, after the initial placebo week (baseline), after three weeks of active treatment, and after the final week on placebo. Assessments of anxiety symptoms, both psychic and somatic, were made by the general practitioner on the Hamilton Anxiety Scale (HAS) (Hamilton, 1959) after one week's treatment with placebo and after three weeks of active medication. The Middlesex Hospital Questionnaire (MHQ) was completed by the patient on admission to the study and after three weeks active treatment. This scale provides a measure of general "emotionality" or "neuroticism" and a profile of six sub-test scores of free-floating anxiety, phobic anxiety, obsessionality, somatic anxiety, depression, and hysteria (Crown and Crisp, 1970).

Subjective impressions of any mood changes were recorded on line analogue rating scales (LARS) consisting of 11 bipolar pairs of adjectives, which were completed by patients at each visit. Any changes in parameters relating to sleep were monitored each

Table 1

Schedule of assessments

Carried out by	Nature	Name	Visit					
			1	2	3	4	5	6
				P	D	D	D	P
Physician	Clinical	Clinical Global Rating Scale (range 0–4)	×	×			×	×
		Hamilton Anxiety Scale (range 0–56)		×			×	
		Middlesex Hospital Questionnaire (range 0–96)	×				×	
Patient	Subjective	Line Analogue Rating Scale (range 0–100)	×	×	×	×	×	×
		Sleep Evaluation Questionnaire (range 0–100)		×	×	×	×	×
Psychologist	Performance	Choice Reaction Time	×	×	×	×	×	×
		Critical Flicker Fusion	×	×	×	×	×	×
		Capsule Count		×	×	×	×	×
		Side-effects		×	×	×	×	×

P = Placebo.   D = Active Drug.

week after admission by the Leeds Sleep Evaluation Questionnaire (LSEQ), a patient completed questionnaire, which records ease of getting to sleep (GTS), quality of sleep (QOS), awakening from sleep (AFS) and behaviour following waking (BFW) (Parrott and Hindmarch, 1980).

The visual choice reaction time (CRT) was used as an index of psychomotor performance. This test measures speed of response to a single stimulus light illuminated at random from a set of six stimulus lights. The total reaction time can be subdivided by means of a computer-assisted apparatus into its recognition and movement components. The mean of 20 stimulus presentations was taken as the response measure. Critical Flicker Fusion Thresholds (CFFT) were also measured at weekly intervals using an apparatus consisting of four light-emitting diodes viewed from a distance of $0·7$ m. The mean of three ascending and three descending presentations as measured by the psychophysical method of limits was recorded (Woodworth and Schlosberg, 1958). All patients received intensive practice on the psychomotor measures on admission to the trial.

In addition to these assessments, letter cancellation and serial subtraction tests were given to those patients capable of completing them at each visit. Any side-effects and a capsule count were also recorded at each test session.

Analysis of Data

Analysis of variance was carried out on the data and 95% confidence intervals computed to test for differences between means (Kirk, 1968).

Results

On opening the randomization code, 23 patients were found to have received treatment with clobazam 10 mg t.d.s. and 24 received diazepam 5 mg t.d.s. Some characteristics of the two study groups are shown in Table 2.

Clinical Rating Scales

At initial assessment (week 1), the two drug groups did not differ significantly on any of the Middlesex Hospital Questionnaire scales or the Clinicians Global Rating. Similarly, at the week 2 baseline, after a week of placebo treatment, there was no distinction between drug groups on either clinical global rating or total ratings on the Hamilton Anxiety Scale, although the diazepam group had significantly higher somatic anxiety ($P < 0·05$) on the HAS at the baseline compared to the clobazam patients. Both clobazam and diazepam significantly reduced the severity of

Table 2

Characteristics of patients in the clobazam and diazepam groups (F=female, M=male)

	Clobazam	Diazepam
Sex	14 F 9 M	14 F 10 M
Anxiety state		
Acute	5	9
Acute on chronic	9	5
Chronic	9	10
Age	44·2	41·5
Marital status		
Divorced	2	3
Single	19	17
Married	3	3
Previous treatment with benzodiazepine	16 no/7 yes	16 no/8 yes
MHQ FFA (week 1)	10·5	11·5

anxiety symptoms ($P < 0·01$) as measured by clinical global rating after three weeks treatment, and anxiety remained reduced after the final placebo week (Fig. 1).

A similar pattern emerges with the HAS ratings, as shown in Fig. 2. After three weeks of active treatment, both drugs significantly reduced total ratings of anxiety ($P < 0·01$) as compared to the week 2 baseline with both psychic and somatic components being reduced.

On the Middlesex Hospital Questionnaire only diazepam significantly reduced scores ($P < 0·01$) on free-floating, phobic and somatic anxiety after three weeks treatment in comparison to the initial assessment at week 1. No significant changes were found on any of the other sub-tests.

Self-rating Scales

On visual line analogue rating scales patients rated themselves as significantly less anxious ($P<0.01$) after a week's treatment with either clobazam or diazepam, in accord with the clinical judgement as measured by CGR and HAS. This self-rated anxiety, however, increased again in comparison with week 3 on the final placebo week (Fig. 3).

After one week's treatment with clobazam patients felt themselves to be significantly

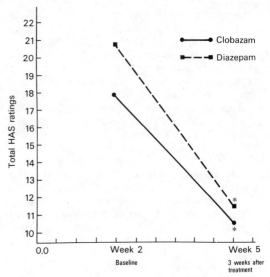

Figure 2. Mean scores of Hamilton Anxiety Scale after one week placebo and three weeks clobazam or diazepam. *Significant difference from week 2.

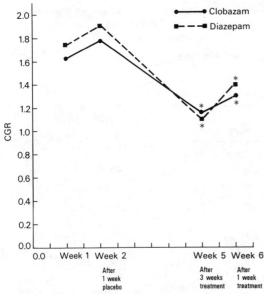

Figure 1. Mean Clinical Global Ratings of anxiety for clobazam and diazepam. *Significant difference from week 2.

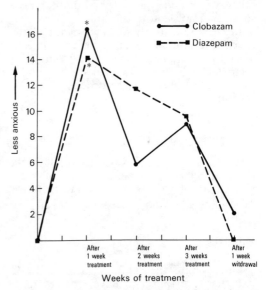

Figure 3. Visual Analogue Scales for anxiety—changes from week 2 baseline for clobazam and diazepam groups. *Significant difference from week 2.

more alert ($P<0.01$) and less tired ($P<0.07$) (see Figs 4 and 5). Patients on clobazam also reported significantly less depression ($P<0.01$) after one week of treatment (Fig. 6) as compared to the week 2 baseline.

The results for the LSEQ are summarized in Table 4. Ease of getting to sleep was significantly improved by both treatments ($P<0.01$), although more consistently by diazepam, while diazepam alone significantly improved the quality of sleep ($P<0.01$). No treatment or time effects were found for awakening from sleep or behaviour following waking.

Psychomotor Measures

Neither the total choice reaction time

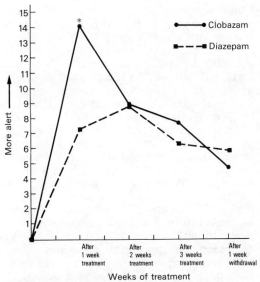

Figure 4. Visual Analogue Scales for alertness—changes from week 2 baseline for clobazam and diazepam groups. *Significant difference from week 2.

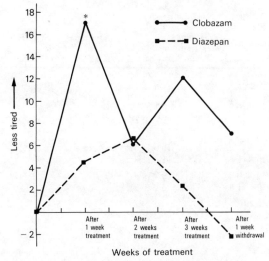

Figure 5. Visual Analogue Scales for tiredness—changes from week 2 baseline for clobazam and diazepam groups. *Significant difference from week 2.

group produced an almost significant difference ($P < 0.08$) between week 3 and week 6 (Table 6).

Since it is known that levels of anxiety can

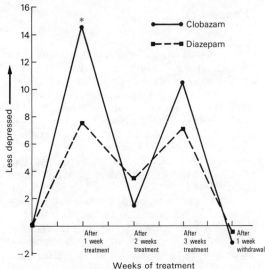

Figure 6. Visual Analogue Scales for depression—changes from week 2 baseline for clobazam and diazepam groups. *Significant difference from week 2.

interfere with psychomotor performance (Clyde, 1981), patients were divided into low (HAS score 0–12), medium (HAS score 13–24) and high anxiety (HAS score 25 and over) groups according to their HAS scores at week 2. A re-analysis was then carried out on total reaction time and critical flicker fusion comparing groups of similar anxiety. The only significant differences to emerge were in the high anxiety group; CFF thresholds were significantly lower in the clobazam group ($P < 0.05$) at all testing sessions, and the clobazam patients TRT at the week 2 baseline was significantly ($P < 0.05$) slower than at week 1 and as compared to the diazepam group at baseline. The means for TRT and CFF according to anxiety level are shown in Table 7.

No results are presented for serial subtraction or letter cancellation tests due to large discrepancies in performance between the two drug groups at baseline.

(TRT) nor the recognition component (RRT) were significantly changed by either drug over the course of the study (Table 5). Critical flicker fusion thresholds were also not affected by either drug, although the gradual rise on the ascending threshold in the clobazam

Side-effects

Reported side-effects are summarized in

Table 8. Slightly more severe complaints of drowsiness and tiredness occurred in the diazepam group.

Discussion

In terms of clinical efficacy as measured by clinical global rating and the Hamilton anxiety scale, clobazam and diazepam clearly show equal anxiolytic activity. This is in accord with the majority of the previous work comparing the effectiveness of clobazam and diazepam in the treatment of anxious patients. Salkind *et al.* (1979) reviewed 28 direct comparisons of the two drugs in anxious patient populations and reported that in 25 of these no significant drug differences in global therapeutic efficacy could be found, whereas, two studies showed clobazam to be superior and in one instance diazepam was more effective in relieving anxiety symptoms. In the present study, the

Middlesex Hospital Questionnaire only indicates diazepam as reducing scores of free-floating, phobic and somatic anxiety. However, this questionnaire was not completed at the week 2 baseline after a week of placebo treatment, but only on admission to the study and, therefore, it cannot be directly compared with the other clinical assessments.

There is no clinical evidence for any rebound of anxiety symptoms after the final placebo week, as the clinical global rating of anxiety remains reduced at week 6, which, for clobazam, is in accordance with the work of Ponciano *et al.* (1981), who found reductions on Hamilton Anxiety scores were maintained one week after cessation of clobazam treatment. At this time, active metabolites of both clobazam and diazepam (Rupp *et al.*, 1979) are present in appreciable quantities. A rebound of symptoms as measured by HAS has been noted two weeks after termination of either clobazam or diazepam treatment (Salkind *et al.*, 1979).

Patient self-rated anxiety, as measured on

Table 3

Clinical assessments. Means (standard error)

Assessment measure	Week number			
	1	2	5	6
Clinical Global Rating				
Clobazam	1·6 (0·1)	1·8 (0·2)	1·2 (0·2)*[a]	1·3 (0·2)*
Diazepam	1·8 (0·1)	1·9 (0·2)	1·1 (0·2)*[a]	1·4 (0·1)*
Hamilton Anxiety Scale				
Total Clobazam		17·8 (1·5)	10·5 (1·4)*	
Diazepam		20·8 (1·8)	11·4 (1·8)*	
Psychic Clobazam		10·7 (0·9)	6·7 (0·8)*	
Diazepam		10·0 (1·0)	6·2 (0·8)*	
Somatic Clobazam		7·2 (0·8)[b]	3·7 (0·7)*	
Diazepam		10·8 (1·1)[b]	5·2 (1·2)*	
Middlesex Hospital Questionnaire				
Free-floating anxiety				
Clobazam	10·5 (0·7)		8·9 (0·7)	
Diazepam	11·5 (0·4)		8·4 (0·8)[a]	
Phobic anxiety				
Clobazam	6·5 (0·8)		6·1 (0·8)	
Diazepam	7·8 (0·6)		6·4 (0·6)[a]	
Somatic anxiety				
Clobazam	7·2 (0·8)		5·5 (0·7)	
Diazepam	8·0 (0·6)		5·5 (0·8)[a]	

*Significant differences from week 2 $P < 0.05$.
[a] Significant difference from week 1 $P < 0.05$.
[b] Significant difference between drugs $P < 0.05$.

Table 4

Leeds Sleep Evaluation Questionnaire. Means (standard error)

	Week number				
	2	3	4	5	6
Getting to sleep					
Clobazam	48·2 (4·1)	54·9 (3·6)	55·6 (2·8)	58·7 (3·3)*	47·3 (2·7)
Diazepam	39·4 (3·2)	57·9 (8·0)*	58·5 (2·7)*	60·2 (2·6)*	52·7 (4·2)*
Quality of sleep					
Clobazam	47·7 (4·4)	52·3 (3·9)	54·9 (3·4)	57·5 (3·8)	45·4 (3·1)
Diazepam	40·0 (3·9)	58·2 (3·7)*	52·9 (4·8)*	57·6 (3·8)*	48·8 (4·0)

*Significant difference from week 2 $P < 0.05$.

visual analogue scales, is largely in accord with the clinicians' judgement, since both drug groups rate themselves as significantly less anxious after one week of treatment, however, their subjective anxiety has returned by week 6. The observation that only patients on clobazam feel themselves to be more alert and less tired after a week's treatment does indicate that the drugs can be differentiated in anxious patients in that clobazam is perceived as less sedating by the patients. It may appear paradoxical that tranquillizing agents can increase arousal, but tiredness and fatigue are part of the anxiety syndrome (Wheeler *et al.*, 1950; Cohen and White, 1951) and are relieved in conjunction with the anxiety. The greater sedation possibly experienced by more patients on diazepam is also indicated by the consistent improvement in quality of sleep in this drug group over the trial period.

A further point of interest arising from patients' self-ratings is the significant reduction in self-rated depression after one week's treatment with clobazam. This suggests some action of clobazam on depressive symptoms, although the elevation of mood does not persist.

The lack of treatment effect on the psychomotor measures agrees with the previous work on normal volunteers for clobazam, but not with that for diazepam (Borland and Nicholson, 1974; Hindmarch, 1979). This absence of performance impairment is consistent with earlier reports (Malpas *et al.*, 1974; Zimmerman-Tansella *et al.*, 1979) that the sedative effects of the benzodiazepines appear to be less easily observed in patient populations than in volunteer subjects. Two previous studies directly comparing clobazam and diazepam in anxious patients produced only slight evidence for diazepam to have

Table 5

Choice Reaction Time. Means (standard error)

	Week number					
	1	2	3	4	5	6
TRT						
Clobazam	776·8	774·4	746·8	754·8	773·3	762·0
	(50·6)	(44·6)	(39·3)	(51·0)	(53·2)	(42·1)
Diazepam	758·4	781·7	742·6	759·7	745·2	734·2
	(39·3)	(39·5)	(34·5)	(39·9)	(30·1)	(30·1)
RRT						
Clobazam	486·7	460·4	450·0	449·5	473·3	476·3
	(31·4)	(25·3)	(23·9)	(28·0)	(32·8)	(35·8)
Diazepam	451·0	470·8	462·0	438·3	440·1	437·2
	(25·8)	(26·4)	(22·0)	(21·7)	(17·7)	(18·2)

Table 6

Critical Flicker Fusion Threshold. Means (standard error)

	Week number					
	1	2	3	4	5	6
Ascending						
Clobazam	29·7	27·6	27·1	27·6	27·8	28·7
	(0·7)	(0·8)	(0·8)	(0·7)	(0·7)	(0·6)
Diazepam	28·0	28·5	28·6	28·5	29·0	29·1
	(0·5)	(0·8)	(0·7)	(0·8)	(0·8)	(0·8)
Descending						
Clobazam	28·6	28·2	28·5	28·3	28·3	29·1
	(0·8)	(0·9)	(0·8)	(0·7)	(0·8)	(0·7)
Diazepam	29·1	29·6	30·2	29·1	29·6	29·7
	(0·6)	(0·7)	(0·6)	(0·6)	(0·8)	(0·6)
Mean						
Clobazam	28·2	27·9	27·8	27·9	28·1	28·9
	(0·7)	(0·8)	(0·7)	(0·6)	(0·7)	(0·5)
Diazepam	28·6	29·0	29·4	28·8	29·3	29·4
	(0·6)	(0·7)	(0·6)	(0·7)	(0·7)	(0·7)

Table 7

Means according to anxiety level

Anxiety level		Total Choice Reaction Time Week number					
		1	2	3	4	5	6
High							
$n=$ 4	Clobazam	840·5	1043·5*[a]	892·25	926·5	887·75	871·25
$n=$ 10	Diazepam	836·7	860·0	821·80	855·8	817·9	770·1
Medium							
$n=$ 14	Clobazam	789·6	722·1	706·0	699·5	752·5	723·3
$n=$ 9	Diazepam	690·9	761·9	701·9	696·6	710·9	733·7
Low							
$n=$ 5	Clobazam	690·0	705·5	744·6	772·4	740·0	769·2
$n=$ 5	Diazepam	723·2	661·0	657·6	680·8	661·4	666·0

Anxiety level	Critical Flicker Fusion Week number					
	1	2	3	4	5	6
High						
Clobazam	25·0*	24·4*	26·0*	25·8*	25·1*	26·2*
Diazepam	29·0	29·3	29·5	29·3	30·7	29·7
Medium						
Clobazam	29·0	28·5	28·6	28·4	28·6	29·6
Diazepam	28·3	29·8	29·6	29·2	29·2	29·5
Low						
Clobazam	28·6	29·0	28·5	28·5	28·8	29·1
Diazepam	28·3	27·1	29·0	27·0	26·8	28·5

*Significant difference between drugs $P < 0.05$.
[a]Significant difference from week 1 $P < 0.05$.

Table 8

Side effects reported in clobazam and diazepam groups

Side-effect	Clobazam			Diazepam		
	Mild	Severity Moderate	Severe	Mild	Severity Moderate	Severe
Loss of libido	—	—	1	—	—	1
Drowsiness	6	3	2	4	5	4
Dizziness	2	—	1	—	1	—
Lack of concentration	1	1	0	0	2	1
Slowed down	1	—	—	1	—	1
Nausea	—	—	—	—	1	1
Loss of memory	—	1		1	—	—
Difficulty in waking	—	—	—	—	—	2
Absent-mindedness	2	—	—	1	—	—

more detrimental effects on performance. Radmayr (1980) noted more pronounced side effects after diazepam (7·5 mg/day/15 mg/day) as compared to clobazam (15 mg/day/30 mg/day), while neither drug affected reaction time or critical flicker fusion thresholds. In the second study, digit symbol substitution test performance was impaired by diazepam 17 mg/day, but not by clobazam 35 mg/day or placebo (Salkind *et al.*, 1979). There are several possible factors to explain why any drug differences in performance are more difficult to detect in patient populations. First, a patient group is much more heterogeneous on characteristics such as age, background, education and physical health than normal volunteer subjects, which leads to greater variation in psychomotor performance. Secondly, much less rigorous control exists over testing conditions in a clinical study, which, again, can result in greater variation due to factors of practice, task motivation and environmental conditions. Thirdly, the opposing influences of drug accumulation and tolerance over the course of a trial obviously produce different effects with chronic administration as compared to acute dosage studies (Wittels and Stonier, 1981). Finally, anxious patients may respond differently than volunteers because of differences in levels of anxiety. High levels of anxiety can interfere with performance (Saranson and Maudler, 1982; Hamilton, 1979), thus alleviation of anxiety can improve performance. Subjects differing in anxiety level have been found to respond differently to clobazam (Clyde, 1981). A very wide range of anxiety was found to exist in the present study group,

from a score of 2 on the Hamilton Anxiety Scale at week 2 to a score of 35 on the scale, which further adds to the variability observed in psychomotor performance. It was attempted to control for the involvement of anxiety by dividing patients into low, medium and high anxiety groups according to their baseline HAS scores and comparing groups of similar anxiety level on psychomotor performance. This was not a very even distribution however, since the diazepam group contained ten high anxiety patients compared to four highly anxious clobazam patients. All that emerged from this analysis was that in the high anxiety group significant differences between the drug groups on CFF thresholds and TRT existed prior to administration of treatments.

It was, therefore, concluded from this study that although clobazam and diazepam are equivalent anxiolytics in general practice in terms of clinical global rating, Hamilton Anxiety Scale and patients' self-ratings of anxiety, there is some indication that clobazam is perceived subjectively as less sedating. No significant differences were found in the psychomotor measures, which may be due to baseline differences between the drug groups, especially in levels of anxiety and the great inter-subject variability in performance.

PART B

Follow-up Survey

Approximately one year after the end of

the original trial, it was decided to investigate the subsequent medical treatment of the study patients, especially with regard to their psychological state, using their medical records. Information was available on 35 of the original 47 patients, the remaining 12 having moved from the area, changed doctors, or their records were otherwise inaccessible. Sixteen of these patients had received diazepam during the trial and 19 were given clobazam. Characteristics of these patients are shown in Table 9.

A note was made of any psychotropic medication or possible psychosomatic illnesses occurring after the patient had finished the trial. A summary of the results for psychoactive prescriptions is shown in Table 10. Equal numbers of patients from both drug groups received no subsequent psychoactive medication according to the records, while slightly more from the diazepam group received further anti-anxiety and hypnotic treatments. The most striking difference, however, is that those patients who had received clobazam were subsequently prescribed a much greater incidence of antidepressant medication. A

Table 9

Follow-up study sample: patient characteristics

	Clobazam	Diazepam
Total	19	16
Sex	8 M 11 F	7 M 9 F
Age	45·1	45·1

total of 42·1% of the clobazam follow-up group were prescribed antidepressant drugs compared to 12·5% of the diazepam follow-up sample.

If the hypnotic and antianxiety categories are grouped together, no cell frequency is less than two and, as such, a chi-square test of association can be done (chi-square = 4·02, $df = 1$, $P < 0.05$). This shows that a significant association exists between patient drug group in the original trial and later prescriptions of psychotropic medication. From inspection of Table 10, this difference does seem to arise from the greater frequency of antidepressant medication in those patients from the clobazam group.

Such a finding could possibly be interpreted by implicating clobazam in the causation of this apparent depression; however, this conflicts strongly with the observation from the original study that patients' self-rated depression was reduced after a week's treatment with clobazam. A more likely explanation is that anxiety-masked depression was present in the clobazam group prior to the clinial trial, even though any suspicion by the clinician of underlying depression was stated explicitly as one of the exclusion criteria. A further indication of this possible initial bias in the clobazam sample is that on admission the diazepam group had higher scores on all sub-tests of the Middlesex Hospital Questionnaire, except for depression on which clobazam patients scored higher.

Several suggestions for the improvement of future clinical trials arise from this follow-up survey and the original study. First, the importance of follow-up studies in checking for any hidden variables which were not obvious at the time of the original trial, but which may emerge later, has been illustrated. Such follow-ups can be used to investigate the

Table 10

A summary of patients receiving psychoactive medication after original trial

Study group	Patients with no psychotropic prescriptions	Patients receiving psychotropic medication			Total
		Antianxiety	Antidepressant	Hypnotic	
Clobazam 30 mg	5 (26·3%)	5 (26·3%)	8 (42·1%)	1 (5·3%)	19
Diazepam 15 mg	5 (31·25%)	7 (43·75%)	2 (12·5%)	2 (12·5%)	16

validity of the initial study results. Second, stricter entrance criteria than clinical judgement are needed to ensure a more homogeneous patient population. A certain level on a scale, such as the Hamilton Anxiety Scale, above which patients have to score to be entered into the trial, should be denoted. In addition, some means of screening out patients with underlying depression should be used if a wholly anxious sample is required. A possible candidate for this function could be the Hopkins Symptom Checklist which has a separate anxiety and depression score (Derogatis *et al.*, 1974). Finally, the large variance in psychomotor measures and the differences between drug groups discovered at baseline provide some justification for pre-test allocation to treatment groups on the basis of psychomotor test scores. This should ensure that each sample contains a similar range of psychomotor ability and should eliminate any initial diferences which can obscure treatment effects on performance measures.

Summary

General practice patients clinically diagnosed as anxious received either clobazam 10 mg t.d.s. or diazepam 5 mg t.d.s. over a three-week period. Clinical ratings of anxiety via a clinical global rating scale (CGR) and the Hamilton Anxiety Scale (HAS) indicated both treatments to be equipotent in alleviating anxiety. Patients' self-ratings of anxiety on line analogue rating scales (LARS) concurred with this anxiolytic equivalence, whilst only patients on clobazam rated themselves as more alert, less tired and less depressed after one week's treatment, which suggests that less sedation was experienced. Psychomotor performance was unaffected by either treatment.

A follow-up survey of the study sample was carried out approximately 12 months after the end of the original trial. Using the available medical records, it was discovered that a significant association existed between the study drug group and subsequent prescriptions of psychotropic medication, with patients in the clobazam group receiving more antidepressant medication after the trial than patients in the diazepam group. Such a finding could indicate a greater incidence of anxiety-masked depression in those patients receiving clobazam.

It is concluded that future clinical trials could be improved by following up the study sample, having more specific entrance criteria than clinical judgement, and ensuring that drug groups are matched initially on psychomotor performance.

Acknowledgements

We would like to thank C. Hollett and B. J. Hickey for their help in analysing the data.

References

Borland R.G., and Nicholson, A.N. (1974). Immediate effects on human performance of a 1,5-benzodiazepine derivative (clobazam) compared with the 1,4-benzodiazepines chlordiazepoxide hydrochloride and diazepam. *British Journal of Clinical Pharmacology* **2**, 215–221.

Clyde, C.A. (1981). The influence of personality on response to low doses of benzodiazepines. *Royal Society of Medicine International Congress Symposium Series* **43**, 74–86.

Cohen, M.E., and White, P.D. (1951). Life situations, emotions and neurocirculatory asthemia (anxiety neurosis, neurasthemia effort syndrome). *Psychosomatic Medicine* **13**, 335–357.

Crown, S., and Crisp, A.H. (1970). "Manual of the Middlesex Hospital Questionnaire." Psychological Test Publications, Barnstaple.

Derogatis, L.R., Lipman, R.S., Rickels, K., Uhlenhuth, E.H., and Covi, L. (1974). The Hopkins Symptom Checklist (HSCL): A self-report symptom inventory. *Behavioural Science* **19**, 1–15.

Hamilton, M. (1959). The assessment of anxiety states by rating. *British Journal of Medical Psychology* **32**, 50–55.

Hamilton, V. (1979). Information processing aspects of neurotic anxiety and the schizophrenias. *In* "Information Processing Approach" (V. Hamilton, and D. Warburton, Eds). Wiley, London.

Hindmarch, I. (1979). Some aspects of the effects of clobazam on human performance. *British Journal of Clinical Pharmacology* **7** (1), 77S–82S.

Kirk, R.E. (1968). "Experimental Design. Procedures for the Behavioural Sciences." Wadsworth Publishing Company, California.

Malpas, A., Legg, N.J., and Scott, D.F. (1974). Effects of hypnotics on anxious patients. *British Journal of Psychiatry* **124**, 482–484.

Parrott, A.C., and Hindmarch, I. (1980). The Leeds Sleep Evaluation Questionnaire in psychopharmacological investigations—a review. *Psychopharmacology* **71**, 173–179.

Ponciano, E., Relvas, J., Mendes, F., Lameiras, A., Vaz Serra, A., and Hindmarch, I. (1981). Clinical effects and sedative activity of bromazepam and clobazam in the treatment of anxious out-patients. *Royal Society of Medicine International Congress and Symposium Series* **43**, 125–131.

Radmayr, E. (1980). Clobazam and diazepam in the treatment of neurotic out-patients. *Therapiewoche* **30**, 117.

Rupp, W., Badian, M., Christ, O., Hajdu, R.D., Kulkarni, R.D., Taeuber, K., Uihlein, M., Bender, R., and Vanderbeke, O. (1979). Pharmacokinetics of single and multiple doses of clobazam in humans. *British Journal of Clinical Pharmacology* **7**, 51S–57S.

Salkind, M.R., Hanks, G.W., and Silverstone, J.T. (1979). Evaluation of the effects of clobazam, a 1,5-benzodiazepine, on mood and psychomotor performance in clinically anxious patients in general practice. *British Journal of Clinical Pharmacology* **7**, 113S–118S.

Saranson, S.B., and Maudler, G. (1952). Some correlates of test anxiety. *Journal of Abn. Soc. Psych.* **47**, 810–817.

Siegfried, K., Koeppen, D., Taeuber, K., Badian, M., Malercyzyk, V., and Sittig, W. (1981). A double-blind comparison of the acute effects of clobazam and lorazepam on memory and psychomotor functions. *Royal Society of Medicine International Congress and Symposium Series* **43**, 13–21.

Steiner-Chaskel, N., and Lader, M.H. (1981). Effects of single doses of clobazam and diazepam on psychological functions in normal subjects. *Royal Society of Medicine International Congress Symposium Series* **43**, 23–32.

Wheeler, E.O., White, P.D., Red, E.W., and Cohen, M.E. (1950). Neurocirculatory asthenia (anxiety neurosis, effort syndrome, neuroasthenia). A twenty year follow-up of 173 patients. *Journal of American Medical Association* **142**, 878.

Wittels, P.Y., and Stonier, P.D. (1981). The effects of benzodiazepines on psychomotor performance in patients. *Royal Society of Medicine International Congress Symposium Series* **43**, 111–118.

Wittenborn, J.R., Flaherty, C.F., McGough, W.E., and Nash, R.J. (1979). Psychomotor changes during the initial day of benzodiazepine medication. *British Journal of Clinical Pharmacology* **7**, 69S–76S.

Woodworth, R.S., and Schlosberg, H. (1958). "Experimental Psychology." Methuen, London.

Zimmermann-Tansella, C., Tansella, M., and Lader, M.H. (1979). A comparison of the clinical and psychological effects of diazepam and amylobarbitone in anxious patients. *British Journal of Clinical Pharmacology* **1**, 605.

Comparison of Drug Treatment (Clobazam) and Relaxation Therapy in the Management of Anxiety. Preliminary communication

D. J. THOMPSON

Airedale General Hospital, Keighley, W. Yorkshire, U.K.

Introduction

This paper represents an interim report of an open study that compares the effectiveness of a benzodiazepine (clobazam) with relaxation training in the treatment of anxiety symptoms.

Benzodiazepines have achieved widespread acceptance for the treatment of anxiety symptoms since their introduction in 1960. Recently, increasing concern has been expressed over the complications of prolonged usage. As a result, the role of benzodiazepines has been reviewed, particularly in the treatment of chronic anxiety symptoms.

Relaxation training was first described in Jacobson (1938). It is a relatively simple technique, which involves muscular exercises designed to relax the patient and induce a state of tranquility. Clinical impressions indicate that relaxation training is an effective treatment for anxiety symptoms, but it is unfortunate that there are few studies that have utilized a patient sample.

One of the first studies is that of Mathews and Gelder (1969) who reported their experience with a sample of 14 patients, all of whom suffered from phobic anxiety. Clinical improvement with relaxation was accompanied by a significant reduction of EMG activity and skin conductance when compared with a control group.

Borkovec and Sides (1979) reviewing 25 investigations of relaxation training, noted that the technique was significantly more effective in the patient sample compared with the normal control group. He also noted that it was more effective when administered "live" rather than in a taped version.

In the present study, the relaxation instructions were administered using an audio-tape, which patients may take home with them. The relaxation tape lasts approximately 14 min and the patient was requested to use the tape twice daily.

Patients and Methods

The patient sample was obtained from out-patients referred to the Psychiatric Department at Airedale General Hospital over the last two years. Sixty consecutive out-patients presenting with symptoms of anxiety were randomized into three different groups: (1) 20 mg clobazam at night; (2) relaxation training; and (3) combined 20 mg clobazam at night and relaxation training.

The patients to be included in the study had to fulfil the criteria of having duration of symptoms greater than one month, and an anxiety score on the Leeds Irritability, Depression, Anxiety Scale (IDA) (Snaith, 1978).

Patients were excluded from the study if they were aged less than 16 or over 65, had a depression score on the IDA greater than seven or, had anxiety symptoms complicated by physical illness. Also excluded were patients with concurrent psychotic or major depressive illness, a significant clinical deterioration requiring additional treatment or intervention, including admission or, who were unable to stop their previous psychotropic medication for a period of one week prior to starting the trial.

Patients satisfying inclusion into the trial were requested to stop any previous psychotropic medication and started on placebo clobazam capsules for one week prior to randomization into the three groups.

Standardization of the treatment between the three groups was effected by limiting the duration of each appointment to 15 min. In addition, patients received a brief typed sheet which summarized our understanding of anxiety and encouraged patients to confront the situations or cognitions that precipitated anxiety symptoms. The programme of treatment consisted of an initial assessment interview when they were started on placebo; they then returned for follow up at one week, three weeks, five weeks, seven weeks and a final appointment at 13 weeks. The active treatment period lasted one month from week one to week five.

Assessments

Patients were assessed using the following instruments:

(1) the Leeds IDA Scale;
(2) Spielberger State and Trait anxiety scale;
(3) a Self-Rating Visual Analogue Scale comprising a somatic symptoms scale and psychological symptoms scale;
(4) Critical Flicker Fusion Threshold (Smith and Misiak, 1976).

Assessments were made at week 0, 1, 3, 5, 7 and 13.

Results

The characteristics of the three samples are presented in Table 1. No marked differences exist on any of the variables between the three groups with the exception of the male/female ratio. It is evident that in the relaxation group there is a relative excess of males over females compared with the other two groups. This may be as a result of the randomization

procedure, which did not include any method of statification for age or sex.

From the results of this study it is evident that the anxiety scores on all the rating instruments have improved over time in the three treatment groups. The data were analysed using non-parametric methods (Kruskal-Wallis one-way analysis of variance). This revealed no significant differences between the three treatments, although there is a trend on all measures favouring relaxation and against the combined clobazam and relaxation group. Clobazam alone keeps an intermediate position.

The depression scale on the IDA shows a similar pattern with no significant difference again between the three groups.

Discussion

In discussing these results, it is worth stating that the study is not yet complete and it is anticipated that 20 patients will be accumulated in each group as in the original design. Furthermore, statistical analyses has only been completed for the IDA data and no information is currently available of the results of the Locus Control enquiry.

The results must, therefore, be treated with some caution. Perhaps the most surprising finding is the failure of the combined clobazam and relaxation group to show a clear superiority. One possible explanation may be an impairment of learning ability due to the benzodiazepine and a subsequent interfer-

Table 1

Demographic data for three groups

	Clobazam (C)		Relaxation (R)		Combined C and R	
Size	17		16		17	
Age	37·1		33·3		34·4	
M/F	2/15		8/8		3/14	
Past psych. history	48·2%		50%		26·2%	
Duration	7·7 ± 6·8 yr		8·0 ± 4·4 yr		13·1 ± 5·9 yr	
Current illness	Phobic anxiety	9	Phobic anxiety	8	Phobic anxiety	6
	Free floating	7	Free floating	4	Free floating	8
	Neurotic dep	1	Neurotic dep	4	Neurotic dep	3
Duration	3·9 ± 4·2 yr		6·0 ± 6·0 yr		2·7 ± 2·9 yr	
Range	5 m–12 yr		3 m–20 yr		3 m–10 yr	

ence in the patient's ability to acquire relaxation skills. Alternatively, benzodiazepines and relaxation treatments are based on entirely different approaches, relaxation being a self-control technique, and benzodiazepines providing the opportunity of anxiety relief through external agents. It is conceivable that the mixture of treatments simply confuses the patient.

Previous studies have indicated benefits from both benzodiazepines and relaxation techniques (Hafner and Marks, 1976; Johnston and Gath, 1973). More recently both treatments have been assigned a more limited role of being purely palliative and of no long-term curative value (Marks, 1981).

In the present study, both treatments are used purely as anxiolytic and combined with a behavioural treatment paradigm, namely confrontation of their anxiety using exposure *in vivo*. In this role, anxiolytics have been shown to produce significant improvements over placebo (Marks *et al.*, 1972). The present study supports these findings. Improvements in the measure of anxiety following a period of active treatment are maintained and enhanced at two months follow up.

References

Borkovec, T. D. and Sides, J. K. (1979). Critical procedural variables related to the physiological effects of progressive relaxation: A review. *Behaviour Research and Therapy* **17**, 119–125.

Hafner, J. and Marks, I. M. (1976). Exposure *in vivo* of agorophobics, contribution diazepam, exposure and anxiety evocation. *Psychological Medicine* **6**, 71–88.

Jacobsen, E. (1938). "Progressive Relaxation." University of Chicago Press, Chicago.

Johnston, D. and Gath, D. (1973). Arousal levels and attribution effects in diazepam assisted flooding. *Brit. J. Psych.* **123**, 463–466.

Marks, I. M. (1981). "Cure and Care of Neurosis." Wiley & Sons, New York.

Marks, I. M. *et al.* (1972). Enhanced extinction of fear by flooding during waning diazepam. *Brit. J. Psych.* **121**, 493–505.

Mathews, A. M. and Gelder, M. G. (1969). Psycho-physiological investigations of brief relaxation training. *Journal of Psychosomatic Research* **13**, 1–12.

Snaith, R. R., Constantopoulos, A. A., Jardine, M. Y. and McGuffin, P. (1978). A clinical scale for the self-assessment of irritability. *British Journal of Psychiatry* **132**(2), 164–171.

Smith, J. M. and Misiak, H. (1976). Critical Flicker Fusion (CFF) and Psychotropic Drugs in normal human subjects—a review. *Psychopharmacology* **47**, 175–182.

Benzodiazepine Misuse in Poly-drug Users

L. FERREIRA, M. J. OLIVEIRA and I. HINDMARCH*

*Centro de Seleccao do Porto, Porto, Portugal and *Human Psychopharmacology Research Unit, Department of Psychology, University of Leeds, Leeds, UK*

Introduction

It is possible to identify two classes of benzo-diazepine abuser. First, there are those individuals who seek out a supply of benzodiazepines to augment an already established pattern of poly-drug use. Secondly, there are those whose use of benzodiazepines is iatrogenic. In this group the use of benzodiazepines originated in the clinical situation, and by persistent and repeated prescribing of the drugs the individual became sufficiently dependent upon them to seek out further supplies on the black market.

Marks (1978) identified 151 cases of benzodiazepine abuse in poly-drug/alcohol abusers. Lader (1981) suggests that such figures could well be under-estimates as it is difficult to know just how many persons become dependent in a medical therapeutic context and then turn to illicit supplies to maintain the habit which has been established.

It has been known for some time that poly-drug abusers have frequent recourse to the use of benzodiazepines and/or alcohol. Adolescent poly-drug abusers aged between 14 and 17 years were shown (Hindmarch, 1972) to be persistent users of nitrazepam and chlordiazepoxide. In the past ten years many more benzodiazepine derivatives have been introduced to the clinical market on a worldwide basis. The widespread clinical use of these drugs is reflected in the numbers of prescriptions issued and it is estimated (Lader, 1978) that one in ten adult males and one in five adult females use benzodiazepines at some time in any one year.

All benzodiazepines, have a profile of anti-anxiety, hypnotic, amnestic, muscle relaxant and anti-epileptic activity. It is difficult to distinguish between the drugs as regards their clinical effectiveness as anxiolytics, hypnotics, etc., but human and animal pharmacological studies have shown that striking differences do exist between the various derivatives with respect to patient tolerability and pharmacokinetic, pharmacodynamic, amnestic, and cognitive effects.

The aims of this present study were two-fold. First, to investigate the pattern of benzodiazepine use in a group of drug-dependent patients. Secondly, to see if any pattern of preference emerges in terms of the derivatives which are used. Any pattern of preference which emerges is to be viewed against the pharmacokinetic and psychopharmacological differences that have been established between the benzodiazepines.

The observations were carried out in Portugal between 1979 and 1980. At that time some 16 benzodiazepine derivatives were available for clinical use. It was assumed that the poly-drug abusers would have equal access to all of these derivatives and the objective of investigating the preference between these derivatives was pursued on this assumption.

Patients and Methods

Between May 1979 and May 1980 the drug-dependent patients attending the Centro de Estudes da Profilaxia da Droga in Oporto were individually interviewed. All patients had confirmed histories of opiate abuse and a serious involvement with many other psychotropics, viz. cannabis, psychostimulants (amphetamine, methylphenidate), sedatives (barbiturates), and hallucinogens (LSD). Details of drugs used and age of first use were collected along with demographic data and medical-legal histories of problems directly associated with drug using behaviour. In addition each patient was shown a list of the 36 proprietary names of medications representing the 16 benzodiazepine derivatives then available in Portugal.

Patients were asked to identify the proprietary names of drugs with which they were acquainted and to rank those drugs, with which they were familiar through direct experience, in order of preference, taking into account the totality of the drug using experience.

Results

Completed interviews were obtained from 95 patients (80 male, 15 female) with a mean age of 21·6 (range 15–38) years. The 16 generic names representing the 36 benzodiazepine medications available in Portugal in 1980 are given in Table 1.

There were ten benzodiazepines consistently identified by the patients and represented by nine generic compounds listed in Table 2.

Of the 95 patients, 63 (66%) had medical complications connected with their poly-drug use and legal problems, because of drug misuse, had involved 67 (71%) of the population although the level of criminality was not high and restricted to minor and petty offences.

Five patients reported no experience of benzodiazepines and a further 13, although admitting use, gave no references. In three cases the benzodiazepines had been prescribed first in a medical therapeutic context and the patients had continued to use them illicitly. The bulk of the population, 90

patients, had no medical history of primary clinical use of benzodiazepines and had only used such substances in an illegal manner.

Table 3 shows the majority of the present sample were illicitly using more than three controlled drugs over and above their admitted experience with benzodiazepines and, therefore, establishes this population as poly-drug users. The mean age of first reported drug experience and the number of people reporting their first experience of named drugs are given in Table 4 along with figures from the total sample showing overall drug experience.

Table 5 presents the number of patients reporting abuse of a named benzodiazepine.

Discussion

The range of controlled substances used by this group of drug dependents clearly identifies them as poly-drug users. Well over two-thirds of the sample had medical and legal complications as a result of their drug using activity, prior to the interviews in which these present data were collected.

Table 2

Benzodiazepines known by poly-drug abusers in Oporto, 1979–1980

Bromazepam	Lorazepam
Chlordiazepoxide	Medazepam
Diazepam	Nitrazepam
Flunitrazepam	Oxazepam
Flurazepam	

Table 1

Benzodiazepines available in Portugal (1979) and Year of Introduction

BZD	Year	BZD	Year
Bromazepam	1975	Estazolam	1977
Camazepam	1977	Flunitrazepam	1976
Chlordiazepoxide	1961	Flurazepam	1973
Clobazam	1978	Lorazepam	1971
Clonazepam	1975	Medazepam	1971
Clorazepate	1972	Nitrazepam	1966
Desmethyldiazepam	1977	Oxazepam	1966
Diazepam	1963	Temazepam	1971

Table 3

The number of different drugs used by patients

Number of different drugs used (excluding Benzodiazepines)	Number of patients reporting use
1	2 (2%)
2	6 (6%)
3	18 (19%)
4	40 (42%)
5	20 (21%)
6	9 (10%)

Table 4

Number of Patients reporting use of controlled drugs, mean age of first use (±S.D.) and number of patients reporting first drug of experience

Type of drug ICD-9	No. patients reporting use	% of sample	First use mean age in years + S.D.	No. patients reporting 1st drug of experience
Cannabis	91	96%	15·3 (2·4)	74
Amphetamines	70	74%	16·7 (2·5)	8
Morphine	95	100%	17·4 (3·3)	4
Hallucinogens	42	44%	16·7 (2·2)	5
Cocaine	33	35%	17·6 (3·1)	1
Barbiturates	46	48%	17·3 (3·1)	2
Others	3	3%	18·0	1

Table 5

The number of patients reporting abuse of a named Benzodiazepine

Benzodiazepine	Number of users
Flunitrazepam	79
Diazepam	17
Lorazepam	10
Flurazepam	8
Bromazepam	7
Oxazepam	4
Nitrazepam	2

The prime reason for this study was an investigation of the preferences shown by this group of drug users for benzodiazepine derivatives and these details of the drug using habits of the sample are given only to establish the poly-drug using nature of the population and the high level of drug using experience. The early mean age of first use of a range of psychoactive drugs was such to suggest that this present population is not naive and that any expressed preferences would be as a result of individual experiences.

Table 5 gives some indication of the number of drug users reporting experiences of named benzodiazepines. Throughout the interview the commercial names as used for these drugs in Portugal were used. A consideration of Table 5 shows that over 80% of the sample reported abuse of flunitrazepam. Although instances of the abuse of oxazepam, bromazepam and nitrazepam were recorded it is apparent that the majority of

benzodiazepine abuse was of flunitrazepam and to a lesser extent of lorazepam, diazepam and flurazepam.

Figure 1 presents an index of the preferences shown by the patients for the drugs they admitted abusing. Each set of preferences for a particular drug are expressed as the percentage of first, second and third rank placings given. The greater the percentage of first choice ratings indicates an overall preference for that drug and implicitly confirms its misuse potential. We have assumed that the individuals in this study have equally free

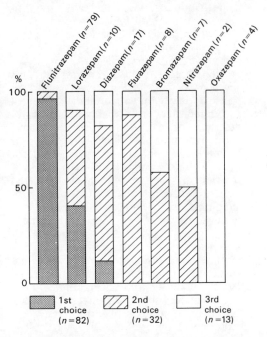

access to each of the benzodiazepines available in Portugal and it is, therefore, interesting to reason why three drugs, i.e. flunitrazepam, lorazepam, and diazepam should be the first choice for use by a population of polydrug abusing patients.

The first argument would be that these drugs are those that have been on the market the longest and are, therefore, more likely to be available and known to the drug using populations. It could certainly be argued that diazepam, lorazepam and nitrazepam were among the earliest drugs to be available in Portugal, but flunitrazepam and bromazepam are, relatively speaking, recently marketed therapeutic agents. There is also the noticeable absence of chlordiazepoxide, which, as one of the longest available drugs, would have to be included if time on the market were the only criteria for determining the preference for a drug.

There is nothing to suggest, in the information we have concerning the black market availability and price of these substances, that flunitrazepam is in any way cheaper or more available than the other drugs found to be amongst the first choice preferences of this group of drug users.

Diazepam could very well be in the top three drugs because of its availability. It exists in Portugal in four commercial forms. Its effects as a powerful sedative, anti-convulsant, sleep inducer, muscle relaxant, and anti-anxiety agent are well known. Woody *et al.* (1975) have reported that narcotic users taking large doses of diazepam often experience a subjective and very pleasant "high" of relaxation. Lader (1981) reports that his patients have described a "rush" effect in response to diazepam with euphoria, flight of ideas, enhancement of confidence, pleasant relaxation, and calmness. These subjective and somatic sensations of well-being could be sufficient to account for the preference for this drug in this population of drug users.

Lorazepam, the second most preferred drug, is a benzodiazepine which has a profound amnestic activity (Siegfried *et al.*, 1981; Paes de Sousa *et al.*, 1981) in both patient and volunteer populations. Thus, lorazepam is widely used as a premedication for procedures such as endoscopies where its soporific and amnestic activities enable the patient to forget the unpleasant, clinical procedures. The drowsiness, stupor, and amnesia produced by high doses of lorazepam could well be one of the reasons why the drug is

popular in this population of drug abusers.

The main and obvious feature of this survey is in the remarkable number of users who indicate their personal first choice and preference for flunitrazepam. The reasons for this drug being the first choice of the majority of benzodiazepine abusers is obviously very complex but its basis may lie in what is known about the pharmacokinetics of the compound. Flunitrazepam is very rapidly absorbed (as are lorazepam and diazepam) and exerts its powerful hypnotic activity very soon after oral ingestion. It also has amnestic activity much the same as that produced by lorazepam, although its retrograde effects are not quite as deep or as complete. High doses of flunitrazepam would produce effects similar to high doses of the other two preferred benzodiazepines. It is, however, likely that the rapid onset of action of this drug is the main reason why it is preferred by the drug abuser. The immediate subjective impression of drug activity or "hit" is probably what places it in the first rank of drugs of choice. Benzodiazepine receptor studies show that flunitrazepam has a higher affinity for the receptor than diazepam, which in turn has a higher affinity than lorazepam. The three drugs together are amongst those that bind most strongly to the receptor and it could be this neurochemical property that accounts for the expressed preference for flunitrazepam, lorazepam and diazepam. (Schacht, personal communication.)

The small number of patients reporting benzodiazepine abuse originating in a therapeutic context tends to support Marks' (1978) contention that there is not a serious problem of benzodiazepine misuse originating in the clinical milieu.

The problems of benzodiazepine abuse in a purely therapeutic situation are usually controlled by the clinical management of the case. Patients who have been prescribed benzodiazepines for a long period of time have their doses gradually reduced in an attempt to wean them off dependency on the drug. However, problems of abuse of benzodiazepines in a population of illicit drug abusers are more difficult to control, but it is not the intention of this paper to offer suggestions relating to the clinical management of either patients or drug abusers who have become dependent upon the benzodiazepine.

This paper has illustrated that from a wide choice of benzodiazepines, experienced drug users select three derivatives and rank the effects of these and their intention to abuse them frequently above all the other available medications.

Assuming that the complex reasons which led to this particular ranking of benzodiazepines can be regarded as some crude index of a differential abuse potential, then it can clearly be seen that not all benzodiazepines have the same abuse characteristics.

We can conclude that although many benzodiazepines share similar clinical profiles of activity they do not all possess the same misuse potential as rated by a group of experienced drug abusers. This conclusion in no way asserts that any other benzodiazepine, not featured on this list, does not possess any abuse potential. All that is claimed is that some drugs are more preferred to others and that such preferences might represent some inate qualities of the derivatives selected.

The clinical implications of such preferences in the management of anxious or sleep disturbed patients is not clear but does, perhaps, indicate the importance of careful clinical control of any patient prescribed benzodiazepines. Certainly no patient should be given a benzodiazepine over a period of time sufficient for him to develop problems of drug dependency. Frequent review of patients' progress in clinical situations where benzodiazepines have to be chronically prescribed might identify problems of drug abuse at an early stage.

Patients treated chronically with large doses of flunitrazepam, lorazepam and diazepam should, according to the findings of this study, have a particular preference for the effects of these drugs which could well pose problems when cessation of treatment is envisaged and problems of misuse and dose escalation considered.

Summary

The aims of the present study were to investigate the pattern of benzodiazepine use in a group of drug-dependent patients and to detect any pattern of drug preference, which could be viewed against pharmacological differences established between the benzodiazepines. The study was conducted between May 1979 and May 1980 in Oporto, Portugal. The results indicate that patients treated chronically with large doses of flunitrazepam, lorazepam or diazepam should have a particular preference for the effects of these drugs which could pose problems when cessation of treatment is envisaged.

References

Hindmarch, I. (1972). Patterns of drug use and attitudes to drug users in a school aged population. In "Student Drug Surveys" (S. Einstein and S. Allen, eds), pp. 77–87. Baywood, New York.

Lader, M. (1978). Benzodiazepines—the opium of the masses? *Neuroscience* **3**, 159–165.

Lader, M. (1981). Benzodiazepine dependence. In "The Misuse of Psychotropic Drugs" (R. Murray *et al.*, eds), pp. 13–16. Gaskell, London.

Marks, J. (1978). "The Benzodiazepines. Use, Overuse, Misuse, Abuse." MTP Press, Lancaster.

Paes de Sousa, M., Figuiera, M.-L., Loureiro, F. and Hindmarch, I. (1981). Lorazepam and clobazam in anxious elderly patients. *Royal Society of Medicine International Congress Symposium Series* **43**, 120–123.

Siegfried, K., Koeppen, D., Taeuber, K., Badian, M., Malerczyk, V. and Sittig, W. (1981). A double-blind comparison of the acute effects of clobazam and lorazepam on memory and psychomotor functions. *Royal Society of Medicine International Congress Symposium Series* **43**, 13–21.

Woody, G. F., O'Brien, C. P. and Greenstein, R. (1975). Misuse and abuse of diazepam: An increasingly common medical problem. *International Journal of Addiction* **10** 843–848.

PART 2

Psychopharmacology and Anti-Epileptic Activity

Psychopharmacology of Clobazam with Special Reference to its Anticonvulsant Activity

H. J. KRUSE

Department of Pharmacology, Hoechst AG, D-6230 Frankfurt am Main 80, West Germany

Summary

In psychopharmacological tests in rats and mice clobazam was on average five times less potent than diazepam (e.g. potentiation of narcosis, prevention of clonic seizures, reduction of shock-induced fighting). With regard to psychomotor side-effects, however, clobazam was 8–10 times less active than diazepam. Clobazam potency was closest to diazepam in antagonizing electroshock seizures (ratio 1·4) and has been additionally tested against chemically induced *tonic* seizures (e.g. pentetrazol, picrotoxin, bicuculline) using standard anticonvulsants as reference drugs. The protective indices (TD_{50}/ED_{50}) were well above 1, ranging from 2·4 (bicuculline) to 23·1 (pentetrazol), and clobazam was superior to all reference drugs both in the extent of its anticonvulsive spectrum and in terms of therapeutic indices. The diazepam/clobazam potency ratios in chemically induced tonic seizures were much below those found against clonic seizures or other tests mentioned above, emphasizing clobazam's anticonvulsant activity profile. The 2,4 di-one-like structure in the 1,5-benzodiazepine molecule is a common element in many classical antiepileptics and may be the chemical correlate of the predominant anticonvulsant activity of clobazam.

Introduction

The 1,5-benzodiazepine clobazam is a well established anxiolytic drug. It has been shown to be about one-half as potent as diazepam in clinical studies, but to produce less psychomotor side-effects at equipotent dose levels (for review see Koeppen, 1979, this volume pp. 207–215; and Brogden et al., 1980).

Moreover, clobazam was found to exert marked anticonvulsant effects against electroshock and various chemoshock seizures in rodents (Barzaghi et al., 1973; Caccia et al., 1980; Shenoy et al., 1982) and also to suppress reflex epilepsy in audiosensitive mice and photosensitive baboons (Chapman et al., 1978; Meldrum et al., 1979).

Nevertheless, the clinical evaluation of clobazam's anticonvulsant potential was neglected for some time until Gastaut and Low (1979) reported it to be effective against all varieties of human epilepsy.

In comparative psychopharmacological studies, carried out in 1980 and presented here, clobazam was on average five times less potent than diazepam. The only exception was in electroshock (ECS) seizures in which the two drugs' potencies differed only by a factor of 1·4 (see Table 1).

Since ECS-induced convulsions are considered an animal model of generalized and partial epileptic seizures, it was tempting to assume that the emphasis of clobazam's clinical profile should be on antiepileptic (anti-grand mal) activity. To test this hypothesis pharmacologically, clobazam was additionally investigated in several chemoshock models, with tonic convulsions induced by pentetrazol, picrotoxin, bicuculline, isoniazid, nicotine, and strychnine.

In addition to diazepam, the clinically well-established antiepileptics phenytoin, carbamazepine and valproate (drugs of choice against generalized and partial seizures) and ethosuximide, clonazepam and valproate (drugs of choice against absence and myoclonic seizures; Porter, 1982), were used as reference drugs.

Material and Methods

Subjects

NMRI male mice (WIGA, Sulzfeld and Iva-

Table 1
Seizure Tests

Convulsing agent	Dose (mg/kg) and route of administration	Seizure type evaluated	Observation time (min)
Electroshock (ECS)	12 or 25 mA, 50 Hz, 200 ms, via corneal electrodes	Tonic	0·1
Pentetrazol (PTZ)	100 i.p.	Clonic	30
	85 s.c.	Clonic	30
	125 s.c.	Tonic	30
Picrotoxin (PTX)	3·5 s.c.	Clonic	45
	15 s.c.	Tonic	45
Bicuculline (BIC)	5 s.c.	Tonic	30
Isoniazid (INH)	300 s.c.	Clonic	60
	600 s.c.	Tonic	60
Nicotine (NIC)	1·5 i.v.	Tonic	0·1
Strychnine (STR)	1·2 s.c.	Tonic	30

mA = milli-amps; ms = milli-seconds; Hz = Hertz; i.p. = intraperitoneal; s.c. = subcutaneous; i.v. = intravenous.

novas, Kisslegg), weighing 20–25 g and Wistar male rats (Ivanovas, Kisslegg), weighing 180–220 g, were used. They were group-housed in perspex cages under a 12 hr light/ 12 hr dark cycle with unlimited access to food and water (except for rats used in the Geller Conflict Test). Experiments were generally carried out between 8:00 and 12:00 h at a room temperature of 21–23°C.

Drugs

The following drugs were used and suspended in 1% methyl cellulose (Tylose): clobazam, diazepam, clonazepam, phenobarbital sodium, phenytoin, carbamazepine, sodium valproate and ethosuximide. All drugs were administered orally in volumes of 10 ml/kg (mice) or 2 ml/kg (rats). Controls received the same volume of vehicle. The tests were carried out at the time of peak effect which was generally at 60 min post-dosing except for phenobarbital (2 hr) and phenytoin (4 hr).

The following auxiliary agents were used and dissolved in distilled water or 0·9% saline: hexobarbital, thiopental, ethanol 96%, pentetrazol, picrotoxin, bicuculline (with 0·1 ml N-HCl added), isoniacid, nicotine, and strychnine nitrate. All doses refer to the salts.

Methods

Rotarod

Mice or rats were selected according to their ability to maintain equilibrium on a slowly revolving wooden rod (mice: 16 r.p.m., diameter 4 cm; rats: 7 r.p.m., diameter 7·5 cm) for more than 60 s ($n = 10$).

If, after drug treatment, the animals fell off the rod within 60 s, they were considered ataxic. The ED_{50} or minimal median "neurotoxic" dose (TD_{50}) was defined as the dose causing ataxia in 50% of the subjects and was calculated by probit analysis.

Traction test

Mice were selected according to their ability to pull themselves up on to a tightrope ("horizontal wire") with their hindpaws within 5 s after grasping the wire with the forepaws ($n = 10$). If, after drug treatment, the animals were unable to climb up within 5 s after being placed on the wire they were considered relaxed in muscle tone. The ED_{50} was defined as the dose causing muscle relaxation in 50% of the subjects and was calculated by probit analysis.

MOTEX Test *(Motility-Exploration)*

The same method was used as described in detail previously (Kruse, 1982). The ED_{50} was defined as the dose reducing the number of explored holes by 50% and was determined graphically.

Induction of ethanol narcosis

Mice were injected with a subthreshold dose of ethanol (2 g/kg i.p.) which produced no anaesthesia in controls ($n = 10$). The ED_{50} was defined as the dose producing anaesthesia in 50% of the subjects and was calculated by probit analysis.

Induction of hexobarbital narcosis

Mice were injected with a subthreshold dose of hexobarbital (15 mg/kg i.v.) which produced no anaesthesia in controls ($n = 10$). The ED_{50} was defined as the dose producing anaesthesia in 50% of the subjects and was calculated by probit analysis.

Prolongation of thiopental narcosis

Mice were injected with an anaesthetic dose of thiopental (25 mg/kg i.v.) and the interval between loss and regaining of the righting reflex ("sleeping-time") was measured ($n = 10$). The ED_{+100} was defined as the dose producing a 100% increase in sleeping-time over controls and was determined graphically.

Shock-induced fighting

Three mice were placed together in a perspex box equipped with a grid floor which measured $15 \times 15 \times 15$ cm^3. A 0·6 mA scrambled footshock was delivered through the grids for a 2 min observation period and the number of fights during this interval was recorded ($n = 9$).

The ED_{50} was defined as the dose reducing the total number of fights by 50% and was determined graphically.

Asphyxia test

The survival time of mice in air-tight closed bottles containing a volume of 250 ml air was measured ($n = 10$). The ED_{+50} was defined as the dose prolonging survival time by 50% over controls and was determined by regression analysis.

Geller conflict test in rats

The method described by Geller and Seifter (1960) and modified after Davidson and Cook (1969) was used ($n = 10$). The ED_{+300} was defined as the dose increasing punished responding by 300% over controls and was determined graphically.

Seizure tests in mice

The test parameters may be gathered from Table 1.

Results and Discussion

The results of clobazam and diazepam in some psychopharmacological tests on tranquilizer effects are summarized in Table 2.

Clobazam was 8–10 times less potent than diazepam in producing unwanted side-effects such as sedation, ataxia, and muscle relaxation (see rotarod-, MOTEX-, and traction-test). In other tests, clobazam proved only 3–7 times less potent than diazepam ($Q =$ potency diazepam/clobazam, in parentheses): induction of ethanol- and hexobarbital-narcosis (3·2 and 3·3 respectively), prolongation of thiopental-narcosis (7·0), prevention of isoniazid-, picrotoxin-, and pentetrazol-induced clonic seizures (4·9, 5·2 and 5·4 respectively), inhibition of shock-induced fighting (4·2), prolongation of asphyxia survival time (5·6), and enhancement of punished responding in Geller's conflict test (7·5).

The potency of clobazam was closest to diazepam in suppression of electroshock seizures ($Q = 1·4$). This favourable ratio was replicated in a second experiment (see Table 3) and also with a higher voltage of ECS (25 mA, 50 Hz, 200 ms). Under the latter conditions clobazam and diazepam yielded ED_{50} values of 13·3 (10·0–17·5) and 8·5 (6·2–11·5) mg/kg p.o., respectively ($Q = 1·6$).

The results of the follow-up studies with chemoshock-induced tonic seizures are presented in Table 3. ED_{50} values in a *clonic*

Table 2

Psychopharmacological profile of clobazam and diazepam

Test (mouse)	ED_{50} (mg/kg p.o.)		Q
	Clobazam	Diazepam	
Rotarod 16 r.p.m. (mouse)	39·3 (17·5–88·2)	5·0 (2·9–8·7)	7·9
Rotarod 7 r.p.m. (rat)	104·0 (56·0–171)	11·5 (8·6–15·3)	9·0
Traction (horizontal wire)	51·9 (39·0–69·1)	5·6 (3·9–8·0)	9·3
MOTEX (inhibition of exploration)	33·0	3·2	10·3
Ethanol narcosis (induction)	13·9 (9·6–20·1)	4·3 (2·8–7·2)	3·2
Hexobarbital narcosis (induction)	12·7 (8·0–20·3)	3·8 (1·9–7·4)	3·3
Thiopental narcosis (prolongation)	7·7 (ED_{+100})	1·1 (ED_{+100})	7·0
Pentetrazol 100 mg/kg i.p. (clonic seizures)	3·9 (3·0–5·0)	0·72 (0·49–1·1)	5·4
Picrotoxin 3·5 mg/kg s.c. (clonic seizures)	4·5 (3·1–6·4)	0·86 (0·52–1·4)	5·2
Isoniazid 300 mg/kg s.c. (clonic seizures)	12·3 (7·0–21·4)	2·5 (1·2–5·3)	4·9
Electroshock 12 mA (tonic seizures)	3·8 (2·4–6·0)	2·7 (1·4–5·0)	1·4
Shock-induced fighting	6·3 (ED_{+50})	1·5 (ED_{+50})	4·2
Asphyxia survival time	22·4 (18·3–29·6)	4·0 (3·0–5·8)	5·6
Geller conflict (rat)	62·0 (ED_{+300})	8·3 (ED_{+300})	7·5

Q: potency ratio diazepam/clobazam (ED clobazam/ED diazepam. i.p. = intraperitoneal; s.c. = subcutaneous; p.o. = per os; r.p.m. = rotations per minute.

seizure test (pentetrazol) and TD_{50} values (impairment of rotarod performance) are given for comparison.

Clobazam reliably and consistently prevented seizures in all models. Its individual maxima of activity were against PTZ and NIC while it exerted its lowest potency against INH and BIC. But even in tests of minimal activity, clobazam's anticonvulsant dose level was still well separated from neurotoxic doses which was not the case for any reference drug.

The rank order of potency for clobazam and the other drugs in the tests employed (tonic seizures only) was as follows:

Clobazam	: PTZ > NIC > PTX > ECS > STR > INH > BIC
Diazepam	: PTZ > NIC > INH > PTX > ECS > STR > BIC
Clonazepam	: PTZ > INH > NIC > ECS > BIC > PTX > STR
Phenobarbital	: PTZ > NIC > PTX > ECS > INH > BIC > STR
Phenytoin	: PTX > ECS > PTZ > BIC > NIC > INH > STR
Carbamazepine:	PTX > ECS > PTZ > BIC > NIC > INH > STR
Valproate	: PTX > PTZ > NIC > ECS > BIC > INH > STR
Ethosuximide	: PTZ > NIC > INH > BIC > PTX > STR > ECS

Phenytoin, carbamazepine and valproate displayed their maximal potency against PTX seizures, with all other drugs maximally potent against PTZ seizures.

Phenytoin, carbamazepine, phenobarbital and valproate (i.e. drugs of choice against generalized and partial epileptic seizures) were even more potent against PTX than ECS seizures. On the other hand, clonazepam and ethosuximide (i.e. drugs mainly active against absence and myoclonic seizures) showed very little activity in suppressing PTX-induced tonic convulsions. Thus, the latter test may be considered an adequate chemoshock model for the prediction of effectiveness against generalized and partial seizures.

More important than mere ED_{50} values are their relationship to neurotoxic dose levels. Therefore, the ratio of TD_{50} to ED_{50} ("Protective Index", P.I.) was calculated and is presented in Table 4. In terms of P.I. values, clobazam was superior to diazepam, clonazepam, phenobarbital, valproate, and ethosuximide in all eight tests and superior to phenytoin and carbamazepine in four tests (see also Figs 1, 2).

Moreover, clobazam had the broadest spectrum of anticonvulsant activity, since most of the reference antiepileptics were inac-

Table 3

Profile of anticonvulsant activity of clobazam and other antiepileptics in mice

Drug	Pretreatment (h)	TD$_{50}$ (mg/kg p.o.) Rotarod	Test; ED$_{50}$ (mg/kg p.o.)							
			ECS 12 mA, 200 ms	Pentetrazol 125 mg/kg	Pentetrazol 85 mg/kg	Picrotoxin 15 mg/kg	Bicuculline 5 mg/kg	Isoniazid 600 mg/kg	Nicotine 1·5 mg/kg	Strychnine 1·2 mg/kg
Clobazam	1	39·3 (17·5–88·2)	8·0 (5·6–11·3)	1·7 (1·4–2·2)	2·3 (1·4–3·7)	4·7 (3·0–7·2)	16·2 (12·9–20·4)	10·7 (6·9–16·6)	2·3 (1·7–3·1)	10·4 (6·4–16·9)
Diazepam	1	5·0 (2·9–8·7)	5·7 (4·2–7·6)	0·41 (0·27–0·62)	0·50 (0·31–0·81)	4·1 (2·5–6·6)	10·0 (7·6–13·2)	2·8 (2·0–4·0)	0·80 (0·47–1·4)	4·9 (2·3–10·0)
Clonazepam	1	0·34 (0·19–0·63)	0·58 (0·32–1·0)	0·038 (0·031–0·047)	0·043 (0·028–0·066)	2·3 (1·2–4·2)	1·0 (0·69–1·5)	0·075 (0·045–0·13)	0·14 (0·10–0·22)	>5
Phenobarbital	2	47·1 (33·2–66·7)	13·8 (10·2–18·7)	6·7 (4·5–9·8)	15·9 (5·7–44·3)	12·2 (9·5–15·7)	20·5 (15·9–26·3)	18·7 (14·0–25·1)	7·6 (6·1–9·5)	46·9 (34·3–64·2)
Phenytoin	4	101 (82·4–125)	6·9 (5·2–9·1)	7·6 (6·1–9·5)	>100	3·6 (2·4–5·3)	10·4 (8·1–13·4)	21·8 (17·0–21·8)	19·8 (13·2–29·6)	>100
Carbamazepine	1	102 (79·6–131)	8·1 (6·5–10·2)	11·2 (9·0–13·9)	>100	7·3 (5·4–9·9)	16·2 (12·9–20·4)	25·0 (19·0–33·0)	18·1 (13·1–25·0)	>100
Valproate	1	477 (318–712)	259 (190–354)	158 (117–214)	264 (212–329)	75·4 (46·2–123)	362 (282–464)	494 (392–622)	168 (125–227)	>800
Ethosuximide	1	906 (341–2400)	>1000	130 (97·5–130)	264 (212–329)	950 (estimate)	836 (477–1460)	568 (443–729)	247 (196–310)	>1000

( ): 95% confidence limits.

Table 4

Protective indices of clobazam and other antiepileptics in tests on anticonvulsant activity in mice

Drug	Test; Protective Index (P.I.)							
	ECS	PTZ (tonic)	PTZ (clonic)	PTX	BIC	INH	NIC	STR
Clobazam	4·9	23·1	17·1	8·4	2·4	3·7	17·1	3·8
Diazepam	0·9	12·2	10·0	1·2	0·5	1·8	6·3	1·0
Clonazepam	0·6	9·0	7·1	0·2	0·3	4·5	2·4	<0·1
Phenobarbital	3·4	7·0	3·0	3·9	2·3	2·5	6·2	1·0
Phenytoin	14·6	13·3	<1·0	28·1	9·7	4·6	5·1	<1·0
Carbamazepine	12·6	9·1	<1·0	14·0	6·3	4·1	5·6	<1·0
Valproate	1·8	3·0	1·8	6·3	1·3	1·0	2·8	<1·0
Ethosuximide	<0·9	6·9	3·4	~1·0	1·1	1·6	3·7	<1·0

P.I. = TD_{50} (rotarod)/ED_{50} (seizure-test).

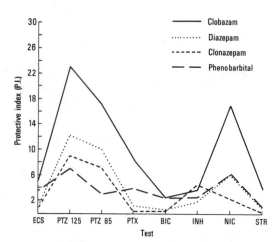

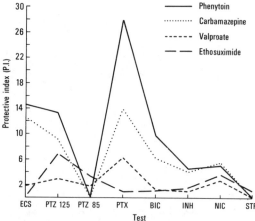

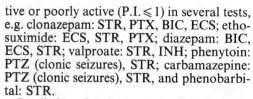

Figure 1. Protective indices (TD_{50} rotarod test/ ED_{50} seizure test) of clobazam, diazepam, clona- zepam, and phenobarbital in tests with tonic extensor convulsions induced by the following treatments: electroshock (ECS), pentetrazol (PTZ 125), picrotoxin (PTX), bicuculline (BIC), isoniazid (INH), nicotine (NIC) and strychnine (STR). PTZ 85: clonic seizures induced by pen- tetrazol.

Figure 2. Protective indices of phenytoin, car- bamazepine, valproate, and ethosuximide in the same tests as in Fig. 1.

protective indices in the tests employed the following rank orders are obtained:

ECS: phenytoin > carbamazepine > clo- bazam > phenobarbital > valproa- te > diazepam > clonazepam > eth- osuximide

tive or poorly active (P.I. ≤ 1) in several tests, e.g. clonazepam: STR, PTX, BIC, ECS; etho- suximide: ECS, STR, PTX; diazepam: BIC, ECS, STR; valproate: STR, INH; phenytoin: PTZ (clonic seizures), STR; carbamazepine: PTZ (clonic seizures), STR, and phenobarbi- tal: STR.

By listing the drugs according to their

PTZ: (tonic seizures) clobazam > phenytoin > diaze- pam > carbamazepine ≥ clonaze- pam > phenobarbital > ethosuxi- mide > valproate

PTZ: (clonic seizures) clobazam > diazepam > clonaze- pam > ethosuximide ≥ phenobar- bital > valproate > carbamazepi- ne ≥ phenytoin

PTX: phenytoin > carbamazepine > clobazam > valproate > phenobarbital > diazepam > ethosuximide > clonazepam

BIC: phenytoin > carbamazepine > clobazam ⩾ phenobarbital > valproate > ethosuximide > diazepam > clonazepam

INH: phenytoin ⩾ clonazepam ⩾ carbamazepine > clobazam > phenobarbital > diazepam ⩾ ethosuximide > valproate

NIC: clobazam > diazepam ⩾ phenobarbital > carbamazepine ⩾ phenytoin > ethosuximide > valproate > clonazepam

STR: clobazam > phenobarbital ⩾ diazepam > phenytoin ⩾ carbamazepine > ethosuximide > valproate > clonazepam

Clobazam is found seven times (i.e. in all tests except for INH seizures) in one of the first three positions, more often than any reference drug.

A final comparison of the potency of clobazam and diazepam in tonic seizure models results in the following ratios (Q according to Table 2, test in parentheses): 1·1 (PTX), 1·4 (ECS), 1·6 (BIC), 2·1, (STR), 2·9 (NIC), 3·8 (INH), and 4·1 (PTZ).

These data show that the potency of clobazam is closer to diazepam in antagonism of tonic seizures than in any other test: against picrotoxin-, electroshock-, bicuculline- and strychnine-induced *tonic* convulsions, clobazam was only 1·1–2·1 times less potent than diazepam. Against *clonic* seizures and in other psychopharmacological tests it was about five (3–7) times less potent and in producing psychomotor side-effects, clobazam was even 8–10 times less active than diazepam.

Conclusion

The emphasis of clobazam's pharmacological profile is on suppression of tonic convulsions (inhibition of seizure spread), but it prevents clonic seizures (elevation of seizure threshold) as well.

In terms of the extent of its anticonvulsant spectrum and therapeutic index, clobazam is superior to 1,4-benzodiazepines (diazepam, clonazepam) and other antiepileptics (phenytoin, carbamazepine, phenobarbital, valproate, ethosuximide).

In clinical studies, effectiveness mainly against generalized tonic-clonic and partial (simple and complex) seizures may be predicted.

Clobazam's (benzodiazepine) *2,4-di-one* (imide-like) structure, which is also found in classic antiepileptics such as barbiturates, hydropyrimidines, hydantoins, oxazolidines, succinimides, acetyl ureas, etc., but not in 1,4-benzodiazepines (Fig. 3), may be the chemical correlate of its predominant anticonvulsant activity.

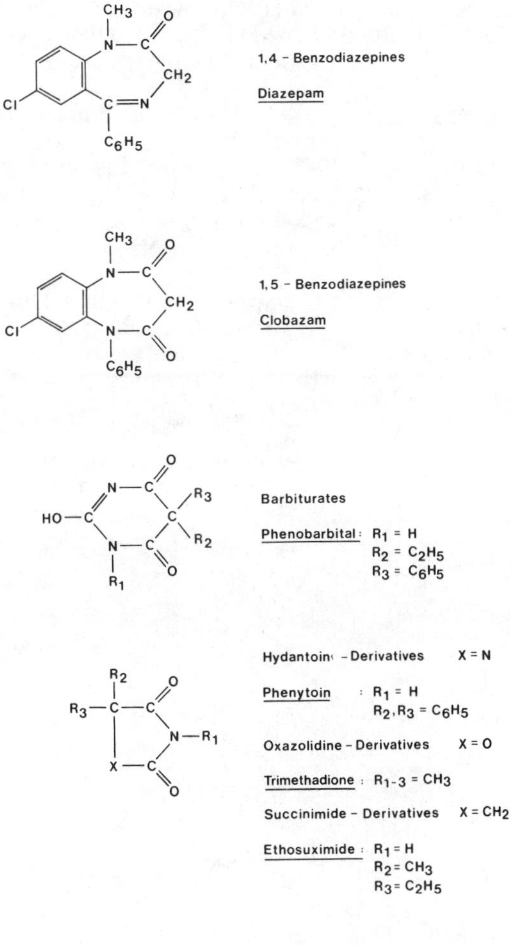

Figure 3. Clobazam and its structural relationship (imide-like structure) to antiepileptics such as barbiturates, hydantoins, oxazolidines, succinimides, etc.

References

Barzaghi, F., Fournex, R. and Mantegazza, P. (1973). Pharmacological and toxicological properties of clobazam, a new psychotherapeutic agent. *Arzeimittel-Forschung* **23**, 683–686.

Brogden, R. N., Heel, R. C., Speight, T. M. and Avery, G. S. (1980). Clobazam: A review of its pharmacological properties and therapeutic use in anxiety. *Drugs* **20**, 161–178.

Caccia, S., Guiso, G., Samanin, R. and Garattini, S. (1980). Species differences in clobazam metabolism and antileptazol effect. *J. Pharm. Pharmacol.* **32**, 101–103.

Chapman, A. G., Horton, R. W. and Meldrum, B. S. (1978). Anticonvulsant action of a 1,5-benzodiazepine, clobazam, in reflex epilepsy. *Epilepsia* **19**, 293–299.

Davidson, A. B. and Cook, L. (1969). Effects of combined treatment with trifluoperazine-Hcl and amobarbital on punished behavior in rats. *Psychopharmacologia* (Berlin) **15**, 159–168.

Gastaut, H. and Low, M. D. (1979). Antiepileptic properties of clobazam, a 1,5-benzodiazepine, gia (Berlin) **1**, 482–492.

Geller, I. and Seifter, J. (1960). The effects of meprobamate, barbiturates, *d*-amphetamine and promazine on experimentally induced conflict in the rat. *Psychopharmacologia* (Berlin) **1**, 482–492.

Koeppen, D. (1979). Review of clinical studies on clobazam. *Br. J. clin. Pharmac.* **7**, 139S–150S.

Kruse, H. J. (1982). Clobazam: Induction of hyperlocomotion in a new nonautomatized device for measuring motor activity and exploratory behavior in mice: Comparison with diazepam and critical evaluation of the results with an automatized hole-board apparatus ("Planche à Trous"). *Drug Dev. Res.* **S1**, 145–151.

Meldrum, B. S., Chapman, A. G. and Horton, R. W. (1979). Clobazam: Anticonvulsant action in animal models of epilepsy. *Br. J. clin. Pharmac.* **7**, 59S–60S.

Porter, R. J. (1982). Clinical efficacy and use of antiepileptic drugs. In "Antiepileptic Drugs" (D. M. Woodbury, J. K. Penry and C. E. Pippenger, eds), pp. 167–175. Raven Press, New York.

Shenoy, A. K., Miyahara, J. T., Swinyard, E. A. and Kupferberg, H. J. (1982). Comparative anticonvulsant activity and neurotoxicity of clobazam, diazepam, phenobarbital, and valproate in mice and rats. *Epilepsia* **23**, 399–408.

Anticonvulsant Benzodiazepines and Performance

C. A. CULL and M. R. TRIMBLE

Department of Neuropsychiatry, The National Hospitals for Nervous Diseases, Queen Square, London WC1N 3BG, UK

Summary

Two studies were carried out comparing the effects of 10 mg clobazam t.i.d. for two weeks versus placebo, and 0·5 mg clonazepam t.i.d. for two weeks versus placebo, in a double-blind cross-over design. Ten and nine healthy male volunteers, respectively, participated in each study. Performance on a series of automated psychological tests was assessed on four occasions: prior to any treatment; at the end of the first two-week treatment period; following a two-week wash-out phase; and again at the end of the second two-week treatment period. Minimal impairment in psychological functioning was found with clobazam, only the more complex tasks of arithmetical ability and immediate recall for words being affected. In contrast, the pattern of findings with clonazepam suggests that it may have adverse effects on a broader range of cognitive functions.

Introduction

The use of benzodiazepines as adjunctive treatment of epilepsy is now becoming accepted, particularly clonazepam and the 1,5-benzodiazepine, clobazam.

Clonazepam has been found to be an effective oral adjunctive treatment in generalized absence seizures (Rey Pias, 1971; Dreifuss and Sato, 1982), myoclonic seizures (Mikkelsen *et al.*, 1976; Nanda *et al.*, 1976; Dreifuss and Sato, 1982), partial seizures (Munthe-Kaas and Strandjord, 1973), and a variety of epileptic phenomena in childhood (Eeg-Olofsson, 1973; Jacobides, 1976).

Clobazam has been found to be of use in refractory epilepsy of all types (Critchley *et al.*, 1981; Martin, 1981), particularly in partial seizures (Gastaut and Low, 1979; Allen *et al.*, 1983), and in primary and secondary generalized seizures in children (Shimizu *et al.*, 1982).

There is some suggestion, from clinical studies, that this latter drug may have fewer side-effects than the 1,4-benzodiazepines (see Trimble, 1983), and in addition, it may have less sedative and cognitive effects than other benzodiazepines.

In contrast to the fairly large amount of information that has been collected concerning the cognitive effects of clobazam, similar reports for clonazepam are scarce. In the one study that has come to light, clonazepam seemed to result in a deterioration of attention and psychomotor function in a group of hyperactive children (Vyborova *et al.* 1979).

The following study was undertaken in an attempt to explore further the effects of these two drugs on various aspects of cognitive functioning.

Method

Subjects

Nineteen healthy male volunteers participated in the study. In group I there were ten subjects, with a mean age of 20·5 years (range 19–25 years), and nine subjects in group II with a mean age of 22·2 years (range 19–33 years). No subjects were taking any other psychoactive medication.

Design (see Fig. 1)

In effect two studies were conducted. Group I subjects received 10 mg clobazam t.i.d., or matching placebo capsules for a period of two weeks, in a double-blind cross-over design, with half the subjects receiving cloba-

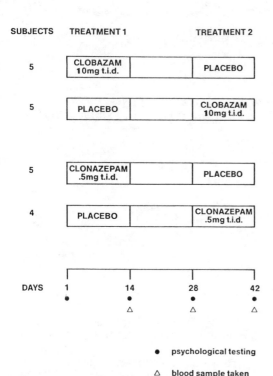

Figure 1. Study design.

with three target digits on the VDU, below which a series of 100 digits are presented, one at a time. For each one, the subject has to give a yes/no response, on a keyboard, as to whether it is the same as any of the target numbers (Fig. 2).

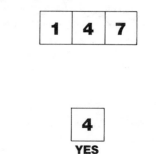

YES

Figure 2. Example of the three-target scanning test.

The second such test uses only one target digit, but is extended into a vigilance task by having 300 items to be responded to (Fig. 3). In addition, a modified version of the Digit Symbol Substitution Test (DSST) was used. In this a symbol is presented to the subject and he has to press the key of the number that goes with the symbol. Fifty items were presented to each subject (Fig. 4).

zam first. A two-week drug-free period was incorporated between the two treatment sessions. The same design was followed for the group II subjects, the only difference being that they received 0·5 mg clonazepam t.i.d.

A battery of psychological tests was administered prior to any treatment, and again at the end of the first treatment period, the drug-free period, and the second treatment period.

2. Mental Speed
As a measure of mental speed, 40 slides of outline drawings of common objects in red or black were presented. For each slide, the subject was asked "Is it red?", referring to the colour of the drawing, or "Is it living?", a question about category membership.

3. Central Cognitive Processing Ability
To investigate central cognitive processing ability, 25 simple addition tasks were pre-

Psychological measures

The tests used were presented via a microcomputer, in conjunction with a carousel projector, so that test stimuli were presented directly on the visual display unit (VDU) or projected on to a screen. For most of the tasks, the method of responding was by key presses.

The areas of cognitive functioning investigated were as follows.

1. Tests of attention and sensory processing
Two of the tests of attention and sensory processing were automated versions of a digit cancellation task. The subject is presented

NO

Figure 3. Example of the one-target scanning test.

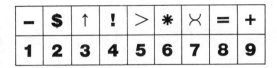

Figure 4. Example of the modified DSST.

sented to the subject, ranging from a single-digit plus a single-digit, to the addition of 2 two-digit numbers. The subjects were asked to perform the calculations mentally, and to press the appropriate keys when they had arrived at an answer.

4. Memory
Two tests of recall memory were used, memory for pictures and memory for words. Twenty pictures were presented to the subjects by means of a projector for an exposure duration of 3 s each. Immediately after, and 1 h after presentation, subjects were asked to recall as many of the test items as they could. A similar procedure was followed for the memory for words task, again using 20 stimuli. Unlike the other tasks, these responses were recorded and scored manually.

5. Perceptuo-Motor Performance
Three simple reaction time tasks were used, as measures of the perceptuo-motor component involved in responses to the previous tasks. These involved pressing a predetermined key in response to a particular stimulus, which was an outline drawing on the VDU for two of the tasks, and the onset of a light stimulus on the projector screen for the third.

With the exception of the memory tasks, response latencies and errors were recorded by the microcomputer and stored on disc, response latency being taken as the performance measure. Different sets of stimuli were used for each of the four testing sessions.

Statistical Analysis

For each of the two groups, a repeated measures analysis of variance was performed to look at treatment and order effects. Where

significant differences were found, an analysis of variance was carried out to compare performance under the two no-drug conditions, to investigate the presence of practice effects. Performance under drug and placebo conditions were then compared by an analysis of covariance, covarying each treatment with the appropriate drug-free session.

PSYCHOLOGICAL MEASURES	CLOBAZAM	CLONAZEPAM
I Attention and Sensory Processing		
3 target scanning		
1 target scanning		
DSST		
II Mental Speed		
Colour	x	
Category		x
III Central Cognitive Processing Ability		
Mental arithmetic		x
IV Perceptuo – Motor Performance		
RT to picture 1		
RT to picture 2		x
RT to light onset	x	x
V Memory		
Pictures : immediate		
: delayed		x
Words : immediate	x	x
: delayed		x

x   no baseline difference

Figure 5. Measures showing differences between the no-drug conditions (x is no difference).

Results

Clobazam

No order effects were found. Significant differences between the two no-drug conditions were found on 10/13 measures, with an improvement over sessions suggesting that a practice effect was present. However, this was taken into account in comparing drug and placebo treatments by the analysis of covariance, in which significant differences were found on only two measures—the mental arithmetic task ($P < 0.01$), and immediate recall for words ($P < 0.001$), in the direction of impairment under the drug condition (see Figs 6 and 7).

Clonazepam

Again, no order effects were found. Significant differences between the two no-drug conditions were found on only 6/13 measures (see Fig. 5). In the drug-placebo compari-

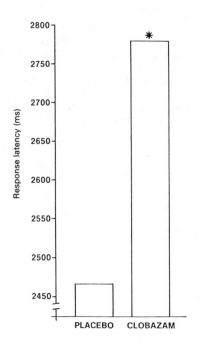

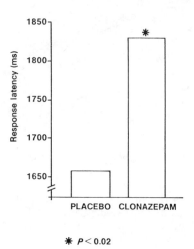

* P < 0.02

Figure 8. Response latencies for the DSST under placebo and clonazepam conditions.

* P < 0.01

Figure 6. Response latencies for the mental arithmetic task, under placebo and clobazam conditions.

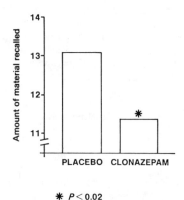

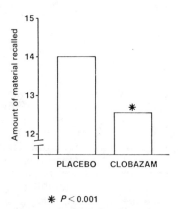

* P < 0.02

Figure 9. Amount of material recalled under placebo and clonazepam conditions for the immediate memory for pictures task.

* P < 0.001

Figure 7. Amount of material recalled under placebo and clobazam conditions for the immediate memory for words task.

mental arithmetic, the three-digit scanning task, decision making for colour, delayed memory for words, and one of the perceptuomotor tasks (Fig. 11).

Discussion

sons, significant differences were found on the DSST ($P < 0.02$) (Fig. 8), immediate memory for pictures ($P < 0.02$) (Fig. 9), and delayed memory for pictures ($P < 0.01$) (Fig. 10). However, borderline probability values of $P < 0.1$ were found on a further five tasks—

It would seem, therefore, that clobazam had little influence on the cognitive functioning of normal volunteers as assessed in this study. Significant impairments in performance were found on only two measures—mental arithmetic and immediate recall for words. This would seem to be in contrast with many of the studies of normal volunteers where no effect or beneficial effects have been reported. But in these studies the majority of post-drug assessments took place either within a few hours after a single dose (Borland and Nicholson, 1974; Gudgeon and Hickey, 1981; Siegfried *et al.*, 1981; Steiner-Chaskel and Lader, 1981; Subhan, 1981), or within only a few days after repeated dosing (Hindmarch *et al.*, 1977; Hindmarch and Parrott, 1978; Hindmarch and Gudgeon, 1980; Robinson *et al.*, 1981), and may bear little relationship to the cognitive sequelae of chronic administration.

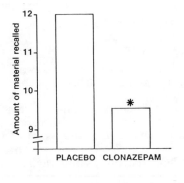

* P < 0.01

Figure 10. Amount of material recalled under placebo and clonazepam conditions for the delayed memory for pictures task.

PSYCHOLOGICAL MEASURES		CLOBAZAM	CLONAZEPAM
I	Attention and Sensory Processing		
	3 target scanning		•
	1 target scanning		
	DSST		x
II	Mental Speed		
	Colour		
	Category		•
III	Central Cognitive Processing Ability		
	Mental arithmetic	xx	•
IV	Perceptuo – Motor Performance		
	RT to picture 1		
	RT to picture 2		•
	RT to light onset		
V	Memory		
	Pictures : immediate		x
	: delayed		xx
	Words : immediate	xxx	
	: delayed		•

xxx	p < 0.001	x	p < 0.02
xx	p < 0.01	•	p < 0.1

Figure 11. Comparison of significant findings.

It is also possible that the significantly beneficial effects of clobazam have been a reflection of practice or learning, as a result of the relatively short time intervals between testing sessions. In the present study, assessments took place at fortnightly intervals and despite an attempt to minimize the contribution of practice by using different stimuli at each session, these effects still occurred to a degree. Similarly, Salkind *et al.* (1979), in an investigation of anxious outpatients, also using a fortnightly test interval, found a significant improvement in the DSST for both a clobazam treated group and a placebo group. In addition, the measures used in the present study were modified for automated administration, and thus may not be comparable with the standard presentation of tests, such as the DSST, used in other studies.

With regard to impairments, these have been found on a numerical task (Hindmarch and Gudgeon, 1980) after three days of drug ingestion, and have also been reported for 40 and 60 mg clobazam following a single dose (Parrott and Munton, 1981). Similarly for memory, impairments after single drug administrations have been found with amounts ranging from 30 to 60 mg (Subhan, 1981).

In the only other comparable study to the present one, that of Thompson and Trimble (1981), no statistically significant treatment effects on memory were found. But they did report that there was a consistent trend towards impaired performance following clobazam.

Our findings would seem to be in keeping with the idea that clobazam, although having some detrimental effects, minimally impairs cognitive functioning.

In contrast, the clonazepam data suggest a very different picture, one of a more general impairing effect. Although only three of the measures showed a statistically significant impairment, namely DSST, and memory for pictures, both immediate and delayed, a number of other tasks did show borderline probability values, which was not the case at all for clobazam (see Fig. 11). Given the small number of subjects, the fairly large number of measures used, and some variable standard deviations in the raw data, it may well be that statistically significant results might emerge if a larger sample were investigated. Further, the fact that comparatively fewer practice effects were found under clonazepam conditions in comparison to clobazam, on exactly the same series of measures, may suggest that clonazepam actually impeded this learning process.

A further factor to be taken into consideration here, with regard to the epileptic patient, is that the amount of clonazepam used in this study was not really equivalent to an anticonvulsant dose. The initial recommended dose is 1·5 mg per day (Browne, 1976), whereas maintenance doses of anything from 2 mg (Rey Pias, 1971) to 12 mg per day (Lance and Anthony, 1977), have been employed in clinical studies of its anticonvulsant properties. It may well be that, as with the other benzodiazepines, a greater degree of impairment will be found with these larger quantities. In contrast, the impairments found with clobazam in this study were for an equivalent anticonvulsant dose.

If impairment occurs at all with clobazam it would seem that it is restricted to those tasks involving a greater complexity of mental processing, as has been suggested by Thompson and Trimble (1981). In contrast, clonazepam would seem to have a wider ranging effect, showing additionally, effects on fairly simple tasks such as our modified DSST. Further investigation with clonazepam is clearly warranted, as our data would seem to suggest that its detrimental effects are more in keeping with those of the 1,4-benzodiazepines rather than the relatively less impairing 1,5-benzodiazepine, clobazam.

References

Allen, J. W., Oxley, J. W., Robertson, M. M., Trimble, M. R., Richens, A. and Jawad, S. S. M. (1983). Clobazam as adjunctive treatment in refractory epilepsy. *British Medical Journal* **286**, 1246–47.

Borland, R. G. and Nicholson, A. N. (1974). Immediate effects on human performance of a 1,5-benzodiazepine (clobazam) compared with the 1,4-benzodiazepines, chlordiazepoxide hydrochloride and diazepam. *British Journal of Clinical Pharmacology* **2**, 215–21.

Browne, T. R. (1976). Clonazepam: a review of a new anticonvulsant drug. *Archives of Neurology* **33**, 326–32.

Critchley, E. M. R., Vakil, S. D., Hayward, H. W., Owen, M. V. H., Cocks, A. and Freemantle, N. P. (1981). Double-blind clinical trial of clobazam in refractory epilepsy. In "Clobazam: The Royal Society of Medicine International Congress and Symposium Series, No. 43" (I. Hindmarch and P. D. Stonier, eds), pp. 159–64. Royal Society of Medicine, London.

Dreifuss, F. E. and Sato, S. (1982). Benzodiazepines: clonazepam. In "Antiepileptic Drugs" (D. M. Woodbury, J. K. Penry and C. E. Pippenger, eds), pp. 737–52. Raven Press, New York.

Eeg-Olofsson, O. (1973). Experiences with Rivotril in treatment of epilepsy—particularly minor motor epilepsy—in mentally retarded children. *Acta Neurologica Scandinavica* **49** (Suppl. 53), 29–31.

Gastaut, H. and Low, M. D. (1979). Antiepileptic properties of clobazam, a 1,5-benzodiazepine, in man. *Epilepsia* **20**, 437–46.

Gudgeon, A. C. and Hickey, B. J. (1981) A dose-range comparison of clobazam and diazepam: 1. Tests of psychological functions. In "Clobazam: The Royal Society of Medicine International Congress and Symposium Series, No. 43" (I. Hindmarch and P. D. Stonier, eds), pp. 1–5. Royal Society of Medicine, London.

Hindmarch, I. and Gudgeon, A. C. (1980). The effects of clobazam and lorazepam on aspects of psychomotor performance and car handling ability. *British Journal of Clinical Pharmacology* **10**, 145–50.

Hindmarch, I. and Parrott, A. C. (1978). The effect of a sub-chronic administration of three dose levels of a 1,5-benzodiazepine derivative, clobazam, on subjective assessments of sleep and aspects of psychomotor performance the morning following night time medication. *Arzneimittel-Forschung* **28**, 2169–72.

Hindmarch, I., Hanks, G. W. and Hewett, A. J. (1977). Clobazam, a 1,5-benzodiazepine, and car driving ability. *British Journal of Clinical Pharmacology* **4**, 573–78.

Jacobides, G. M. (1976). A comparative study of clonazepam in Greek children and adolescents. In "Epileptology" (D. Janz, ed.), pp. 159–64. Georg Thieme, Stuttgart.

Lance, J. W. and Anthony, M. (1977). Sodium valproate and clonazepam in the treatment of intractable epilepsy. *Archives of Neurology* **34**, 14–17.

Martin, A. A. (1981). The anti-epileptic effects of clobazam: a long-term study in resistant epilepsy. In "Clobazam: The Royal Society of Medicine International Congress and Symposium Series, No. 43" (I. Hindmarch and P. D. Stonier, eds), pp. 151–57. Royal Society of Medicine, London.

Mikkelsen, B., Birket-Smith, E., Brandt, S., Holm, P., Lund, M., Thorn, I., Vestermark, S. and Olsen, P. Z. (1976). Clonazepam in the treatment of epilepsy: a controlled clinical trial in simple absences, bilateral massive epileptic myoclonus, and atonic seizures. *Archives of Neurology* **33**, 322–25.

Munthe-Kaas, A. W. and Strandjord, R. E. (1973). Clonazepam in the treatment of epileptic seizures. *Acta Neurologica Scandinavica* **49** (Suppl. 53), 97–102.

Nanda, R., Keogh, H. D., Lambie, D., Johnson, R. H., Melville, I. D. and Morrice, G. D. (1976). The effects of clonazepam upon epilepsy control and plasma levels of other anticonvulsants. In "Epileptology" (D. Janz, ed.), pp. 145–51. Georg Thieme, Stuttgart.

Parrott, A. C. and Munton, A. (1981). Comparative effects of clobazam and diazepam on psychological performance under different levels of background noise. In "Clobazam: The Royal Society of Medicine International Congress and Symposium Series, No. 43" (I. Hindmarch and P. D. Stonier, eds), pp. 51–57. Royal Society of Medicine, London.

Rey Pias, J. M. (1971). Estudio clinico-electroencefalografico de un nuevo antiepileptico derivado de las benzodiacepinas: el clonazepan. *Archives of Neurobiology* **34**, 487–98.

Robinson, R., Gudgeon, A. C. and Hindmarch, I. (1981). Oxazolam, ketazolam and clobazam compared with placebo on tests of psychomotor function. In "Clobazam: The Royal Society of Medicine International Congress and Symposium Series, No. 43" (I. Hindmarch and P. D. Stonier, eds), pp. 59–65. Royal Society of Medicine, London.

Salkind, M. R., Hanks, G. W. and Silverstone, J. T. (1979). Evaluation of the effects of clobazam, a 1·5 benzodiazepine, on mood and psychomotor performance in clinically anxious patients in general practice. *British Journal of Clinical Pharmacology* **7** (Suppl. 1), 113s–118s.

Shimizu, H., Abe, J., Futagi, Y., Onde, S., Tagawa, T., Mimaki, T., Yamatodani, A., Kato, M., Kamio, M., Sumi, K., Sugita, T. and Yabuuchi, H. (1982). Antiepileptic effects of clobazam in children. *Brain and Development* **4**, 57–62.

Siegfried, K., Koeppen, D., Taeuber, K., Badian, M., Malerczyk, V. and Sittig, W. (1981). A double-blind comparison of the acute effects of clobazam and lorazepam on memory and psychomotor functions. In "Clobazam: The Royal Society of Medicine International Congress and Symposium Series, No. 43" (I. Hindmarch and P. D. Stonier, eds), pp. 13–21. Royal Society of Medicine, London.

Steiner-Chaskel, N. and Lader, M. H. (1981). Effects of single doses of clobazam and diazepam on psychological functions in normal subjects. In "Clobazam: The Royal Society of Medicine International Congress and Symposium Series, No. 43" (I. Hindmarch and P. D. Stonier, eds), pp. 23–32. Royal Society of Medicine, London.

Subhan, Z. (1981). A dose-range comparison of clobazam and diazepam: ii. effects on memory. In "Clobazam: The Royal Society of Medicine International Congress and Symposium Series, No. 43" (I. Hindmarch and P. D. Stonier, eds, pp. 7–12. Royal Society of Medicine, London.

Thompson, P. J. and Trimble, M. R. (1981). Clobazam and cognitive functions: effects in healthy volunteers. In "Clobazam: The Royal Society of Medicine International Congress and Symposium Series, No. 43" (I. Hindmarch and P. D. Stonier, eds), pp. 33–38. Royal Society of Medicine, London.

Trimble, M. R. (1983). Benzodiazepines in epilepsy. In "Benzodiazepines Divided: A
    Multidisciplinary Review" (M. R. Trimble, ed.), pp. 277–89. John Wiley and
    Sons Ltd, London.
Vyborova, L., Balastikova, B., Drtilkova, I. and Nahunek, K. (1979). Clonazepam and
    dithiaden in hyperkinetic children. *Activitas Nervosa Superior* (Praha) **21**,
    155–56.

Rectal Absorption of Clobazam: Pharmacokinetic Aspects and Possible Use in Epilepsy

I. B. DAVIES,* A. W. PIDGEN, J. MCEWEN,† J. D. ROBINSON, S. E. WALKER
and P. D. STONIER

*Department of Clinical Pharmacology, Hoechst U.K. Ltd., Walton Manor,
Milton Keynes, Buckinghamshire, U.K.*

Summary

The pharmacokinetics of clobazam and its major active metabolite N-desmethylclobazam were studied after single doses of clobazam (30 mg) in each of three formulations (oral capsule, suppository, rectal solution) given to six normal subjects in a balanced three-way cross-over study. The rectal solution was absorbed rapidly with virtually no lag time and its initial rate of absorption was quicker than for the capsule, although time to peak concentrations were not significantly different between capsule and solution; absorption from the suppository was slow. Area under the curve to infinity was similar for all formulations. N-desmethylclobazam plasma concentrations, peak concentrations, time to peak, and area under the curve to the last measured time point were similar for all formulations. Clobazam rectal solution gave, rapidly, adequate plasma clobazam concentrations sustained for 6 h after dosing; therefore, rectal solution could be rapidly effective and long-lasting in treatment of epileptic fits.

Introduction

Benzodiazepines such as diazepam and clonazepam are useful in acute treatment of epileptic fits (Howard *et al.*, 1968) and as adjunctive treatment to prevent fits when given in chronic treatment with other anticonvulsant drugs (Beaumont, 1982). Treatment of fits by intravenous administration of

anticonvulsants may be difficult, as in children (Dhillon *et al.*, 1982), or in severely epileptic adults who have frequent fits. Rectal administration of diazepam has been used in the treatment of fits in children (Dhillon *et al.*, 1982) and the use of rectal administration of clonazepam has been studied in adults (Jensen *et al.*, 1983).

able in Britain for treatment of anxiety and adjunctive treatment of epilepsy (Martin, 1981). Clobazam is relatively insoluble and therefore cannot be given by intravenous or intramuscular injection. Therefore, rectal formulations of clobazam were studied to find if rectal absorption of clobazam occurred quickly enough to justify clinical trials of rectal clobazam in epileptic patients. N-desmethylclobazam is a major active metabolite of clobazam and has anticonvulsant activity (Fielding and Hoffmann, 1979) and, therefore, plasma concentrations of N-desmethylclobazam were also measured after rectal clobazam administration.

Subjects and Methods

Six normal subjects (four male, two female: weight 56·2–86 kg, age 26–45 years) were given clobazam (30 mg) as a single dose of each of three formulations, oral capsule, rectal suppository or solution, according to a balanced cross-over design. Medication was given at 0800 h on the study day after an overnight fast since 2200 h. Two weeks were allowed between each administration. Suppositories and rectal solution were self-administered by subjects according to individual verbal instructions. Rectal solution was

* *Present address:* Charterhouse Clinical Research Unit, St. Bartholomews Hospital, London, UK.
† *Present address:* Drug Development Scotland Ltd, Ninewells Hospital & Medical School, Dundee, UK.

contained in a 10 ml polypropylene syringe with a soft polyethylene applicator; allowance was made for the deadspace in the rectal solution container so that the correct dose was instilled into the rectum. Venous blood (5 ml) was taken before dosing and after dosing of 5, 10, 20 min and then at 0·5, 1, 1·5, 2, 2·5, 3, 4, 6, 8, 10, 24, 30, 96 and 164 h. Plasma concentrations of clobazam and norclobazam were measured by the Analytical Department, Hoechst U.K. Ltd, using, respectively, gas chromatography with nitrogen detection (sensitivity 20 ng/ml, inter-assay and intra-assay coefficients of variation, about, 10% and 6–7% respectively) or HPLC (sensitivity 6 ng/ml, inter- and intra-assay coefficients of variation approximately 4–5%).

The study was approved by the Hoechst U.K. Ethics Committee and subjects gave informed signed consent. The study was conducted according to the Declaration of Helsinki.

Pharmacokinetic analysis of clobazam and *N*-desmethylclobazam plasma concentrations was carried out using a bioavailability programme for a Hewlett Packard MX(E) minicomputer (Ings *et al.*, 1980). Data were tested for homogeneity of variance and normality of distribution and then by analysis of variance with pairwise comparisons.

Results

Clobazam pharmacokinetics

Clobazam absorption was faster from the rectal solution than from the rectal suppository or the oral capsules; this was emphasized by the initial 2 h plasma concentration-time profile (Fig. 1). Clobazam was detectable in plasma 5 min after administration of rectal solution; 10 min after dosing the concentration was 131 ± 48 ng/ml and after 20 min exceeded 200 ng/ml. However, there was no significant difference between time to peak plasma clobazam concentrations between the rectal solution and the capsule, but time to peak values for these formulations were less than for the suppository (Table 1). Peak plasma concentrations were greater after the capsule than the rectal formulations (Table 1, Fig. 1). However, bioavailability as measured by AUC to infinite time and terminal half-life was similar for all three formulations (Table 1, Fig. 2). The elimination phase for clobazam with all formulations was prolonged (Fig. 3).

N-desmethylclobazam pharmacokinetics

There was a delay of about 4 h for the capsule and about 6–8 h for the rectal formulations before *N*-desmethylclobazam, the major metabolite of clobazam, appeared in plasma (Fig. 3). Peak plasma concentrations were similar for all formulations; there was a trend for the time to peak concentration to be longer for the suppository (Table 2). The AUC to last measured time point was similar for all formulations (Table 2). The prolonged

Table 1

Clobazam pharmacokinetic parameters

Parameter	Oral capsule	Rectal solution	Rectal suppository
Time to peak (h)	$1·39 \pm 1·38$	$1·67 \pm 0·41$	$4·33 \pm 2·96$
Peak level (ng/ml)	$702·5 \pm 183·6$	$410·4 \pm 110·8$	$281·6 \pm 86·6$
Terminal half-life (h)	$31·7 \pm 11·7$	$32·3 \pm 11·8$	$32·9 \pm 11·1$
$AUC_{0-\infty}$	13275 ± 2913	13742 ± 3468	12190 ± 3487

All values mean $\pm$ SD for inter-individual variation.

Time to peak less for capsule than solution ($P < 0·05$) or suppository ($P < 0·05$) and less for solution than suppository ($P < 0·05$). Peak level greater for capsule than solution ($P < 0·05$) or suppository ($P < 0·001$) and greater for solution than suppository ($P < 0·05$).

$AUC_{0-\infty}$ area under curve from time 0 to infinity.

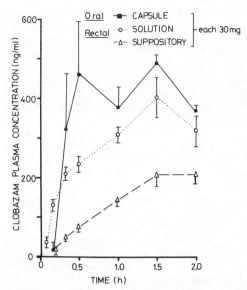

Figure 1. Plasma clobazam concentrations
0–2 h after administration of clobazam (30 mg)
as an oral capsule (■), rectal suppository (△),
or rectal solution (○); values are mean±stan-
dard deviation for six subjects in each case.

elimination phase and relatively short
duration of sampling (Fig. 3) prevented calculation of elimination half-life and AUC to
infinity values; however, the elimination half-
life approximated 40–60 h for all formulations in those subjects for whom an estimate
of elimination half-life was possible.

Discussion

Route of administration and clobazam pharmacokinetics

In spite of similarity in peak plasma concentration and time to peak values for oral capsule and rectal solution of clobazam, the
initial absorption rate of clobazam was faster
from the rectal solution than from the capsule
(Fig. 1). The faster initial absorption from the
rectal solution may reflect the simplicity of
absorption across a single type of epithelium
in comparison with the more complex process
of oral absorption, where tablet or capsule
disintegration/dissolution and gastric empty-
ing time are initially rate-limiting to the
absorption process (Beckett, 1978). However,
the eventual peak concentration with the oral

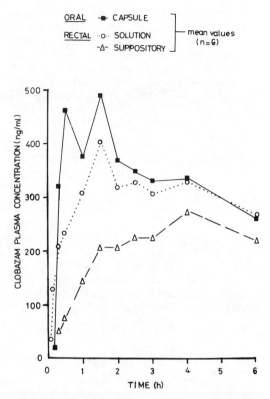

Figure 2. Plasma clobazam concentrations
0–6 h after administration of capsule, suppository or rectal solution, symbols as in Fig. 1.
Values are means for six subjects in each case.

capsule was greater than with either rectal
formulation, probably reflecting the 10^4-fold
greater absorptive surface area in the small
intestine compared with the rectum (de Boer
et al., 1982). Formulation is a critical factor
in determining rate of drug absorption from
the rectum and this may explain the slower
rate of absorption from the rectal suppository than from the solution (de Boer et al.,
1982). Drug absorption from the rectum occurs via the haemorrhoidal venous system
which partially bypasses the liver and could
result in differences in bioavailability for
drugs which are metabolized by the liver (de
Boer et al., 1982). However, AUC values for
clobazam from oral and rectal routes were
similar; in contrast, rectal diazepam administration may produce higher blood diazepam concentrations than with oral diazepam
(Schwartz et al., 1966). Diazepam, too, is
absorbed at an initially faster rate from a
rectal solution than from solid oral dosage

forms (Moolenaar *et al.*, 1980; Mattila *et al.*, 1981). A striking feature of this study was the smaller variability in plasma clobazam concentrations after rectal administration; presumably the simpler process of rectal absorption was affected by fewer variables than oral gastro-intestinal absorption and so produced greater homogeneity of plasma clobazam profiles after rectal administration. The route of administration in this study did not influence elimination half-life values which were similar to one previous study (Greenblatt *et al.*, 1981) but shorter than in one other (Vallner *et al.*, 1978).

Route of administration and N-desmethylclobazam kinetics

Similar peak plasma concentrations of *N*-desmethylclobazam, the major and active metabolite of clobazam (Fielding and Hoff-

man, 1979; Aucamp, 1982) occurred after all formulations (Table 2, Fig. 3). However, there was a trend for a slower rate of appearance of *N*-desmethylclobazam in blood after rectal administration, especially for the suppository (Table 2, Fig. 3). The slower rate of *N*-desmethylclobazam appearance after the rectal route may result from the drug initially bypassing the liver where *N*-desalkylation of clobazam occurs. The long time to peak for *N*-desmethylclobazam (Fig. 3) and the long time to reach steady state described previously (Rupp *et al.*, 1979) may also reflect biliary excretion of a glucuronide—possibly of hydroxylated norclobazam—with enterohepatic recycling for the 3-hydroxy metabolite of *N*-desmethyldiazepam (Garattini *et al.*, 1973). In this study, the elimination half-life of *N*-desmethylclobazam could not be determined accurately for all subjects, but the approximate value of 40–60 h was similar for all formulations and was similar to that described previously (Rupp *et al.*, 1979).

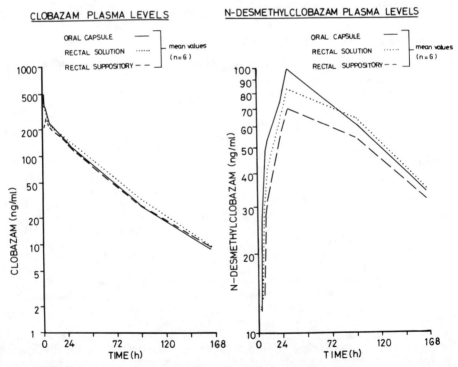

Figure 3. Plasma clobazam (left panel) or N-desmethylclobazam (right panel) concentrations for 0–164 h after administration of clobazam (30 mg) as an oral capsule (–), rectal solution (......), or rectal suppository (– – – –). Lines represent mean values for six subjects in each case. Individual time points are represented by points of inflexion of the lines.

Table 2

N-desmethylclobazam pharmacokinetics

Parameter	Oral capsule	Rectal solution	Rectal suppository
Time to peak (h)	$39 \cdot 0 \pm 28 \cdot 1$	$39 \cdot 0 \pm 28 \cdot 1$	$51 \cdot 0 \pm 34 \cdot 9$
Peak concentration	$92 \cdot 0 \pm 27 \cdot 5$	$84 \cdot 0 \pm 17 \cdot 2$	$74 \cdot 1 \pm 21 \cdot 0$
AUC_{O-T} (ng ml^{-1}h)	9329 ± 2297	9682 ± 3142	8302 ± 3322

AUC_{O-T} is area under curve from time 0 to last measured time point (164 h). No statistically significant differences found for any parameter or formulation.
Note: plasma concentration profiles did not allow for calculation of elimination half-life or AUC to infinite time.

Potential use of rectal clobazam for treatment of epilepsy

Clobazam was absorbed rapidly with virtually no lag time from the rectal solution and gave plasma clobazam concentrations above 200 ng/ml 30 min after administration; the concentrations were sustained at 200–300 ng/ml for 8–10 h after administration (Figs 1–3). There is little information about the relationship between plasma clobazam concentrations and anticonvulsant effects in epileptic patients or between plasma and brain or cerebro-spinal fluid clobazam concentrations in animals. A similar situation obtains for diazepam (Booker and Celesia, 1973). In rat brain, clobazam concentration was about one-third of that in blood, while in dogs brain and blood clobazam concentrations were similar (Volz et al., 1979). In treatment of acute fits with a rectal formulation of a benzodiazepine, obviously rapid absorption would be needed; in this study, absorption of clobazam from the rectal solution was sufficiently rapid to justify further evaluation of the formulation in epileptic patients. Rectal solutions of diazepam and clonazepam also may be absorbed sufficiently rapidly to be of use in treating acute fits (Moolenaar et al., 1980; Jensen et al., 1983). Rectal diazepam solutions have been successful in children as premedication before operations (Mattila et al., 1981) and to treat convulsions (Augrell et al., 1981) and to treat convulsions (Augrell et al., 1975; Knudsen, 1977, 1979, 1981; Munthe-Kaas, 1980; Dhillon et al., 1982). The sustained plasma concentration of clobazam found in this study may also be of use, for it is a common clinical observation that after a single intravenous dose of a benzodiazepine to stop fits, a further dose is necessary a short time later, possibly resulting from a rapid decrease in plasma/brain concentrations. Repeated use of a benzodiazepine over a short period of time or sustained plasma concentrations carry a theoretical risk of respiratory depression; however, in three studies with rectal diazepam this was not reported (Munthe-Kaas, 1980; Knudsen, 1981; Mattila et al., 1981).

N-desmethylclobazam is an active anticonvulsant and accumulates after repeated dosing with clobazam (Rupp et al., 1979). The slow rate of appearance of N-desmethylclobazam after the rectal solution would be unlikely to be of importance in immediate anti-convulsant effect, although norclobazam could contribute to a more prolonged anti-convulsant action after multiple doses of clobazam. The entry into plasma of both clobazam and N-desmethylclobazam after the rectal suppository was probably too slow to be of potential use for acute treatment of fits; this has been the experience with suppositories of diazepam (Augrell et al., 1975; Knudsen, 1977; Munthe-Kaas, 1980; Dhillon et al., 1982).

References

Augrell, S., Berlin, A., Ferngren, H. and Hellström, B. (1975). Plasma levels of diazepam after parenteral and rectal administration in children. *Epilepsia* **16**, 277–283.
Aucamp, A. K. (1982). Aspects of the pharmacokinetics and pharmacodynamics of benzodia-

zepines with particular reference to clobazam. *Drug Development Research* Suppl. 1, 117–126.

Beaumont, G. (1982). Benzodiazepine therapy in epilepsy. *Psychiatry in Practice* **1**, 50.

Beckett, A. H. (1978). Bioavailability of drugs. In "Drug Metabolism in Man" (J. W. Gorrod and A. H. Beckett, eds), pp. 25–60. Pharmaceutical Soc., Taylor and Francis Ltd, London.

Booker, H. E. and Celesia, G. (1973). Serum concentrations of diazepam in subjects with epilepsy. *Archives of Neurology* **29**, 191–194.

de Boer, A. G., Moolenaar, F., de Leede, L. G. J. and Breimer, D. D. (1982). Rectal drug administration: clinical pharmacokinetic considerations. *Clinical Pharmacokinetics* **7**, 285–311.

Dhillon, S., Ngwane, E. and Richens, A. (1982). Rectal absorption of diazepam in epileptic children. *Archives of Disease in Childhood* **57**, 264–267.

Fielding, S. and Hoffman, I. (1979). Pharmacology of antianxiety drugs with special reference to clobazam. *British Journal of Clinical Pharmacology* **7**, 7S–16S.

Garattini, S., Marcucci, F., Morselli, P. L. and Musini, E. (1973). The significance of measuring blood levels of benzodiazepines. In "Biological Effects of Drugs in Relation to Their Plasma Concentrations" (D. J. Davies and B. N. C. Pritchard, eds), pp. 211–225. British Pharmacological Society, Macmillan Ltd, London.

Greenblatt, D. J., Divoll, M., Puri, S. K., Ho, I., Zinny, M. A. and Shader, R. I. (1968). Clobazam kinetics in the elderly. *British Journal of Clinical Pharmacology* **12**, 631–636.

Howard, F. M. Jr, Seybold, M. and Reiher, J. (1968). The treatment of recurrent convulsions with intravenous injection of diazepam. *Medical Clinics of North America* **52**, 977–987.

Ings, R. M. J., Pidgen, A. W. and Johnson, D. (1980). Analysis of bioavailability studies. In "Abstracts of World Congress on Clinical Pharmacology and Therapeutics" (P. Turner and C. Padgham, eds), Abstracts 0416. Macmillan Ltd, London.

Jensen, P. K., Abild, K. and Pulsen, M. N. (1983). Serum concentration of clonazepam after rectal administration. *Acta Neurologica Scandinavica* **68**, 417–420.

Knudsen, F. U. (1977). Plasma diazepam in infants after rectal administration in solution and by suppository. *Acta Paediatrica Scandinavica* **66**, 563–567.

Knudsen, F. U. (1979). Rectal administration of diazepam in solution in the acute treatment of convulsions in infants and children. *Archives of Disease in Childhood* **54**, 855–857.

Knudsen, F. U. (1981). Successful intermittent diazepam prophylaxis in febrile convulsions: preliminary results of a prospective, controlled study. In "Advances in Epileptology—XIIth Epilepsy International Symposium" (M. Dam, L. Gram and J. K. Penry, eds), pp. 165–168. Raven Press, New York.

Martin, A. A. (1981). The antiepileptic effects of clobazam: a long-term study in resistant epilepsy. In: Clobazam: International Congress and Symposium Series No. 43 (P. D. Stonier and I. Hindmarch, eds), pp. 151–157. Royal Society of Medicine, London.

Mattila, M. A. K., Ruoppi, M. K., Ahlström-Bengs, E., Larni, H. M. and Pekkola, P. O. (1981). Diazepam in rectal solution as premedication in children with special reference to serum concentrations. *British Journal of Anaesthesia* **53**, 1269–1272.

Moolenaar, F., Bakker, S., Visser, J. and Huizinga, T. (1980). Biopharmaceutics of Rectal Administration of Drugs in Man. IX. Comparative biopharmaceutics of diazepam after single rectal, oral, intramuscular and intravenous administration in man. *International Journal of Pharmaceutics* **5**, 127–137.

Munthe-Kaas, A. W. (1980). Rectal administration of diazepam: theoretical basis and clinical experience. In "Antiepileptic Therapy: Advances in Drug Monitoring" (S. I.

Johanessen, ed.), pp. 381–389. Raven Press, New York.

Rupp, W., Badian, M., Christ, O., Hajdu, P., Kulkarni, R. D., Taeuber, K., Uihlein, M., Bender, R. and Vanderbeke, O. (1979). Pharmacokinetics of single and multiple doses of clobazam in humans. *British Journal of Clinical Pharmacology* **7**, 51S–57S.

Schwartz, D. B., Vecchi, M., Ronco, A. and Kaiser, K. (1966). Blood levels after administration of diazepam in various forms. *Arzneimittel-Forschung* **16**, 1109–1110.

Vallner, J. J., Needham, T. E., Jun, H. W., Brown, W. J., Stewart, J. T., Kotzan, J. A. and Honigberg, I. L. (1978). Plasma levels of clobazam after three oral dosage forms in healthy subjects. *Journal of Clinical Pharmacology* **18**, 319–324.

Volz, M., Christ, O., Kellner, H.-M., Kuch, H., Felhaber, H.-W., Gantz, D., Hadju, P., and Cavagna, F. (1979). Kinetics and metabolism of clobazam in animals and man. *British Journal of Clinical Pharmacology* **7**, 41S–50S.

Clobazam in Resistant Epilepsy—A Long-term Study

A. A. MARTIN

Department of Electroencephalography, Lancaster Moor Hospital, Lancaster, U.K.

Clobazam has been used as adjunctive therapy in a cohort of patients with epilepsy of mixed types and aetiology since August 1979. The first report on the results of treatment has been published (Martin, 1981), and the cohort has continued under study until the present time, a period of 51 months (4·25 years).

Of the initial cohort of 54 patients with resistant epilepsy, five were withdrawn due to inadequacy of the follow-up and a further patient died of intercurrent illness unrelated to epilepsy; thus, 48 patients have been followed up for at least 48 months (four years).

In all these patients clobazam was prescribed as additional therapy to standard anticonvulsants, consisting mainly of one or more of the following drugs: phenobarbitone, phenytoin, carbamazepine, and sodium valproate.

The dosage regimen of clobazam has mainly involved the administration of single daily doses before retiring to bed, in initial doses of 10–20 mg, increasing by 10 mg at monthly intervals until control of seizures is achieved. Of those patients who have been seizure-free for periods of one year or more, namely 17 (34%), 15 have received 10–30 mg daily, one has received 40 mg daily, and one 50 mg daily. No patient has received more than 80 mg.

In those patients in whom addition of clobazam led to a substantial seizure-free period, a reduction or discontinuation of other medication was achieved without loss of control.

Of the 17 patients who have been seizure-free for one year or more, six (12% of cohort) continue to be seizure-free after four years, four (8%) after three years, three (6%) after two years and four (8%) after one year.

One patient in the latter group, on 30 mg clobazam daily, developed a grossly abnormal EEG and was found at surgery to have a glioma, but has continued to be seizure-free.

Over the period of follow-up of four years, there have been no significant adverse side-effects attributable to clobazam apart from reports which have been infrequent and mild. Favourable side-effects have related mainly to an improved sense of well-being, better performance at work and study and expressed relief of freedom from seizures coupled with a growth in confidence as time passes, this latter effect probably enhanced by the discontinuation or reduction of basic medication where this has been possible. It appears unlikely that drug tolerance will occur in those 13 patients in this group who have been seizure-free for two years or more (26% of cohort).

Of the remaining 31 patients in the cohort 12 (25%) have shown a substantial reduction in seizure frequency, both when assessed against pre-study baseline seizure frequency and in the occurrence of freedom from seizures during the study of 5–11 months. In such cases tolerance was assumed to have occurred and clobazam was discontinued for 4–6 weeks. Resumption of treatment was sometimes but not always successful in producing a further period of freedom from seizures of several months.

In seven patients (14%) there was either moderate reduction in seizure frequency or a change in seizure pattern, e.g. from major to minor seizures, but no prolonged seizure-free period.

In 12 patients (25%) there was no change in overall fit frequency or clinical condition.

Summary

In a cohort of 48 patients with resistant epilepsy studied for up to four years, clobazam was shown to be substantially or moderately effective adjunctive therapy in 75% of cases, with 17 patients (34%) remaining seizure-free for 1–4 years and continuing.

Reference

Martin, A. A. (1981). The anti-epileptic effects of clobazam: a long-term study in resistant epilepsy. In "Clobazam" (I. Hindmarch and P. D. Stonier, eds), pp. 151–157. International Congress and Symposium Series, Number 43. Royal Society of Medicine, London.

A Long-term Study of the Efficacy of Clobazam as an Antiepileptic Drug. Short Report.

J. W. ALLEN,* S. JAWAD, ** J. OXLEY, * and M. TRIMBLE***

* Chalfont Centre for Epilepsy, Chalfont St. Peter, Gerrards Cross, Bucks, U.K.,
** Department of Pharmacology and Therapeutics, Welsh National School of
Medicine, Heath Park, Cardiff, U.K. and *** National Hospital for Nervous
Diseases, Queen Square, London WC1N 3BG, U.K.

Introduction

The benzodiazepines have a well established role in the treatment of epilepsy (Browne and Penry, 1983). Recently (Allen et al., 1983), we have reported the 1,5-benzodiazepine clobazam to be an effective drug in the short-term treatment of intractable epilepsy. We now present the results of a long-term study on the antiepileptic properties of clobazam at 12 months.

Patients, Methods and Results

Fifty-two residents at the Chalfont Centre for Epilepsy (aged 16–69 years) with at least four fits per month were studied. Baseline fit frequencies were monitored over one month by attendant staff and 10–30 mg clobazam was then added to each patient's regime, which otherwise remained constant. Those subjects showing a 50% reduction in fit frequency were included in the long-term study as "responders", and seen at monthly intervals by the investigating physician.

Fasting blood samples were taken at regular intervals for the measurement of antiepileptic drug levels, including clobazam and desmethylclobazam. Tolerance was defined as a return to baseline fit frequency. Clobazam was discontinued by making reductions of 10 mg at weekly intervals.

Twenty-six subjects "responded", 13 failed to respond to 30 mg daily, and 13 were withdrawn because of adverse effects. Of the 26 "responders", 20 (77%) developed tolerance to the antiepileptic effects at a median of 3·5 months (range 1–8 months), three (11·5%) showed no tolerance, and three (11·5%)

dropped out (two due to adverse effects and one was lost to follow-up), as shown in Fig. 1.

The respective antiepileptic drug levels (mean ± SD, μmol/l) for the 1–2 month period prior to and at the development of tolerance were: phenytoin 48·7 ± 8·2 and 46·3 ± 9·2; carbamazepine 27·5 ± 3·2 and 26·9 ± 2·9; phenobarbitone 93·3 ± 28·0 and 88·3 ± 13·0; sodium valproate 492·0 ± 106·9 and 495·0 ± 119·6; clobazam 0·3 ± 0·3 and 0·27 ± 0·3; and desmethylclobazam 61·6 ± 35·2 and 62·1 ± 32·7.

Comment

One of the problems of using the benzodiazepines in the chronic treatment of epilepsy is the development of tolerance, again highlighted in this study. Nevertheless, a substan-

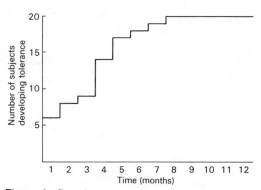

Figure 1. Development of Tolerance.

tial proportion of previously intractable patients benefitted from a period of improved seizure control lasting at least three months, and in a small proportion a longer-lasting benefit was achieved. Gastaut and Low (1979) also recorded a high incidence of tolerance (50% of his subjects developed "exhaustion" within 45 days), and Martin (1981) reported a median time to tolerance of 6·5 months. The tolerance in this study cannot be explained by changes in the levels of concomitant antiepileptic drugs, clobazam or desmethylclobazam, which did not vary significantly. Twenty-nine per cent of subjects were withdrawn at some stage because of adverse effects (mainly sleepiness, unsteadiness and irritability). This compares with none reported by Martin (1981) and 5% by Gastaut and Low (1979). The different populations studied may explain the discrepancy. Although withdrawal fits were a problem in some patients, they occurred less frequently than in our previous study, and status epilepticus was not encountered. This may have been due to the more prolonged period of clobazam withdrawal.

The usefulness of clobazam in the long-term treatment of severe epilepsy is limited by the development of tolerance, the occurrence of adverse effects, and a liability to withdrawal fits. It is, however, suggested that for a small proportion of those who respond initially, clobazam is effective on a long-term basis and its trial in otherwise intractable cases, especially with partial seizures, is advocated. Further work is required to establish the cause of tolerance and its appropriate management. The drug should be used with caution, particularly in severely handicapped patients, and with adequate follow-up to ensure that it is discontinued carefully if it becomes ineffective.

References

Browne, T. R. and Penry, J. K. (1983). Benzodiazepines in the treatment of epilepsy: A review. *Epilepsia* **14**, 277–310.
Allen, J. W., Oxley, J.l Robertson, M., Trimble, M., Richens, A. and Jawad, S. (1983). Clobazam as adjunctive treatment in refractory epilepsy. *Br. Med. J.* **286**, 1246–1247.
Gastaut, H. and Low, M. D. (1979). Antiepileptic properties of clobazam, a 1,5-benzodiazepine, in man. *Epilepsia* **20**, 437–446.
Martin, A. A. (1981). The antiepileptic effects of clobazam: A long term study in resistant epilepsy. In "Clobazam" (I. Hindmarch and P. D. Stonier, eds), pp. 151–157. International Congress and Symposium Series, Number 43. Royal Society of Medicine, London.

The Treatment of Elderly Patients with Clobazam: A Multi-centre Clinical Trial. Short Report.

F. NOEL

Laboratoires Diamant, Tour Roussel-Nobel, Cedex 3, 92080 Paris la Defense, France

Introduction

The efficacy and clinical safety of clobazam (5 mg t.d.s.) used to treat anxiety in elderly patients was evaluated in a randomized double-blind placebo-controlled trial over four weeks.

Patients and Methods

Ten physicians took part in the study and enrolled elderly patients who presented with anxiety, either free of, or associated with, other psychiatric illness including depressive disorders, psychosomatic syndromes or behavioural disturbances. The patients were free from dementia or severe organic disease.

Patients were randomized to treatment groups with either placebo or 5 mg clobazam t.d.s. for four weeks. Other psychotropic drugs were permitted only in specific cases, e.g. antidepressants, and treatment for concurrent organic disease was also permitted.

Assessments were performed on admission to the study and after one and four weeks of treatment. A ten-item symptom rating scale suitable for the elderly was used and anxiety, depressive troubles, psychosomatic troubles, psychomental deficiency, asthenia, apathy, restlessness, psychopathic disorders, aggressiveness, headache, sleep disturbances and anorexia were rated on a four-point scale. The sum of scores constituted a global score. An overall assessment of efficacy was made by the investigator at the end of the trial according to a four-point scale (excellent, good, poor, absent). Side-effects were assessed by using a checklist together with an overall physician assessment of tolerability (excellent, moderate, poor).

Results

One hundred and fifty-four patients were admitted to the study; 95 women and 59 men with an age range of 58–94 years (mean $69 \cdot 6 \pm 9 \cdot 7$ years). There were 120 outpatients and 34 inpatients. The demographic data of the patients randomized into two groups of 77 did not differ significantly. Of the patients 111 suffered a concurrent medical illness, the most frequent being arterial hypertension (29 cases), cardiovascular diseases (28) and gastrointestinal disorders (23). The psychiatric back grounds of the two groups were similar with the onset of anxiety symptoms occurring on average two years prior to the study (range 15 days to 20 years; 45% ranged from 2–6 months). Seventy-four patients had received previous psychotropic medication mainly anxiolytic drugs with a good result in 46%.

The two treatment groups did not differ significantly in severity of symptoms prior to the trial. The reduction in global symptom rating was significantly different between the group in favour of clobazam.

Although the mean severity of each item was reduced in the two groups, the reduction was greater in the clobazam group. The physicians' overall efficacy assessment showed that this was "excellent" or "good" in 53% of the clobazam group compared with 31·5% of the placebo group, a difference which was statistically significant.

Twenty-three patients discontinued treatment before the end of the fourth week due to lack of efficacy (four clobazam, six placebo), or side-effects (four clobazam, eight placebo), and one patient had a severe organic disease requiring admission to hospital. Side-effects to clobazam were drowsiness (three cases, day 7) and muscular weakness (one case, day 7), and to placebo, were drowsiness (four cases, day 7), dizziness (one case, day 4) and excitement/insomnia (one case, day 4). Some of these symptoms were present before commencement of treatment and represented either part of the clinical symptomatology or were induced by previous psychotropic drugs. There was no significant difference between the two groups with respect to global side-effect scores, nor in the overall assessment by the physician with tolerability assessed as "perfect" in 82% of patients in each group.

Blood pressure and pulse rate were recorded before and at the end of the study in 72 patients on clobazam and 71 on placebo with stable values being recorded throughout.

It is concluded that 15 mg clobazam daily in divided dosage is an effective and well tolerated treatment of anxiety in elderly patients.

Clobazam in Drug Resistant Epilepsy: An Open Prospective Study. Preliminary Communication.

N. CALLAGHAN and T. GOGGIN

Department of Neurology, Cork Regional Hospital, Wilton, Cork, Ireland

Summary

Clobazam was added to anticonvulsant treatment in 33 patients with drug-resistant epilepsy. Ten patients suffered from generalized seizures and 23 patients from partial seizures. Sixty-six per cent of patients with generalized seizures and 49% with partial seizures improved for a period of six months. Improvement was maintained in 57% of patients with generalized seizures and 33% of patients with partial seizures over a period of 12 months. Thirty-five per cent of all patients who improved initially maintained improvement for periods which ranged from 15–18 months. Exhaustion occurred in 25% of patients over a period which ranged from 6–12 months. Improvement in EEG abnormalities occurred only in two patients. The drug was tolerated well by most patients. It was possible to reduce the prescribed number of anticonvulsant drugs from three to two drugs in five patients and to reduce the dose of other anticonvulsant medications in four patients.

Introduction

The 1,4-benzodiazepines are established as anticonvulsants. Side-effects may occur which includes psychomotor impairment, together with relapses at intervals of weeks or months following initial seizure control (Edwards and Eadie, 1973; Browne, 1976; Korttila and Linnoila, 1975). Clobazam, a 1,5-benzodiazepine, has been found to have anticonvulsant activity (Gastaut, 1981), but the effects may be short-lived in some patients due to tolerance and exhaustion of efficacy. exhaustion of efficacy.

It has been established that seizure control is achieved in many patients on monotherapy especially if progress is monitored with blood levels (Reynolds and Chadwick, 1976; Callaghan et al., 1978, 1983; Feely et al., 1979). However, in some of these patients monotherapy may fail to control seizures and, when polypharmacy is prescribed, the response is not always satisfactory. Martin (1981) in an open study and Critchley et al. (1981) in a double-blind trial have shown that clobazam improves seizure control in some patients with resistant and refractory epilepsy when added to other anticonvulsant drugs. We report the results of an open study carried out to evaluate the anticonvulsant properties of clobazam when added to other drugs in patients with refractory seizures.

Patients and Methods

Thirty-three patients attending a seizure clinic were selected for this study. Details of patients' age, duration of epilepsy, duration of treatment, and seizure frequency prior to entry to the study are summarized in Table 1. Seizure frequency, which was based on assessment over a six-month period prior to entry into the study, was greater at a significant level for patients with partial seizures. As shown in Table 2a, ten patients were taking monotherapy. All of these had been treated with more than one anticonvulsant drug as monotherapy in an attempt to improve seizure control and failed to respond, despite optimal levels of the drugs. The drugs documented in Table 2a are the drugs prescribed as monotherapy before clobazam was added to the treatment. As shown in Table 2b, 23 patients were taking multiple drugs; 12 of these patients had initially been treated with monotherapy but had failed to respond. A second drug was then added in an attempt to improve seizure control. Satisfactory res-

Table 1

Demographic Data

n	Age (Yr) ±SD (Range)	Duration of epilepsy (Yr) ±SD (Range)	Baseline seizure frequency (per month) ±SD (Range)	Duration of treatment (months) ±SD (Range)
		1. All patients		
33	24·5± 9·7 (12–54)	12·8±7·7 (2–35)	70±158 (1–914)	14·5±6·0 (1–20)
		2. Patients with generalized seizures		
21	24·9± 8·9 (14–48)	12·9±7·5 (4–35)	35± 43 (1–152)	14·9±6·1 (2–20)
		3. Patients with partial seizures		
12	23·2±11·5 (12–54)	12·4±8·2 (2–30)	139±249 (9–914)*	13·8±6·0 (1–20)

* Partial seizures more frequent than generalized: $P < 0.001$.

ponse was not obtained despite optimal levels of carbamazepine, sodium valproate, phenytoin and phenobarbitone either ingested or derived from primidone. Eleven patients in the polytherapy group had been taking multiple drugs when initially referred to the seizure clinic. An attempt to rationalize drug treatment by reducing the number of drugs prescribed was not successful. The levels of the drugs were then adjusted to achieve optimal levels for the drugs prescribed and patients continued to have frequent seizures.

Twenty-one patients suffered from primary generalized tonic clonic seizures and 12 patients from partial seizures. Eight patients had partial complex seizures with secondary generalized attacks and four patients, simple partial seizures with secondary generalized attacks.

An electroencephalogram was carried out on all patients prior to entry into the study. Nineteen patients had bilateral generalized seizure discharges, eight patients focal spike discharges with associated bilateral generalized seizure discharges, and six patients, bilateral paroxysmal slow activity.

Clobazam was prescribed initially in a dose of 10 mg per day. The patients were then seen at intervals of two weeks and at each visit details were obtained about seizure control and side-effects. A specimen of blood was taken for estimation of clobazam levels. If control was not satisfactory, the dose of clobazam was increased by 10 mg until the patients achieved good control. In patients who achieved good control, further upward dose adjustments were carried out at monthly intervals. Depending upon seizure response and patients' requirements, the maximal dose

Table 2

Concomitant medication

(a) Monotherapy Drug	Number of patients
Carbamazepine (CBZ)	7
Phenytoin	2
Sodium valproate	1
Total	10

(b) Polytherapy Drugs	Number of patients
CBZ + phenytoin	4
CBZ + phenobarb.*	5
CBZ + valproate	5
CBZ + primidone	3
CBZ + nitrazepam*	2
Phenytoin + phenobarb.*	2
CBZ + primidone + valproate*	2
Total	23

*Polytherapy as initial treatment; others—preceded by monotherapy.

of the drug was based on the dose which the patient could tolerate without side-effects. Response to treatment was evaluated as follows, based on assessment over a minimal period of three months.

Excellent response—Complete freedom from seizures

Good response —Greater than 50% reduction in seizure frequency

Poor response —No improvement or less than 50% reduction in seizure frequency.

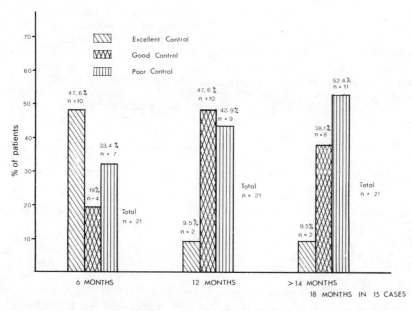

Figure 1. *Changes in Control: generalized seizures.*

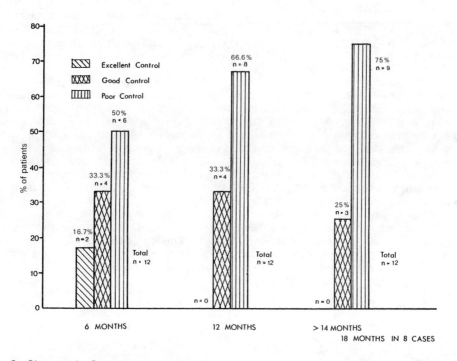

Figure 2. *Changes in Control: partial seizures.*

Results

The response to treatment for patients with generalized seizures is summarized in Fig. 1, and for patients with partial seizures in Fig. 2. The improvement which occurred at six months for all types of seizures was not maintained at 12 months when control deteriorated in 58% of patients with generalized seizures and 16% of patients with partial seizures. Further deterioration occurred in 19% of patients with generalized seizures and 8% of patients with partial seizures over a period which ranged from 15–18 months. Sixty per cent of all patients improved over a period of six months; 50% of those who improved had deteriorated at 12 months and 65% had deteriorated at 18 months. Thirty-five per cent maintained improvement.

The drug was generally well tolerated with mild/moderate side-effects occurring in seven patients (drowsiness (2), headache (1), dry mouth (1), apprehension (1), lightheadedness (1), sweating (1)) and severe side-effects in three patients (drowsiness (2), dry mouth (1)). The drowsiness which occurred in four patients was dose related and severe drowsiness occurred when a dose in excess of 40 mg per day was prescribed.

Discussion

In this study we have shown that the addition of clobazam to established anticonvulsant treatments improved seizure control in some patients with drug-resistant seizures. A total of 35% of patients maintained improvement for periods which ranged from 15–18 months. In keeping with the findings of Gastaut (1981) exhaustion occurred in 25% of patients. Gastaut has shown that while a reduction in antiepileptic effect occurred before three months of treatment in 50% of patients, it sometimes developed during the first week or even during the first days. In our study, however, improvement was maintained over an initial period of six months

before exhaustion occurred in some patients. Other patients maintained improvement for 12 months before deterioration in seizure control occurred. It has been suggested (Martin, 1981) that in view of the long half-life of clobazam and its active metabolite, desmethylclobazam, it might be possible to delay or avoid exhaustion by prescribing relatively small doses of the drug initially with further increments if necessary. It is therefore possible that a policy to increase gradually the dose according to the patient's requirements postponed the onset of exhaustion in our patients.

It has been shown (Martin, 1981) that as the dosage of clobazam was increased, seizure control improved and it was possible to reduce the dose of other anticonvulsant drugs and to discontinue some drugs. Our attempt to rationalize polytherapy by discontinuing some anticonvulsant drugs proved disappointing. It was only possible to reduce polytherapy from three-drug combinations to a two-drug combination in five patients, and to reduce the dose of anticonvulsant drugs in four other patients, three taking carbamazepine and one taking primidone. Although Gastaut (1981) found that better response occurred in patients with partial complex seizures, we could not find any difference between the response of patients with partial complex attacks and simple partial seizures.

The overall effect of clobazam on EEG abnormality was disappointing as improvement in the EEG occurred only in two patients. There was no parallel between EEG changes and clinical improvement in the great majority of cases. Gastaut (1981) has shown that improvement in the electroencephalogram was parallel with clinical improvement in the great majority of patients.

This study therefore confirms previous observations that clobazam improves seizure control in some patients with drug-resistant epilepsy. While improvement was associated with increase in polytherapy in many patients and the introduction of polytherapy in the management of others, the addition of clobazam to treatment was not associated with unsatisfactory side-effects.

References

Barzaghi, F., Fournex, R. and Mantegazza, P. (1973). Pharmacological and toxicological properties of clobazam, a new psychotherapeutic agent. *Arzneimittel Forschung* **23,** 683–686.
Browne, T. R. (1976). Clonazepam. *Arch. Neurol.* **30,** 326–332.
Callaghan, N., O'Callaghan, M., Duggan, B. and Feely, M. (1978). Carbamazepine as a single drug in the treatment of epilepsy. *J. Neurol. Neurosurg. Psychiat.* **41,** 907–912.
Callaghan, N., Kenny, R. A., O'Neill, B., Crowley, M. and Goggin, T. (1983). A comparative study between carbamazepine, phenytoin and sodium valproate as monotherapy in previously untreated and recently diagnosed patients with epilepsy. A Preliminary Communication. *Brit. J. Clin. Practice* (Suppl.) **27,** 7–9.
Critchley, E. M. R., Vakil, S. D., Hayward, H. W., Owen, M. V. A., Cox, A. and Freemantle, N. P. (1981). Double-blind clinical trial of clobazam in refractory epilepsy. In "Clobazam" (I. Hindmarch and P. D. Stonier, eds), pp. 159–164. International Congress and Symposium Series, Number 43. Royal Society of Medicine, London.
Edwards, V. E. and Eadie, M. J. (1973). Clonazepam—a clinical study of its effectiveness as an anticonvulsant. *Proc. Aust. Assoc. Neurol.* **10,** 61–66.
Feely, M., Duggan, B., O'Callaghan, M. and Callaghan, N. (1979). The therapeutic range for phenytoin: A reappraisal. *Irish Jnl of Med. Sci.* **2,** 44–49.
Gastaut, H. (1981). The effects of benzodiazepines on chronic epilepsy in man (with particular reference to clobazam). In "Clobazam" (I. Hindmarch and P. D. Stonier, eds), pp. 141–150. International Congress and Symposium Series, Number 43. Royal Society of Medicine, London.
Korttila, K. and Linnoila, M. (1975). Psychomotor skills related to driving after intermuscular administration of diazepam and meteridine. *Anaesthesiology* **42,** 685–691.
Martin, A. A. (1981). The antiepileptic effects of clobazam—a long study in resistant epilepsy. In "Clobazam" (I. Hindmarch and P. D. Stonier, eds), pp. 151–157. International Congress and Symposium Series, Number 43. Royal Society of Medicine, London.
Reynolds, E. H. Chadwick, D. W. (1976). One drug (phenytoin) in the treatment of epilepsy. *Lancet* **1,** 923–926.

Blood Levels of Clobazam and its Metabolites and Therapeutic Effect

T. GOGGIN and N. CALLAGHAN

Clinical Investigation Unit, Cork Regional Hospital, Wilton, Cork, Ireland

Summary

In a clinical study of clobazam (10–40 mg daily) in 33 poorly controlled epileptic outpatients (Callaghan and Goggin, this volume, pp. 143–147), serum levels of concomitant anticonvulsants were monitored before and during the study for a period of 18 months. Serum levels of clobazam and N-desmethylclobazam were monitored monthly where possible. Increase in concomitant anticonvulsant levels were observed at fixed dose during treatment with clobazam, without accompanying clinical toxicity except in patients taking phenytoin. Correlation of clobazam dose and serum level was linear in individual patients although inter-individual differences were observed. Excellent clinical outcome was associated with low doses of clobazam and this was reflected in serum levels of drug and metabolite. When the drug/metabolite ratio was correlated with control of seizures, it appeared that more rapid metabolism of the parent drug was associated with greater control, suggesting a therapeutic significance for the metabolite, N-desmethylclobazam. The clinical value of serum monitoring of clobazam and N-desmethylclobazam is questioned.

Introduction

Since the original observation of Gastaut (1978) the 1,5-benzodiazepine clobazam has been of considerable interest in the control of seizures in patients with epilepsy. Some studies (Martin, 1981; Gastaut and Lowe, 1979) have been of open design and long duration whilst others (Critchley et al., 1981; Allen et al., 1983) have been double-blind in design. All these studies have involved patients with refractory epilepsy which have proven resistant to a battery of accepted anticonvulsant medication as monotherapy or in combinations. All studies are in agreement that a short-term benefit in 50% or more of patients is achieved. However, long-term studies suggest that tolerance or exhaustion is apparent in up to 35% after treatment in excess of six months.

Studies of the effect of clobazam on the serum levels of other anticonvulsant drugs have been published (Vakil et al., 1981; Cocks et al., this volume, pp. 155–157). Monitoring of clobazam levels and its N-desmethyl metabolite in patients with epilepsy has also been undertaken (Cano et al., 1981), but this type of data is comparatively rare.

As part of a study to evaluate clobazam as an anticonvulsant in 33 poorly controlled patients who had failed to respond to therapeutic levels of other anticonvulsants (Callaghan and Goggin, this volume, pp. 143–147), we assessed the relationship of seizure control or seizure type to the serum levels of clobazam and its N-desmethyl metabolite.

In monitoring the levels of other anticonvulsant drugs, both prior to and during clobazam treatment, it was possible to assess any drug interaction which occurred.

Patients and Methods

The 33 patients involved fell into two main groups: ten patients on monotherapy who had failed on carbamazepine, phenytoin and sodium valproate, and 23 patients on polytherapy who had failed on numerous combinations. All patients were poorly controlled at the beginning of the study.

Serum levels of anticonvulsant drugs were assessed at fixed dose, and the three estimates at monthly intervals just prior to clobazam treatment were used as a baseline.

Patients were given clobazam at a dose of 10 mg initially. This was adjusted upward to a maximum of 40 mg in 10 mg increments as indicated from clinical assessment.

In an attempt to standardize sampling time, patients were instructed to take the final dose of each drug 3–4 h prior to a 1400 h seizure clinic. Fasting serum samples were collected at the clinic for the purposes of analysis.

A method was developed using high performance liquid chromatography in reverse phase mode with ultra violet detection at 232 nm for simultaneous analysis of clobazam and its *N*-desmethyl metabolite.

The levels of other anticonvulsants were evaluated by established techniques using high performance liquid chromatography (Kabra *et al.*, 1977) and gas chromatography (Chard, 1976).

Results

The dose of clobazam used (mg/kg/day) was analysed according to seizure control and seizure type (Table 1). Patients who achieved excellent control (free from seizures) did so at a significantly lower dose of clobazam compared with the good (> 50% seizure reduction) and poor (no change) seizure control groups ($P < 0.005$).

Thirty-six per cent of patients maintained excellent control for the first six months assessment period, whilst only 6% maintained this degree of improvement in the second and third assessment periods from 6–12 and 12–18 months. No patient who deteriorated

regained excellent control following upward dose adjustment.

Analysis of dose used in patients who achieved excellent or good seizure control according to partial or generalized seizure type revealed no significant differences between the groups.

A linear relationship between clobazam dose (mg/kg/day) and serum level (ng/ml) was shown in individual patients (Fig. 1), although large inter-individual differences were demonstrated.

Analysis of serum levels of clobazam and *N*-desmethylclobazam by seizure control and type is shown in Table 2. A similar pattern emerges as with dose analysis. The 36% of patients with excellent control at low dose had levels in the range 20–150 ng/ml clobazam and 300–2100 ng/ml *N*-desmethylclobazam, which were significantly lower than levels in the good and poor seizure control groups, with levels of 100–350 ng/ml clobazam and 1000–3500 ng/ml *N*-desmethylclobazam.

Furthermore, the ratio clobazam/*N*-desmethylclobazam was lower in excellent responders compared with the other two categories of seizure control, suggesting a faster metabolism in the former group (Table 2).

There were no significant differences in levels of drug, metabolite or ratio when analysed according to seizure type (Table 2).

Drug interactions were assessed in each of the three six-month follow-up periods (0–6, 6–12, and 12–18 months) compared with baseline levels. Patients whose dosage of concomitant anticonvulsant medication was

Table 1

Clobazam dosage, seizure type and control

	n	Mean dose (mg/kg/day)	± SD	Range
All patients	33	0·33	0·19	0·11–0·97
Seizure control[a]				
Excellent	12	0·23*	0·09	0·11–0·39
Good	8	0·41	0·20	0·15–0·73
Poor	13	0·51	0·20	0·29–0·97
Seizure type[bc]				
Generalized	14	0·32	0·17	0·11–0·60
Partial	6	0·38	0·21	0·15–0·73

[a] At 6 months. Excellent = seizure free; good = > 50% reduction; poor = no change or < 50% reduction.
[b] At baseline.
[c] Excellent and good control.
* Excellent < good or poor $P < 0.005$.

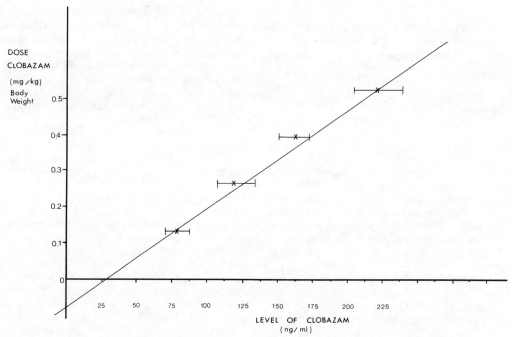

Figure 1. Relationship of dose (mg/kg) and clobazam serum levels (ng/ml) in one patient.

Table 2

Relationship of seizure control and type to serum levels of clobazam and metabolite

Serum Level by Seizure Control	n	Clobazam Mean ± SD (ng/ml)	Range	N-Desmethylclobazam Mean ± SD (ng/ml)	Range	No. of estimates	Ratio Clob/N-Dclob
Excellent	12	77·2± 70·2	(24·8–289·9)	1061·7± 282·5	(309–2137·7)	56	0·07
Good	8	162·6±121·4	(27·2–782·6)	1747·3±1047·7	(131·9–5900)	86	0·09
Poor	13	195·6±108·1	(24·6–523·1)	1890·7± 836·9	(549·4–4131·6)	62	0·11
Serum level by seizure type[a]							
Generalized	14	123·1±108·5	(26·4–782·6)	1450·8± 898·0	(190·9–5900·0)	106	0·08
Partial	6	132·8± 89·3	(24·8–386·3)	1524·5± 907·6	(131·9–4461·0)	42	0·09

Clobazam levels: excellent control < good or poor control; $P < 0.001$.
N-Desmethylclobazam levels: excellent control < good or poor control; $P < 0.005$.
[a] excellent and good control.

altered from baseline were excluded from this analysis. Increases of 25% over baseline serum levels were observed as follows:

(a) 28·6% of patients taking carbamazepine either as monotherapy or polytherapy;
(b) 62·5% of patients taking phenytoin;
(c) 12·5% of patients taking sodium valproate; and
(d) 14·3% of patients taking phenobarbitone.

Clinical toxicity was associated only with increases in phenytoin levels. Four patients had levels > 100 μmol/l of phenytoin during clobazam treatment. Increases in phenytoin levels occurred within weeks of starting clobazam treatment, whereas increases in other drug levels were observed only in the long term.

Discussion

In this clinical study of the adjunctive treatment with clobazam in poorly controlled chronic epileptic patients, detailed analysis has been made of clobazam dosage and serum levels of parent drug and the N-desmethyl metabolite according to responder type and seizure pattern. In addition the effect of clobazam on serum levels of concomitant anticonvulsant levels has been monitored.

It appears that, regarding the dose of clobazam used, two distinct groups of patients emerge: those patients who maintained excellent control for six months (36%) at doses from 0·11–0·39 mg/kg/day, and patients who did not achieve excellent control initially or who deteriorated subsequently and in whom a higher dose range (0·15–0·97 mg/kg/day) was employed.

This second group may be subdivided into those patients in whom no response was achieved at any dose, and patients initially with excellent control at low dose who derived limited benefit from upward dose adjustment once excellent control was lost.

Despite the linearity in individual patients between dose and serum level of drug, this relationship showed considerable inter-individual variation, since the metabolic rate differed. This may be due to different effects of various drug combinations used as suggested by Cano et al. (1981). However, no such evaluation of the effects of combination treatment on clobazam and N-desmethylclobazam levels was possible in the present study, since no clobazam monotherapy control group was included. Nevertheless, consideration of drug/metabolite ratios suggested that more rapid metabolism was associated with greater seizure control. This may have been coincidental in that as the dose of clobazam was raised, the rate of metabolism slowed as it approached saturation. However, it may also suggest a therapeutic significance for the metabolite.

Although interesting patterns developed with regard to the relationship of serum levels and seizure control, tolerance developed in many patients and only 6% maintained excellent control for the 18 month period. Changes in this pattern with time does not allow an optimal range of serum levels to be determined for clobazam in chronic usage. The value to the clinician of routine monitoring of clobazam and N-desmethylclobazam levels is therefore limited. Side-effects, which were rarely severe, were dose-related and serum level was only of secondary importance.

The implications of this study for the clinician are clear. Clobazam will be effective initially when used at low dose and this will give rise to low serum levels of the drug and metabolite. Some patients may remain seizure-free in the longer term if it is possible to maintain them on low doses. This was the case in two patients in this study who maintained excellent control for 18 months at doses of 0·15 and 0·16 mg/kg/day, with corresponding serum levels of clobazam ($35·5 \pm 10·0$ ng/ml, $n = 20$ and $50·7 \pm 30·7$, $n = 14$) and of the metabolite N-desmethylclobazam ($371·5 \pm 121·7$ and $1416·7 \pm 240·3$ ng/ml), respectively.

The sub-group of patients who derived limited value from upward dose adjustment (33% of all patients maintained good control for a period of 18 months) tended to have more rapid metabolism than their counterparts in whom an increased dose was ineffective. However, this point would require further investigation.

The remaining patients (60%) either never responded or had deteriorated to their initial condition after six months treatment. Upward dose adjustment with elevated serum levels in these patients was without effect.

Whilst the effect of drug interactions cannot be ruled out as a contributory factor to control, only one patient had an increase in serum level of other drugs from sub-therapeutic levels. This patient was on combination therapy of phenytoin and carbamazepine and his levels of carbamazepine were in the high optimal range. In other cases, rationalization of treatment, dose reduction, or withdrawal of certain drugs, proved successful.

Note: To convert ng/ml to nmoles/l
    Clobazam × 3·33
    N-desmethylclobazam × 3·50

Therapeutic ranges of other anticonvulsants:

Carbamazepine	15–40 μmoles/l
Phenytoin	40–80 μmoles/l
Phenobarbitone	20–110 μmoles/l
Valproate	300–750 μmoles/l
Primidone	10–50 μmoles/l

Acknowledgements

The authors would like to express their thanks to Hoechst UK Ltd for supporting this study and Miss Heather O'Donovan for secretarial assistance. We would also like to thank Mrs B. Goggin for typing this manuscript.

References

Allen, J. W. and Oxley, J. (1983). Clobazam as adjunctive treatment in refractory epilepsy. *British Medical Journal* **286**, 1246–1247.

Cano, J. P., Bun, H., Iliadis, A., Dravet, C., Roger, J. and Gastaut, H. (1981). Influence of anti-epileptic drugs on plasma levels of clobazam and *N*-desmethylclobazam: Application of research on the relationship between doses, plasma levels and clinical efficiency. In "Clobazam" (I. Hindmarch and P. D. Stonier, eds), pp. 169–174. International Congress and Symposium Series, Number 43. Royal Society of Medicine, London.

Chard, C. R. (1976). A simple method for the determination of epilim in serum. In "Clinical and Pharmacological Aspects of Sodium Valproate (Epilim) in the Treatment of Epilepsy" (N. J. Legge, ed.), p. 89. MCS Consultants, Tunbridge Wells.

Critchley, E. M. R., Vakil, S. D., Hayward, H. W., Owen, M. V. H., Cocks, A. and Freemantle, N. P. (1981). Double blind clinical trial of clobazam in refractory epilepsy. In "Clobazam" (I. Hindmarch and P. D. Stonier, eds), pp. 159–163. International Congress and Symposium Series, Number 43. Royal Society of Medicine, London.

Gastaut, H. (1978). Proprietes anti-epileptiques exceptionalles d'une benzodiazépine nouvelle. *La Vie Medicale* **38**, 5175.

Gaustaut, H. and Low, M. (1979). Anti-epileptic properties of clobazam a 1,5-benzodiazepine in Man. *Epilepsia* **20**, 437.

Kabra, K., Pokar, M., Stafford, B. E. and Matron, L. J. (1977). Simultaneous measurement of phenobarbital, phenytoin, ethosuximide, primadone and carbamezepine in serum by High Performance Liquid Chromatography. *Clin. Chem.* **23**, 1284.

Martin, A. A. (1981). The anti-epileptic effects of clobazam: A long term study in resistant epilepsy. In "Clobazam" (I. Hindmarch and P. D. Stonier, eds), pp. 151–157. International Congress and Symposium Series, Number 43. Royal Society of Medicine, London.

Vakil, S. D., Critchley, E. M., Cocks, A. and Hayward, H. W. (1981). The effects of clobazam on blood levels of phenobarbitone, phenytoin and carbamazepine. In "Clobazam" (I. Hindmarch and P. D. Stonier, eds), pp. 165–167. International Congress and Symposium Series, Number 43. Royal Society of Medicine, London.

The Effect of Clobazam on the Blood Levels of Sodium Valproate

A. COCKS, E. M. R. CRITCHLEY, H. W. HAYWARD and D. THOMAS

Department of Biochemistry, Royal Infirmary, Blackburn, U.K., Department of Neurology, Royal Infirmary, Preston, U.K. and Langho Epilepsy Centre, Blackburn, U.K.

Summary

The combined use of clobazam and sodium valproate in the treatment of chronic, refractory epilepsy was examined in six volunteers, all of whom showed an improvement in fit control on the combination. The patients were at first stabilized on 1500–2000 mg sodium valproate daily. The addition of 20 mg clobazam daily, later 40 mg daily, was accompanied by an increase in valproate levels, and these levels remained elevated in four patients for 3–5 weeks after stopping clobazam. Four patients became ataxic when sodium valproate was combined with 40 mg clobazam daily.

Introduction

The anticonvulsant properties of clobazam, a 1,5-benzodiazepine, were first demonstrated by Barzaghi *et al.* (1973) in mice and by Gastaut (1978) in man. The efficacy of clobazam in refractory epilepsy has been confirmed in double-blind clinical trials by Critchley *et al.* (1981) and Allen *et al.* (1983). In a further study, Vakil *et al.* (1981) showed that the addition of clobazam (20 mg daily) caused no significant increase or decrease in the blood levels of phenobarbitone, phenytoin or carbamazepine. The present study was designed to examine the interaction of clobazam and sodium valproate.

Patients and Methods

Six residents of an epileptic centre consented to participate in a study of the effect of clobazam on blood levels of sodium valproate. The average age of the group was 47 years (37–61 years), three were male and three female. Five were receiving sodium valproate 2000 mg/24 h and one, with the highest blood levels throughout, was receiving 1500 mg/24 h.

Throughout the study, twice-weekly samples were taken for anticonvulsant blood level determinations. After a three-week run-in period, 20 mg clobazam was added to the patients' therapy and continued for four weeks. At the end of this time the dosage was increased to 20 mg twice daily for two weeks. The clobazam dosage was then reduced over a period of three weeks and discontinued. Valproate blood levels were monitored for a further period of five weeks. The staff of the centre kept a day-by-day log of all fits and behavioural changes. The course of the study is summarized in Fig. 1.

In recording the number of fits no distinction was made between mild and severe attacks. However, several patients had severe fits during the period of observation and it was considered ethically necessary to treat severe fits with oral diazepam (10 mg p.r.n.). Each dose was recorded in respect of the

Figure 1. Study plan

Weeks	Run in	20 mg Clobazam	40 mg Clobazam	Withdrawal	Washout
	3	4	2	3	5

timing of blood samples. The subsequent blood levels of valproate were examined independently and no noticeable change was recorded following diazepam administration. As an addendum to the original protocol, we gave 600 mg carbamazepine daily to two patients at the end of the study because fit control was still unsatisfactory. At the same time we reduced the sodium valproate to 1000 mg daily. Further valproate blood levels were taken over a two-week period.

Results

Although no formal statistical tests were thought appropriate, because of the small number of patients, tables are given which summarize the change in plasma level and fit frequency (Tables 1 and 2). Data from the first week of each dose period were excluded allowing the plasma levels and fit frequencies to stabilize before inclusion in the analysis. Data corresponding to a dosage taken for only week one is not represented in this report. The fit frequency is shown in each section standardized over a theoretical period of 28 days.

All patients showed an improvement in fit control with the introduction of clobazam but four patients (three female, one male) became unsteady on the higher dosage, developing a toxic-confusional state. However, less severe changes in behaviour were also noted with 20 mg clobazam daily. Three patients were mildly lethargic and sleepy, two were occasionally confused and incontinent, and one, P.D., became aggressive and unpredictable. Another patient, W.F., became less confused and lethargic whilst on clobazam and T.W., who remained otherwise well throughout, became mildly depressed during the period of clobazam withdrawal.

All six patients showed an increase in valproate levels when taking 20 mg clobazam daily and four showed a further rise when the dosage was increased to 40 mg daily. In only two patients did the valproate levels return approximately to their baseline values or below after clobazam withdrawal.

Discussion

The value of clobazam as an anticonvulsant is clearly demonstrated in the small group of patients studied, four of whom also showed a rebound increase in fits with clobazam with-

Table 1

Table of fit frequencies (standardized) and valproate blood levels (μmol/litre)

Patient	Valproate alone	Valproate + 20 mg clobazam	Valproate + 40 mg clobazam	Clobazam withdrawal	Valproate alone	Valproate + carbamazepine
P.F. 50 yr: F	$\frac{57^*}{478}$	$\frac{28}{666}$ (39%)	$\frac{0}{636}$ 33%)	$\frac{9}{479}$ (0%)	$\frac{4}{509}$ (6%)	
D.R. 57 yr: F	$\frac{27}{516}$	$\frac{17}{705}$ (37%)	$\frac{0}{780}$ (51%)	$\frac{40^*}{982}$ (90%)	$\frac{52^*}{-}$	$\frac{0^{**}}{411}$ (−20%)
P.D. 38 yr: F	$\frac{16}{493}$	$\frac{1}{571}$ (16%)	$\frac{0}{-}$	$\frac{14^*}{769}$ (56%)	$\frac{14^*}{624}$ (27%)	
B.T. 43 yr: M	$\frac{10}{339}$	$\frac{4}{356}$ (5%)	$\frac{0}{454}$ (34%)	$\frac{13}{463}$ (37%)	$\frac{17}{342}$ (1%)	$\frac{3^{**}}{249}$ (−27%)
W.F. 61 yr: M	$\frac{7}{288}$	$\frac{3}{320}$ (11%)	$\frac{0}{410}$ (42%)	$\frac{0}{150}$ (−48%)	$\frac{5}{365}$ 27%)	
T.W. 37 yr: M	$\frac{8}{464}$	$\frac{2}{550}$ (19%)	$\frac{0}{560}$ (21%)	$\frac{4}{571}$ (23%)	$\frac{12}{592}$ (28%)	

*diazepam given p.r.n.
**valproate reduced.

Key: $\dfrac{\text{standardized fit frequency (28 days)}}{\text{mean valproate level (}\mu\text{mol/litre) (\% change from baseline)}}$

Table 2

Mean blood levels of clobazam and desmethyl-clobazam (ng/ml)

Patient	Valproate and 20 mg clobazam daily	Valproate and 40 mg clobazam daily	Valproate and clobazam withdrawal (30/20 mg daily)
P.F.	195	446	157
	321	945	290
D.R.	270	434	127
	281	1391	253
P.D.	261	—	205
	383	—	626
B.T.	286	614	278
	515	1497	853
W.F.	175	619	261
	354	1448	1097
T.W.	225	709	289
	310	1021	521

Key: $\dfrac{\text{Clobazam}}{\text{Desmethylclobazam}}$ ng/ml.

drawal. In contrast to the use of clobazam with phenobarbitone, phenytoin and carbamazepine (Vakil *et al.*, 1981), the combination with sodium valproate proved unsatisfactory. This is related in part to the fact that high doses of valproate were necessary in our patients with long standing epilepsy in order to obtain partial fit control, and in part to a further increase in valproate levels (maximum 39%, average 23%) with the introduction of 20 mg clobazam. Two observations remain unexplained: (a) the combination of valproate with larger doses of clobazam (40 mg) seemed particularly toxic to females; and (b) there appeared to be a cumulative and prolonged effect of clobazam upon valproate metabolism in some patients, possibly resulting from an inhibition of hepatic induction.

Acknowledgements

We wish to thank the residents and staff of Langho Centre, Blackburn, Lancs for their help and cooperation, and Miss E. M. Thomas for a detailed biometric assessment of the data.

References

Allen, J. W., Oxley, J., Robertson, M. M., Trimble, M. R., Richens, A. and Jawad, S. S. M. (1983). Clobazam as adjunctive treatment in refractory epilepsy. *British Medical Journal* **286**, 1246–1247.

Barzaghi, F., Fournex, R. and Mantegazza, P. (1973). Pharmacological and toxicological properties of clobazam. *Arzneimittel-Forschung* **23**, 683.

Critchley, E. M. R., Vakil, S. D., Hayward, H. W., Owen, M. V. H., Cocks, A. and Freemantle, N. P. (1981). Double-blind clinical trial of clobazam in refractory epilepsy. In "Clobazam" (I. Hindmarch and P. D. Stonier, eds), pp. 159–163. International Congress and Symposium Series, Number 43. Royal Society of Medicine, London.

Gastaut, H. (1978). Propriétés anti-épileptiques exceptionalles d'une benzodiazépine nouvelle. *La Vie Médicale* **38**, 5175.

Vakil, S. D., Critchley, E. M. R., Cocks, A. and Hayward, H. W. (1981). The effect of clobazam on blood levels of phenobarbitone, phenytoin and carbamazepine (preliminary report). In "Clobazam" (I. Hindmarch and P. D. Stonier, eds), pp. 165–167. International Congress and Symposium Series, Number 43. Royal Society of Medicine, London.

Plasma Levels and Pharmacokinetics of Clobazam and N-Desmethylclobazam in Epileptic Patients

H. BUN, Ph. COASSOLO, F. GOUEZO, J. P. CANO, C. DRAVET*
and J. ROGER*

*INSERM SC N° 16, Faculté de Pharmacie, Marseille, France, and * Centre Saint-Paul, Bd Sainte Marguerite, Marseille, France*

Summary

The authors have investigated the pharmacokinetic behaviour of clobazam and N-desmethylclobazam in epileptic patients undergoing polytherapy. They emphasized the inter-subject variations, and the influence of the associated epileptic treatment on some pharmacokinetic variables.

The authors have studied the influence of the doses of some antiepileptic drugs, such as phenytoin, carbamazepine, valproic acid, and phenobarbital, on clobazam pharmacokinetics in patients. Significant positive or negative correlations between these variables are reported.

Introduction

Clobazam is a 1,5-benzodiazepine with anxiolytic properties (Brogden *et al.*, 1980) which has been used in the treatment of various forms of epilepsy (Gastaut and Low, 1979). Several studies of the pharmacokinetics of clobazam in healthy volunteers were performed, either after a single dose administration (Vallner *et al.*, 1978, 1980; Greenblatt *et al.*, 1981) or after administration of repeated doses (Rupp *et al.*, 1979; Levy *et al.*, 1983). To date, however, there is little information on the pharmacokinetics of clobazam in epileptic patients. The purpose of this work was, therefore, to follow the evolution of plasma levels of clobazam and its main metabolite, N-desmethylclobazam, and study the pharmacokinetics of these compounds during long-term treatment of epileptics undergoing polytherapy. There were two facets to this work. The first was a study in a large number of patients, of the influence of various antiepileptic comedications on the clobazam and N-desmethylclobazam plasma concentrations (study A). The second was a pharmacokinetic study with modelling of the kinetic behaviour of these compounds and evaluation of the various parameters of the model (study B).

Patients and Methods

Study A

Two hundred and thirty patients were entered into this study. They were aged from one to 58 years and received, during long-term treatment, doses of clobazam ranging from 0·2 to 2 mg/kg/day associated or not with other anti-epileptic drugs (only nine of the 230 patients were undergoing clobazam monotherapy).

Blood samples were taken 3 h after the daily oral intake of clobazam (time close to the t_{max} for clobazam). The doses of the antiepileptic drugs (phenytoin (PH), carbamazepine (CBZ), valproic acid (VA), and phenobarbital (PB)) associated with clobazam were noted.

Study B

The pharmacokinetics of clobazam and N-desmethylclobazam in patients receiving polytherapy were studied after a single dose (S.D.), repeated doses (R.D.), and after discontinuation of the treatment (wash-out, W.O.).

Owing to the difficulties in obtaining a homogeneous group of patients, the criteria for eligibility were the following:

—possibility of therapeutic follow-up (hospitalized or ambulatory patients),

—acceptance of the protocol,
—presence of serious epilepsy with frequent convulsions enabling a good assessment of the effect of the drug, and
—absence of recent clobazam treatment on entering the trial.

A group of 17 patients, aged from six to 32 years, was selected by the above criteria. These cases presented different types of epilepsy, nine of which were partial epilepsy, one a primary generalized epilepsy, and seven secondary generalized epilepsy, five of which presented with the Lennox–Gastaut syndrome.

For single-dose (S.D.) and after discontinuation of repeated administration (W.O.) blood samples were collected before clobazam intake, then 0·5, 1, 2, 3, 6, 12, and 24 h later and, finally, once a day until complete elimination. During multiple dose administration (R.D.), sampling was done twice a day; before and 3 h after the morning intake of clobazam on days 1, 2, and 7, then once a

week for a three-month period. For some patients, the timing of collection was modified in relation to their clinical state. Due to therapeutic requirements, only a limited number of the patients could be included in each of these groups (Table 1).

Analytical method

The plasma concentrations of clobazam and its N-desmethyl metabolite were determined by a gas-liquid chromatographic method previously described (Cano et al., 1979).

Statistical analysis

Study A
Two types of correlation were computed:

(a) by linear regression by the method of least squares with two variables according to the formula $y = a + bx$, taking into account only the plasma level relationship (of clobazam and N-desmethylclobazam) = f (dose of clobazam administered);
(b) by multiple regression of the general equation:
$$y = a + b_1 x_1 + b_2 x_2 + \ldots + b_n x_n.$$

The latter mode of treatment amounts to considering that maximal plasma concentration of clobazam, C (CLO) (or plasma concentration of N-desmethylclobazam 3 h after intake, C (NCO)), depends on the direct sum of the respective contributions of the clobazam doses and each of the other associated anti-epileptic drugs according to the formula:

C(CLO) or C(NCLO) =
    $a + b_1 q_1(\text{CLO}) + b_2 q_2(\text{PH}) + b_3 q_3(\text{CBZ})$
    $+ b_4 q_4(\text{VA}) + b_5 q_5(\text{PB}).$
where $q_1, q_2, \ldots, q_5$ are the administered doses for the various components.

Study B
A three-compartment model was proposed (Bun et al., 1982) (Fig. 1) to describe absorption (K_a), distribution (K_{13}, K_{31}), metabolism (K_{12}), and excretion (K_1, K_2) of orally administered clobazam. This mathematical model is expressed by a set of state differential equations. So it was possible to treat simultaneously the clobazam and N-desmethylclobazam concentration-time curves as responses of the same pharmacokinetic process.

Table 1

Clobazam administration protocols; antiepileptic comedications

Patients	S.D.	R.D.	W.O.	Comedications
ARN	+	+		VA, PRI
CHA	+	+		PB
FOU(1)	+			–
FOU(2)	+			VA
HOU	+			CBZ
MED	+			CBZ, PRI
BAI		+		VA, CBZ, PRI
BOY		+		CBZ, PB
GAN		+	+	CBZ, PB
LEF		+		VA, PB
MAZ		+	+	VA
MAZ		+	+	VA
PAU		+		CBZ, PB
PIO		+		VA, PB
PUE		+		PB
REY		+		PB
SIS		+		CBZ
AMI			+	CBZ, PH
VOG			+	CBZ, PB

SD = single dose; RD = repeated dose; WO = washout after repeated dosage. VA = sodium valproate; PRI = primidone; PB = phenobarbitone; CBZ = carbamazepine; PH = phenytoin.

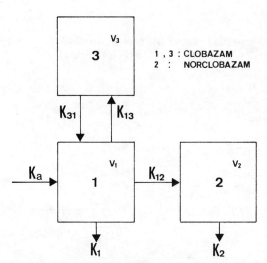

Figure 1. Three compartment model for the CLO(1)-NCLO(2) system including a distribution compartment of CLO(3).

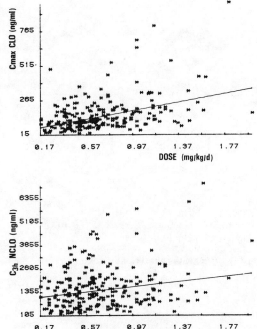

Figure 2. Correlation between plasma concentrations of CLO(A) or NCLO(B) and clobazam doses administered.

Results and Discussion—Study A

Correlation coefficients between clobazam and N-desmethylclobazam plasma levels and administered doses

Simple linear regression
Significant correlations between the dose of clobazam administered and the plasma levels (3 hr after intake) of clobazam ($r = 0.41$, $P < 10^{-9}$) and N-desmethylclobazam ($r = 0.20$, $P < 10^{-2}$) were found (Fig. 2). This analysis did not take into account the associated drugs administered daily.

The data given in the literature on this subject are very divergent. Some authors agree that there is a linear relationship between these two variables (Vallner *et al.*, 1980; Rupp *et al.*, 1979), but these studies were carried out in healthy subjects. Others found non-significant correlations (Tedeschi *et al.*, 1981), but these results were for patients receiving polytherapy.

Multiple regression
The results obtained are summarized in Table 2A for clobazam and Table 2B for N-desmethylclobazam.

For clobazam, the maximal plasma concentration (C_{max}) increased significantly in function of the dose q_1 ($P < 10^{-3}$). The influence of the doses of other anti-convul-sants was variable: VA and PB (doses q_4, q_5) had a significantly negative action on the C_{max} of clobazam, whereas PH and CBZ (q_2, q_3) did not have a significant action on this parameter.

A similar interpretation can be advanced for N-desmethylclobazam. Thus, the plasma concentration of this metabolite 3 h after clobazam intake (C_{3h}) increased in function with doses of CLO (q_1), PH (q_2) and CBZ (q_3), and decreased with VA doses (q_4). In contrast, PB doses (q_5) had no significant action on the N-desmethylclobazam C_{3h}.

Such an interpretation of the multiple regression results suggests the following:

(1) by enhancing N-desmethylclobazam formation, PH and CBZ may play the role of enzyme inducers;
(2) VA, which had negative effects on the clobazam C_{max} and, above all, on the N-desmethylclobazam C_{3h} might enhance biotransformation of N-desmethylclobazam into a probably hydroxylated N-desmethylclobazam derivative;
(3) PB, which had a negative influence on

Table 2

Multiple regression with plasma concentrations of clobazam (A) or N-desmethyl-clobazam (B) versus doses of clobazam and various other anti-convulsant drugs

A.

	Regression coefficients	Standard deviation		Partial correlation coefficients*	
b_1	3·30	0·68	q_1 (CLO)	0·22	$P < 10^{-3}$
b_2	−0·20	0·07	q_2 (PH)	−0·12	$P < 10^{-1}$
b_3	−0·06	0·02	q_3 (CBZ)	−0·06	N.S.
b_4	−0·06	0·01	q_4 (VA)	−0·19	$P < 10^{-2}$
b_5	−0·37	0·11	q_5 (PB)	−0·22	$P < 10^{-3}$

a = 143·8 ± 21·0 ng/ml
Multiple correlation coefficient ± 0·45, $P < 10^{-9}$
F test 10·95, $P < 5 \cdot 10^{-4}$

* of C_{max} CLO with comedications doses $q_1, \ldots q_5$.

B.

	Regression coefficients	Standard deviation		Partial correlation coefficients*	
b_1	22·53	5·81	q_1 (CLO)	0·26	$P < 10^{-4}$
b_2	2·72	0·58	q_2 (PH)	0·25	$P < 10^{-4}$
b_3	0·65	0·16	q_3 (CBZ)	0·30	$P < 10^{-5}$
b_4	−0·50	0·11	q_4 (VA)	−0·39	$P < 10^{-9}$
b_5	−1·70	0·96	q_5 (PB)	−0·01	N.S.

a = 820·8 ± 177·0
Multiple correlation coefficient ± 0·5649, $P < 10^{-9}$
F test 20·06, $P < 5 \cdot 10^{-4}$

* of C_{3h} NCLO with comedications doses $q_1, \ldots q_5$.

the clobazam C_{max} but seemed to have no action on the C_{3h} of the desmethylated metabolite, might enhance direct clobazam biotransformation, probably hydroxylation, which is consistent with its role as an enzyme inducer of oxidative processes.

Results and Discussion—Study B

Test dose administration: plasma levels of CLO and NCLO

Figure 3 shows the evolution in time of plasma concentrations of clobazam and *N*-desmethylclobazam in a patient who had received a single, oral dose of 25 mg of cloba-

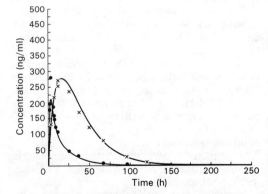

Figure 3. *Administration of a test dose of clobazam; experimental values for CLO (●——●) and NCLO (x——x) and simulated curves.*

zam, with chronic administration of 50 mg/day of PB. The good agreement observed between the experimental values and the simulated curves shows that the model devised for clobazam and N-desmethylclobazam is valid.

Pharmacokinetic variables

The variables estimated from S.D. and W.O. kinetics in various patients are listed in Table 3. Despite considerable intersubject variations, comparison of the means of the variables for S.D. and W.O. could be made. Some variables, particularly V_1, seemed to remain stationary, whereas others, such as K_2 in particular, dropped from S.D. to W.O.

The variables calculated for the kinetics in S.D. and W.O. are listed in Table 4. These various parameters seemed to remain stationary from S.D. to W.O. (except the half-life of elimination of N-desmethylclobazam). The significance of these comparisons is again impaired by the great variance of the experimental values which can be partly ascribed to the heterogeneity of the sample with regard to age, type of epilepsy and comedication. Also, the data from which the S.D. and W.O. variables were determined were not collected in the same subjects, so that examination of the evolution of these variables between S.D.

and W.O. does not demonstrate whether or not the kinetic behaviour of clobazam is stationary.

Comparison of the various pharmacokinetic parameters obtained in the same patient (FOU ...) after administration of a single oral dose of 35 mg of clobazam, given as monotherapy or associated with chronic administration of 1200 mg/day of VA, allows assessment of the effect of this comedication on the kinetic behaviour of clobazam. Thus most of the parameters clearly differed (Tables 3 and 4) according to the protocol employed. In particular, it can be noticed that chronic administration of V.A. resulted in marked reduction in the half-lives of clobazam and N-desmethylclobazam elimination as well as a very great increase in clobazam clearance. This is manifested by plasma levels of clobazam which are much lower in polytherapy; whereas the level of the desmethylated derivative did not seem to be affected by this comedication since the formation of this metabolite is slow.

It is interesting to compare the pharmacokinetic parameters obtained in the epileptic patients undergoing polytherapy after administration of a single dose of clobazam with those found in the literature for healthy volunteers (Vallner *et al.*, 1980; Greenblatt *et al.*, 1981; Tedeschi *et al.*, 1981; Rupp *et al.*, 1979; Levy *et al.*, 1983) on monotherapy. In

Table 3

Estimated pharmacokinetic parameters of clobazam and N-*desmethylclobazam*

	Patients	V_1 (1)	K_1+K_{12} (h^{-1})	K_2 (h^{-1})	$K_{12}{}^{V_1}/{}_{V_2}$ (h^{-1})	C_{10} (µg/ml)	C_{20} (µg/ml)	K_a (h^{-1})
	ARN	169·5	0·21	0·06	0·50	—	—	0·79
	CHA	52·1	0·13	0·05	0·20	—	—	0·41
T.D.	MED	145·1	0·05	0·01	0·13	—	—	2·04
	HOU	151·2	0·06	0·04	0·53	—	—	1·01
	FOU(1)	79·6	0·02	0·05	0·07	—	—	1·59
	FOU(2)	168·3	0·12	0·33	0·33	—	—	1·11
	Mean	127·6	0·10	0·09	0·29			1·16
	(±s.d.)	(45·2)	(0·06)	(0·11)	(0·18)			(0·53)
	AMI	128·4	0·04	0·01	—	0·00	1·84	3·34
	VOG	217·1	0·06	0·01	—	0·03	0·51	12·39
W.O.	GAN	378·6	0·04	0·05	0·58	0·04	0·92	3·77
	MAZ	31·9	0·04	0·02	0·06	—	0·92	1·83
	MAZ	201·4	0·04	0·02	0·01	0·15	0·84	18·85
	Mean	191·5	0·04	0·02	0·21	0·06	1·00	8·04
	(±s.d.)	(114·2)	(0·01)	(0·02)	(0·26)	(0·06)	(0·44)	(6·55)

Table 4

Calculated pharmacokinetic parameters of clobazam and N-desmethylclobazam

	Patients	Cl CLO (l/h)	Cl_1/Cl_2 NCLO	$T\frac{1}{2}$ CLO (h)	$T\frac{1}{2}$ NCLO (h)
T.D.	ARN	34·9	8·4	3·4	11·6
	CHA	7·0	4·0	13·9	13·9
	MED	7·5	10·1	13·4	53·3
	HOU	9·3	13·9	11·3	18·1
	FOU(1)	1·7	1·2	31·7	13·1
	FOU(2)	21·0	1·0	5·6	2·1
	Mean	13·6	6·4	13·2	18·7
	(±s.d.)	(11·2)	(4·7)	(9·1)	(16·2)
W.O.	AMI	5·3	—	16·6	91·4
	VOG	1·9	—	11·6	93·5
	GAN	14·2	11·7	18·4	14·0
	MAZ	1·2	2·8	18·4	33·2
	MAZ	7·5	0·5	18·7	42·1
	Mean	8·2	5·0	16·7	54·8
	(±s.d.)	(4·8)	(4·8)	(2·7)	(32·0)

healthy subjects, the half-lives of the apparent elimination phase vary, depending on the authors, between 18 and 25 h and between 36 and 46 h, respectively, for clobazam and N-desmethylclobazam, while the total plasma clearance for clobazam is close to 2·5 l/h. It can therefore be noted that, in epileptic subjects, there is a very marked increase in clobazam clearance. There is also a reduction in the β-half-lives of clobazam and its metabolite, and as a corollary, the plasma levels of clobazam are lower and there is faster elimination of both components.

Observation of the kinetics obtained during repeated administration of clobazam allows two groups of patients to be distinguished: one group with stable clobazam and N-desmethylclobazam plasma levels and another in which these levels fluctuate greatly, although, in some cases, the doses had to be increased during treatment for therapeutic reasons.

The mathematical model, previously shown to be valid for single dose administration, was used to simulate the evolution in time of theoretical clobazam and N-desmethylclobazam concentrations during chronic administration. Such a simulation was based on parameters determined during either the S.D. or the W.O. The pharmacokinetic behaviour of these two components was confirmed to be stationary in some subjects throughout the whole duration of treatment. This observation is supported by the good relationship which existed between the experimental data for these subjects and the curve simulated from the W.O. parameters (Fig. 4). Conversely, in other patients, the kinetic behaviour of clobazam varied and only seemed to be correct at the beginning of chronic administration, whilst N-desmethylclobazam was clearly variable.

In conclusion, the main characteristics of the pharmacokinetic behaviour of clobazam and its metabolite can be stressed. It can be emphasized that the pharmacokinetic variables of these two components present considerable intersubject variations. Furthermore, the value of some variables is influenced by the nature of the comedication, the pathological state and, in some subjects, by the time of determination during chronic treatment.

Acknowledgements

This study was performed in collaboration with Diamant Laboratories (92800 PUTEAUX, France). The authors are very grateful to Dr A. Iliadis for mathematical treatments and helpful discussions, and to M. Giocanti for her technical assistance.

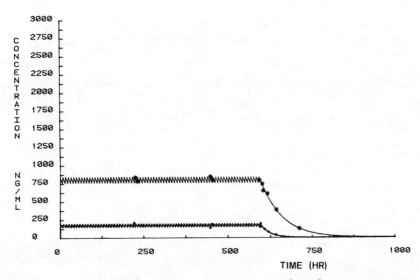

Figure 4. Experimental values of CLO (•——•) and NCLO (*——*) and simulation (——) of repeated doses before the wash-out experiment, from which kinetic parameters were computed.

References

Bun, H., Iliadis, A., Bruno, R., Cano, J. P., Dravet, C. and Roger, J. (1982). Contribution of simulation in the study of the time-dependence and clinical response of clobazam. Workshop on the metabolism of antiepileptic drugs. (In press.)

Brogden, R. N., Heel, R. C., Speight, T. M. and Avery, G. S. (1980). Clobazam: a review of its pharmacological properties and therapeutic use in anxiety. *Drugs* **20,** 161–178.

Cano, J. P., Lindoulsi, T., Sumirtapura, Y., Bun, H., Gouezo, F. and Viala, A. (1979). Considérations générales sur la méthodologie et les cinétiques de deux benzodiazépines: le clonazépam (Rivotril^R) et le clobazam (Urbanyl^R). *Lyon Médicale* **242,** 535–544.

Gastaut, H. and Low, M. D. (1979). Anti-epileptic properties of Clobazam, a 1,5-benzodiazepine in man. *Epilepsia* **20,** 437.

Greenblatt, D. J., Divoll, M., Puri, S. K., Ho, I., Zinny, M. A. and Shader, R. (1981). Clobazam kinetics in the elderly. *Br. J. Clin. Pharmac.* **12,** 631–636.

Levy, R. H., Lane, E. A., Guyot, M., Brachet-Liermain, A., Centraud, B. and Loiseau, P. (1983). Analysis of parent drug-metabolite relationship in the presence of an inducer. *Drugs metab. Dispos.* **11,** 286–292.

Rupp, W., Badian, M., Christ, O., Hajdu, P., Kulkarni, R. D., Taeuber, K., Uihlein, M., Bender, R. and Vanderbeke, O. (1979). Pharmacokinetics of single and multiple doses of clobazam in humans. *Br. J. Clin. Pharmac.* **7,** 51S—57S.

Tedeschi, G., Riva, R. and Baruzzi, A. (1981). Clobazam plasma concentrations: pharmacokinetic study in healthy volunteers and data in epileptic patients. *Br. J. Clin. Pharmac.* **11,** 619–622.

Vallner, J. J., Needham, T. E., Jun, H. W., Brown, W. J., Stewart, J. T., Kotzan, J. A. and Honigberg, I. L. (1978). Plasma levels of clobazam after three oral dosage forms in healthy volunteers. *J. Clin. Pharmac.* **18,** 319–324.

Vallner, J. J., Kotzan, J. A., Stewart, J. T., Honigberg, J. L., Needham, T. E. and Brown, W. J. (1980). Plasma levels of clobazam after 10, 20 and 40 mg tablet doses in healthy subjects. *J. Clin. Pharmac.* **20,** 444–451.

Clobazam in Drug-resistant Patients with Complex Focal Seizures—Report of an Open Study

P. WOLF

Freie Universität Berlin, Berlin, West Germany

Summary

An open follow-up study of 34 patients taking clobazam for 30 months or longer is reported. Ten per cent of patients had a sustained satisfying response to the drug, although a higher percentage (41%) had a shorter good result showing a 75% or better reduction of seizures. There was no clear relationship of serum levels of clobazam or desmethylclobazam to the therapeutic response. If either the clobazam level exceeds $0.6 \mu g/ml$ or the desmethylclobazam level $8 \mu g/ml$, it is likely that the patient will develop signs of toxicity.

Introduction

Clobazam as a drug for epileptic patients has held our interest since the first announcement by Gastaut (1978) that this was an excellent antiepileptic drug. We first conducted an open study, and then a double-blind placebo controlled study, which is about to be terminated and cannot yet be reported. The first report on our open study, which included 26 patients, was given before the German branch of the International League against Epilepsy (Wolf et al., 1981), and a second, the cohort having been expanded to 34 subjects, at the Epilepsy International Symposium 1981, Kyoto (unpublished). In this paper we wish to report the outcome for these 34 patients who, if they are still on clobazam, have been taking it for at least 30 months.

Material and Methods

All patients had uncontrolled seizures at the onset of clobazam treatment. In 29 patients the drug had been administered for the control of seizures, but in the other five as a tranquilizer, for various reasons.

The great majority of the patients had complex focal seizures (Table 1). Generalized tonic-clonic seizures, where they had been present, were already controlled in all but three cases. All patients had proved resistant to routine antiepileptic drugs in maximal, serum level controlled monotherapy or combination treatment. In three patients, the drug history included ineffective treatment with clonazepam.

Table 1

Seizure types of the 34 patients

Seizure type	N
Complex focal (with grand mal = 15)	27
Absences & grand mal	3
Absences & complex focal & grand mal	2
Grand mal only	1
Other	1

Clobazam was added to the previous medication which was not changed. The initial daily dose was 10–20 mg. If there was no clear effect or initial seizure control was followed by a relapse, the dose was augmented unless there were side-effects that prevented it. The highest dose was 130 mg or 2.0 mg/kg. In the five cases where the drug had been prescribed as a tranquillizer, however, the dose was not raised when no anti-epileptic action was observed.

Result

The patients were followed for various periods, the longest follow-up at this moment being 63 months. Initially, seven of these patients responded to clobazam by complete seizure control, and a further seven by more than 75% reduction of seizure frequency. However, relapse occurred in spite of constant medication in all but two patients. The relapses occurred after a seizure-free period that varied between ten days and five months.

At present, seven patients are still on clobazam medication (Table 2). In four of them, the reason for this is its continuing antiepileptic effect; in another two, it is the psychopharmacological action. The last patient, the one who receives the highest dose, has as many seizures as ever but wishes to remain on the drug because he finds the seizures shorter and less distressing than before.

Of the four patients whose seizures still respond to clobazam, one case is not striking because the seizure frequency is just about 50% of the pretreatment frequency. The three others, however, are really satisfying. Their histories are as follows:

(1) K.H., a female now 23 years old had been suffering, since age ten, from focal complex seizures that included a very distressing automatism of vomiting. That the seizures were indeed epileptic was proved by video evaluations showing very typical oral automatism preceding the vomiting. The seizures recurred almost daily, often several times a day, at unpredictable times, and were, in the eyes of most people, a socially unacceptable behaviour. On account of this, and because her intellectual performance was slightly below average, nobody would have her as an apprentice.

Treatment with phenytoin, sodium valproate and primidone had not led to any noticeable improvement, and her medical and social situation was rather poor, when at age 19, clobazam was added to a previous dose of 350 mg phenytoin (serum levels approx. 30 μg/ml).

She had her last vomiting seizure in January 1980, at a clobazam dose of 20 mg, which was then augmented to 40 mg. She went on having isolated auras two to five times a month. Very rarely, less often than once a month, an aura is followed by a short lapse of consciousness without vomiting. Three years ago, she entered professional training which is successfully ongoing.

(2) C.H., a male now 29 years old had his first complex focal seizures at the age of seven, and thereafter virtually every day.

The seizures resisted the repeated and intense therapeutic efforts of experienced epileptologists. There was one seven-week period of seizure control with 400 mg phenytoin, at age 14, but intoxication followed, and dose reduction resulted in relapse. Also, later, the patient was drug-resistant according to the most rigid standards. Clonazepam and nitrazepam were among the drugs that had been without effect.

Again, the most annoying consequence of the seizures was failure to acquire an adequate social position although, in this case, this seemed more due to direct interference of the disease with the young man's scholastic performance.

At age 25, when also mephenytoin therapy (600 mg) had proved inefficient, 10 mg of clobazam were added, and his seizure frequency reduced to 1–6 per month, and when the dose was raised to 20 mg, he became seizure-free.

Twelve months later, slow and stepwise decreases of the mephenytoin dose was begun, but at 200 mg/day, he had a few isolated

Table 2

State of therapy at present in seven patients who still receive clobazam. For details see text

Patients	Sex	Dose		100%	auras only	Seizure control		None	Escape?
		Highest	Present			90%	50%		
R.S.	F	80 mg	20 mg				+		+
K.H.	F	40 mg	20 mg			+			+
C.H.	M	20 mg	20 mg		+				?
U.G.	F	20 mg	10 mg	+					−
H.W.	F	20 mg	20 mg					+	+
K.A.	M	130 mg	120 mg					+	−
L.N.	M	100 mg	20 mg					+	+

auras, and since then he is continuously on 300 mg mephenytoin and 20 mg clobazam.

It was not easy for him to adjust to the life of a healthy person, but luckily his parents were cooperative, and he did succeed. He is an office clerk now, has made friends, and lives by himself. I am afraid he is not always compliant which has, at intervals of months, led to some isolated auras, and a year ago, he had a rather humid night together with some friends which precipitated the one and only complex focal seizure with the present therapy. Thus, he is not 100% seizure-free.

(3) U.G., a woman now aged 62, saw us at age 56 because of four generalized tonic-clonic seizures she had had during the previous 12 months. It turned out that she had been having dreamy states for about 20 years which she had regarded as a curiosity rather than a disease. They would recur in clusters at intervals that could last some months.

Her story is rapidly told. It was easy to control the grand mal seizures, but the dreamy states were resistant to both phenytoin and carbamazepine at maximal doses. Phenobarbital could not be raised above a serum level of 25 µg/ml because she complained of intolerable sedation and would not accept an increase. The same happened with primidone. She has now been completely seizure-free for three years with a treatment of 500 mg primidone plus 20 mg clobazam.

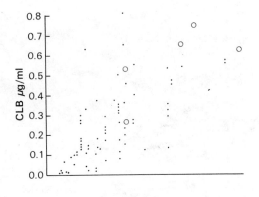

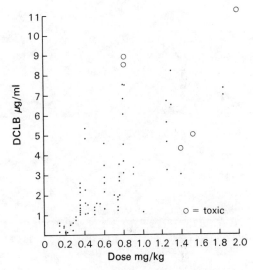

Figure 1. Clobazam doses and serum levels of clobazam (CLB) and desmethylclobazam (DCLB).

Drug Regimens and Serum Levels

During the first years of the study, drug levels of both clobazam (CLB) and desmethylclobazam (DCLB) were repeatedly determined. There was a reasonable but not a very close relation between dose and serum levels of both substances (Fig. 1).

In five patients, five or more drug levels at constant medication were measured (Fig. 2). The data showed rather unstable values both for CLB and DCLB which was unexpected, especially for the metabolite with its long serum half-life. There was, however, no indication that such fluctuations influenced the therapeutic efficiency. Further, relapses at constant medication could not be explained by decreasing drug levels (Wolf *et al.*, 1981).

It has been reported (Gastaut and Low, 1979) that in patients with initial response and later relapse, augmentation of dosage would result in renewed seizure control. With our patients, the same happened but would invariably be followed by repeated relapse. Thus, long-term seizure control was never obtained in any patient who once had a relapse with constant medication.

An important question concerning any drug is its therapeutic range. The typical toxic signs (sedation and irritability) were encountered at various different levels of the drug and its metabolite, and they do not seem to make sense if each substance is looked at separately (Fig. 1). However, if the levels of both compounds are considered together, it transpires that if either the CLB level passes 0·6 or that of DCLB 8 µg/ml, it is very likely that the patient will have clinical signs of toxicity. Thus, if a suspicion of toxicity arises,

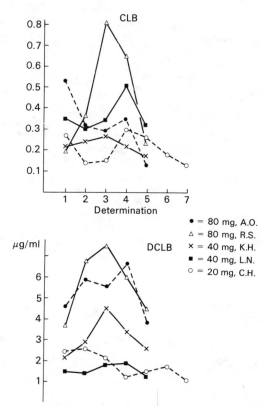

Figure 2. Fluctuation of serum levels of clobazam (CLB) and desmethylclobazam (DCLB) in
five patients with five or more determinations at
constant drug dose.

• = 80 mg, A.O.
△ = 80 mg, R.S.
× = 40 mg, K.H.
■ = 40 mg, L.N.
○ = 20 mg, C.H.

Table 3

Problems with clobazam
therapy

"Escape" phenomenon	Ten patients
Toxicity (sedation, irritability) likely if CLB > 0·6 or DCLB > 8 μg/ml	
Untoward effects	
Possible grand mal precipitation	Two patients
Psychosis with seizure control	One patient
Withdrawal problems	
Seizure precipitation	Nine patients
Possible withdrawal psychosis	One patient
Drug interaction	
CBZ levels raised	One patient

dual adverse reaction was a psychosis developing with seizure control in a patient that
presumably previously had an instance of
forced normalization when she was treated
with primidone. There were, further, two
possible cases of grand mal precipitation.

In all our patients, clobazam was, and is
still, administered together with other
anti-epileptic drugs; interactions with these
seemed to be extremely uncommon. In one of
our patients there was an interaction with
carbamazepine, the levels of which were considerably increased (Wolf et al., 1981).

As with all benzodiazepines, the drug was
difficult to withdraw. Seizure precipitation
was a common problem even if at the time of
withdrawal no anti-epileptic effect could be
demonstrated. There was one case of possible
withdrawal psychosis.

determination of both substances is required
for verification.

In this study, we could not find any relation of the levels of either CLB or DCLB to
the therapeutic efficiency. The three patients
who responded best required only small
doses and had drug levels in the lowest
range. As this seems to indicate that the
antiepileptic action of CLB depends on the
individual response rather than dosage, and
as we were unable to demonstrate that any
of our patients had in the long-run any
benefit from a daily dose exceeding 20 mg,
we reduced the dose for all but one of the
patients who took more than this (Table 2).
This was indeed possible without clinical
deterioration.

Problems with Clobazam (Table 3)

Apart from dose-related effects, one indivi-

Conclusions

In this study, the initial antiepileptic action of
clobazam was remarkable in a cohort that
consisted mostly of drug-resistant patients
with complex focal seizures. The big disad-
vantage of the drug is the frequent relapses
that occur with constant medication. The
consequence of these is that only 10% of our
patients had a decisive long-term benefit from
the drug.

This is a small proportion, and for a
patient in whom a seizure-free period of
some weeks and months had raised hopes, it
is a most upsetting experience to see the
seizures reappear. We therefore feel that clobazam should only be tried in patients who

are resistant to all conventional medications and are so handicapped by the seizures that it is justified to take the chance of relapse occurring.

These risks can be diminished if it is kept in mind that the drug helps at small doses if it helps at all, and there is no reason for dosages in the subtoxic range. The problem of withdrawal seizures after an unsuccessful trial, however, remains, and at this moment we have no indication that this can be avoided by small dose regimens. We hope to get further information on this from the controlled study.

References

Gastaut, H. (1978). Essai préliminaire d'une benzodiazépine en épileptologie. *Nouv. presse méd.* **7**, 2400.

Gastaut, H. and Low, M. D. (1979). Antiepileptic properties of clobazam, a 1,5-benzodiazepine, in man. *Epilepsia* **20**, 437–446.

Wolf, P., Beck-Mannagetta, G., Meencke, J., Röder, U. U., Rohland, C. and Schmidt, D. (1981). Erfahrungen mit der Anwendung von Clobazam (Frisium) als Antiepileptikum. In "Epilepsie 1980. Psychosoziale Aspekte, posttraumatische Epilepsien, medikamentöse Behandlung, diagnostische Methoden" (H. Remschmidt, R. Rentz and J. Jungmann, eds), pp. 164–171. Thieme, Stuttgart and New York.

Low-dose Clobazam as Adjunctive Treatment in Chronic Epilepsy

A. WILSON, C. I. DELLAPORTAS and F. CLIFFORD ROSE

Department of Neurology, Charing Cross Hospital, London, W6 8RF, U.K.

Summary

This study is a double-blind comparison of two doses of clobazam and placebo when added to the anticonvulsant regimen of epileptic patients treated on an outpatient basis. The study included 31 patients who received at least two antiepileptic drugs together for a mean period of 15 years and who, despite optimum levels of antiepileptic medication, still required better control of their seizures. The patients were followed up six months prior to entering the trial and then were randomized into three groups (10 mg clobazam, 20 mg clobazam, and placebo) and followed up for a further six months. Comparing the seizure frequencies recorded during the two six-month periods, the two clobazam-treated groups showed a statistically significant improvement whilst the placebo group did not. There was no evidence to suggest that the addition of clobazam significantly affects the serum levels of standard anticonvulsants taken concurrently.

Introduction

The management of chronic epilepsy is still a considerable clinical challenge. Prescription of a single drug, titrating dose against serum levels, is the treatment of choice, but its value in chronic patients has not yet been fully evaluated. Benzodiazepines have an established role in the treatment of epileptic seizures, especially in the management of status epilepticus either intravenously or per-rectum. Several 1,4-benzodiazepines have been evaluated as oral therapy in long-term management of intractable seizures and have been proved to possess remarkable anticonvulsant properties (Browne and Penry, 1975; Killam and Suria, 1980).

More recently 1,5-benzodiazepines have been introduced, and it is claimed they possess less side-effects but retain therapeutic anticonvulsant potential (Chapman et al., 1979). Clobazam is one of these, where the nitrogen atoms are in the 1 and 5 positions and a ketogroup occupies the 4th position while the rest of the molecule is homologous with diazepam.

Although clobazam was initially introduced as an anxiolytic drug, Gastaut (1978) found a favourable and rapid therapeutic response in 80% of patients in all forms of epilepsy. Equally enthusiastic was Escobado et al. (1978) and Loiseau (1979) who found it most valuable in the control of complex partial seizures. Critchley et al. (1981) showed that in a double-blind controlled cross-over trial, 18 out of 27 inpatients had definite improvement in fit control whilst on 20 mg clobazam compared with placebo, and similar results were reported by Allen et al. (1983).

This paper reports on a double-blind trial of clobazam versus placebo as adjunctive therapy in outpatients with chronic, poorly controlled epilepsy.

Patients and Methods

Thirty-one patients with a mean age of 30 (range 17–56), attending the epilepsy outpatient clinic at Charing Cross Hospital, with uncontrolled seizures at a frequency of four or more per month took part in this trial. Patients with "unstable" forms of epilepsy, such as expanding space occupying lesions, cortical atrophy, and cerebral infarction were excluded from the study, as were those suffering from alcoholism or drug dependency, those taking benzodiazepines or other psychotropic drugs, and those with liver disease. Pregnant women were also excluded.

These patients were on two anticonvulsant drugs whose serum levels were within the optimum therapeutic range. No changes of these were made. They were followed-up in the clinic for a period of six months, being seen approximately every six weeks. At each attendance, serum levels were obtained and a careful record of their seizures kept. Following the six-month observation period the patients were randomized to treatment with clobazam or placebo. One-third received 10 mg clobazam, another third received 20 mg clobazam and the remainder placebo. In all three groups, clobazam or placebo was given in an identically matched capsule as a single dose at night. Compliance for clobazam was assessed by the tablet counting technique.

Two patients had to be withdrawn: one was lost to follow-up and the other developed liver failure for which he had to be admitted to hospital and his treatment discontinued. Of the remaining 29 patients (Table 1), nine took 10 mg clobazam, 11 took 20 mg clobazam, and nine took placebo. Seventeen were male and 12 female and the mean age of all three groups was approximately 30 years. The length of history of epilepsy was approximately 16 years; eight patients had generalized seizures, whilst the remaining 21 had partial seizures with or without secondary generalization. The EEG showed a non-specific abnormality in four patients, generalized paroxysmal abnormality in 20, and a focal paroxysmal abnormality in five patients.

The anticonvulsant affect of the study treatment was investigated by analysis of seizure frequency during the six months prior to entry and the seizure frequency during the six months of the study. Changes in frequencies within a patient were analysed within treatment groups and between treatment groups.

Poor, Good and Excellent control principles were also considered, these being defined as:

Poor control   —reduction in seizure frequency <25% of baseline frequency.
Good control   —reduction in seizure frequency ⩾25% and <50% of baseline frequency.
Excellent control—reduction of seizure frequency ⩾50% of baseline frequency.

Results

The total seizures recorded during the six months prior to the study and those recorded

Table 1

Patients, length of history, type of seizure, and EEG abnormalities

	Placebo	10 mg Clobazam	20 mg Clobazam	Total
Number of patients	9	9	11	29
Age (years)				
Mean	31	31	30	30
S.D.	13	13	12	
Range	(17–54)	(19–51)	(17–56)	(17–56)
Sex				
Male	5	5	7	17
Female	4	4	4	12
Length of history (years)	16·5	17·9	16	16·8
Type of seizure				
Generalized	4	2	2	8
Partial, with or without secondary generalization	5	7	9	21
EEG:				
Normal or non-specific abnormality	1	1	2	4
Generalized paroxysmal abnormality	7	7	6	20
Focal paroxysmal abnormality	1	1	3	5

during the six months of the study are given for each patient in Table 2.

In considering the three treatment groups independently, all show a tendency for improvement in fit control during the study period, but only the two clobazam treatment groups show a statistically significant treatment effect ($P \leqslant 0.02$ for the 10 mg clobazam group and $P \leqslant 0.01$ for the 20 mg clobazam group; Wilcoxon Matched Pairs Signed-Ranks test).

In comparing the change in frequencies made within each of the three treatment groups no statistically significant difference is found (Kruskal-Wallis One-Way Analysis of Variance test).

Table 3 summarizes the levels of control observed. Again it can be seen that the cloba-

Table 2

Seizure Frequencies
(each line corresponds to one patient)

	Seizure type*	Prior to study (6 months)	During study (6 months)	Difference	Reduction (%)
Placebo	G	7	5	2	29
	P	180	150	30	17
	G	4	3	1	25
	P	30	34	−4	−13
	P	15	9	6	40
	P	17	15	2	12
	P	12	10	2	17
	P	14	15	−1	−7
	P	16	10	6	38
Median		15	10	2	17
Range		4–180	3–150	−4–30	−13–40
10 mg Clobazam	P	66	64	2	3
	G	3	0	3	100
	G	4	1	3	75
	P	43	28	15	35
	P	32	24	8	25
	P	41	29	12	29
	P	68	24	44	65
	G	2	2	0	0
Median		36·5	24	5·5	32
Range		2–68	0–64	0–44	0–100
20 mg Clobazam	P+G	182+4	173+5	8	4
	P	15	2	13	87
	P	56	30	26	46
	P	11	2	9	82
	P	25	20	5	20
	P+G	24+4	11+6	11	39
	P	650	50	600	92
	P	22	16	6	27
	P	40	46	−6	−15
	P+G	42+5	30+3	14	30
	G	13	11	2	15
Median		28	20	9	30
Range		11–650	2–178	−6–600	−15–92

*G = generalized seizures and P = partial seizures.

Table 3

Summary of seizure control. Three treatment groups

	Placebo	Clobazam 10 mg	Clobazam 20 mg
Number of patients with poor control (%)	5 (56)	2 (24)	4 (36)
Number of patients with good control (%)	4 (44)	3 (38)	4 (36)
Number of patients with excellent control (%)	nil	3 (38)	3 (28)
Total	9	8	11

Table 4

Mean standard anticonvulsant levels (mmol/l) (each line corresponds to one patient)

	Phenytoin		Phenobarbitone		Carbamazepine		Sodium valproate		Primidone	
	Prior to study	During study	Prior to study	During study	Prior to study	During study	Prior to study	During study	Prior to study	During study
Placebo	—	—	33·0	24·0	8·3	9·1	—	—	6·7	6·3
	23·0	6·0	—	—	5·4	12·3	25	12	—	—
	—	—	—	—	5·6	3·2	90	115	—	—
	—	—	—	—	3·7	1·5	75	97	—	—
	9·2	5·5	9·0	17·0	—	—	—	—	—	—
	—	—	—	—	4·5	6·1	70	35	—	—
	—	—	—	—	8·0	3·5	58	38	—	—
	17·0	16·5	—	—	—	—	90	42	—	—
	8·0	9·0	—	—	—	—	80	53	—	—
Clobazam 10 mg	—	—	23·5	35·5	—	—	80	62	3·5	7·2
	22·4	25·0	22·0	14·8	—	—	—	—	5·5	6·2
	—	—	40·5	42·0	6·8	4·5	—	—	—	—
	15·8	11·0	28·4	25·0	—	—	57	78	—	—
	—	—	35·0	42·0	—	—	75	93	—	—
	23·0	13·3	47·0	18·8	5·0	6·2	—	—	—	—
	14·5	17·0	—	—	6·8	3·2	—	—	—	—
	17·0	13·2	—	—	—	—	76	72	—	—
Clobazam 20 mg	13·0	14·8	—	—	11·0	12·5	—	—	—	—
	6·2	6·0	—	—	—	—	49·5	57	—	—
	—	—	—	—	9·5	11·0	—	—	—	—
	—	—	46·0	23·0	—	—	79	92	—	—
	11·5	13·0	—	—	—	—	90	83	—	—
	16·0	6·2	27·0	15·0	—	—	23	20	—	—
	—	—	37.0	18.0	10.0	10.5	—	—	12.0	5.6
	26·0	21·0	—	—	—	—	75	43	—	—
	—	—	—	—	6·4	770	35	—	—	—
	20·8	23·6	53·5	55·0	9·0	12·0	—	—	12·9	9·0
	13·0	14·5	—	—	6·5	4·3	—	—	—	—

zam treatment groups appear to respond more to treatment than the placebo group. The difference in response is most evident at 50% reduction in seizure level (i.e. poor and good control vs. excellent control).

Generalized and partial seizures were also considered separately. No conclusions could be made about the change in seizure frequency for generalized seizures because of the limited amount of data available. The results of the analysis of partial seizures is similar to those obtained from the analysis of the combined seizures.

Anticonvulsant serum levels recorded during the six months prior to entry into the study, and those recorded during the six months of the study are listed in Table 4, with summary statistics in Table 5.

There is no evidence to suggest that the addition of clobazam significantly affects the anticonvulsant serum levels.

Discussion

These data indicate the effectiveness of cloba-

zam in the management of poorly controlled epileptic seizures, and compare with the results of open studies by Gastaut (1978) who reported a 76% improvement in patients with severe epilepsy, and the double-blind studies of Critchley *et al.* (1981) and Allen *et al.* (1983). We observed an almost 50% reduction of total seizures in both groups of patients on clobazam, and have shown that the treatment effect of the two groups who received the active drug is statistically significant when compared to the placebo group. The improvement was maintained throughout the six-month period, suggesting that the anticonvulsant properties of clobazam continue in some patients for long periods, as noted by Gastaut (1981). We also observed that the addition of clobazam had no significant effect on the serum levels of the anticonvulsants taken concurrently.

Our results encourage the use of 1,5-benzodiazepines in the treatment of epilepsy and further trials are indicated with larger numbers of patients and for longer periods in order to achieve a more reliable and accurate assessment.

Table 5

Mean standard anticonvulsant levels (mmol/l)

	Phenytoin		Phenobarbitone		Carbamazepine		Sodium valproate		Primidone	
	Prior to study	During study	Prior to study	During study	Prior to study	During study	Prior to study	During study	Prior to study	During study
Placebo										
Mean	14·3	9·3	21·0	20·5	5·9	6·0	69·7	56·0	6·7	6·3
S.D.	7·0	5·1	17·0	4·9	1·9	4·1	22·7	36·7	—	—
Range	8–23	5·5–16·5	9–33	17–24	3·7–8·3	1·5–12·3	25–90	12–115	—	—
n	4	4	2	2	6	6	7	7	1	1
Clobazam 10 mg										
Mean	18·5	15·9	32·7	29·7	6·2	4·6	72·0	76·3	4·5	6·7
S.D.	3·9	5·5	9·9	11·8	1·0	1·5	10·2	13·0	1·4	0·7
Range	14·5–23	11–25	22–47	14·8–42	5–6·8	3·2–6·2	57–80	62–93	3·5–5·5	6·2–7·2
n	5	5	6	6	3	3	4	4	2	2
Clobazam 20 mg										
Mean	15·2	14·2	40·9	27·8	8·7	9·6	64·4	55·0	12·5	7·3
S.D.	6·5	6·7	11·4	18·5	1·9	3·2	24·3	28·0	0·6	2·4
Range	6·2–26	6–23·6	27–53·5	15–55	6·4–11	4·3–12·5	23–90	20–92	12–12·9	5·6–9
n	7	7	4	4	6	6	6	6	2	2

Acknowledgements

We are grateful to Miss E. M. Thomas for carrying out the statistical analysis, Drs M. Espir and S. D. Shorvon for advice and help, and Mrs C. Carter for preparing the manuscript.

References

Allen, J. W., Robertson, M. M., Oxley, J., Trimble, M. R. and Richens, A. (1983). Clobazam as adjunctive treatment for refractory epilepsy. *British Medical Journal* **286,** 1246–1247.
Browne, T. and Penry, K. (1975). Benzodiazepines in the treatment of epilepsy: A review. *Epilepsia* **14,** 277–281.
Chapman, A. G., Horton, R. W. and Meldrum, B. S. (1979). Anticonvulsant action of a 1,5-benzodiazepine, clobazam, in reflex epilepsy. *Epilepsia* **19,** 293–299.
Critchley, E. M. R., Vakil, S. A. and Hayward, H. L. (1981). Double-blind trial of clobazam in refractory epilepsy. In "Clobazam" (I. Hindmarch and P. D. Stonier, eds), pp. 159–163. International Congress and Symposium Series, Number 43. Royal Society of Medicine, London.
Escobedo, F., Otero, E., Chaparro, M., Flores, T. and Rubio-D, F. (1978). "Experience with Clobazam as Another Antiepileptic Drug." Epilepsy International Symposium, Vancouver.
Gastaut, H. (1978). Exceptional anti-epileptic properties of a new benzodiazepine. *La Vie Medicale* **88,** 5175–5181.
Gastaut, H. (1981). The effect of benzodiazepines on chronic epilepsy in man. In "Clobazam" (I. Hindmarch and P. D. Stonier, eds), pp. 141–150. International Congress and Symposium Series, Number 43. Royal Society of Medicine, London.
Killam, E. K. and Suria, A. (1980). Benzodiazepines. In "Antiepileptic Drugs: Mechanism of Action" (H. Glaser, K. Penry and D. Woodbury, eds). Raven Press, New York.
Loiseau, P. (1979). Étude des anti-epileptiques actuellement utilises. *La revue du practicien* **29,** 4465–4467.

Clobazam in Catamenial Epilepsy. Short Report

M. FEELY, R. CALVERT, J. HOWE and J. GIBSON

Leeds General Infirmary and St. James's University Hospital, Leeds, UK

We have previously reported on the efficacy of clobazam in a short-term, placebo-controlled, cross-over study in catamenial epilepsy (Feely *et al.*, 1982). In that investigation we found that clobazam, in doses of 20 or 30 mg/day, suppressed exacerbations of epilepsy associated with menstruation while producing few side-effects. We now report our long-term experience of using intermittent clobazam therapy in catamenial epilepsy. By confining treatment to ten days around menstruation we hope to avoid the development of tolerance, which has been seen in many patients during chronic therapy (Gastaut and Low, 1979).

For the purposes of this communication we have confined our observations to those women in whom we had been able to demonstrate clearly the efficacy of clobazam in the initial placebo-controlled investigation. In one such patient clobazam 20 mg proved unacceptably sedative and 10 mg/day was ineffective. We have treated the remaining 13 patients with clobazam 20 or 30 mg daily for ten days around menstruation, in successive menstrual cycles. While an increase in seizure frequence between periods of clobazam ther-

apy has caused us to abandon treatment in three patients, overall seizure frequency was greatly reduced in most patients and we have not seen the development of tolerance to the antiepileptic effect of clobazam in any of these patients (Feely and Gibson, 1984). This is despite the fact that three patients have been successfully treated, with freedom from seizures at menstruation, for three years. Two others did equally well until pregnancy made treatment inappropriate and the remaining patients were followed for between six and 13 months. In all these patients we continued conventional antiepileptic therapy, without change, throughout the period of the investigation.

Many women have an increase in seizure frequency just before and during the menses (Newmark and Penry, 1980). When such exacerbations are severe, additional treatment, using hormones, diuretics or increased doses of conventional antiepileptics, may be given. These measures have been largely unsatisfactory (Newmark and Penry, 1980). We believe that clobazam can greatly help some of these women.

References

Feely, M., Calvert, R., and Gibson, J. (1982). Clobazam in catamenial epilepsy: a model for evaluating anticonvulsants. *Lancet* **ii**, 71–73.

Feely, M., and Gibson, J. (1984). Intermittent clobazam for catamenial epilepsy: avoid tolerance. *Journal of Neurology, Neurosurgery and Psychiatry* (in press).

Gastaut, H., and Low, M.D. (1979). Antiepileptic properties of clobazam, a 1,5-benzodiazepine, in man. *Epilepsia* **20**, 437–46.

Newmark, M.E., and Penry, J.K. (1980). Catamenial epilepsy: a review. *Epilepsia* **21**, 281–300.

Clobazam as Adjunctive Therapy in Chronic Epilepsy: Clinical, Psychological and EEG Assessment

D. F. SCOTT and A. MOFFETT

EEG Department, Section of Neurological Sciences, The London Hospital, Whitechapel, London, U.K.

Summary

The addition of clobazam, generally 20 mg, at night to the pre-existing anticonvulsant regime, usually sodium valproate and carbamazepine, led to a marked improvement in over half of a group of 60 patients with a chronic seizure disorder, be it of focal or generalized type. Results were similar in 12 patients, a subgroup of a more detailed investigation including EEG, and psychological variables who have been studied, so far, for approximately six months. Three were seizure-free, and there was improvement in the EEG. Psychological tests selected to measure both beneficial and unwanted effects showed reduction in anxiety with improvement in alertness and performance. Few complaints were reported by the patients and this was confirmed on self-rating scale assessments. These findings indicate the value of this 1,5-benzodiazepine in chronic epilepsy and the fact that it is well tolerated.

Introduction

The use of oral benzodiazepine compounds in the treatment of chronic epilepsy has been a subject of interest because, in spite of the introduction of sodium valproate and the wider availability of drug level assessment of anticonvulsants, there remains a group of patients in whom seizures are poorly controlled. Our recent double-blind study (Moffett and Scott, 1983) has shown the value of one benzodiazepine compound, namely lorazepam, in this group of patients. Clobazam, the subject of the present communication, offers an alternative, as it has been reported by the similarly controlled studies of Critchley *et al.* (1981) and Allen *et al.* (1983) to be effective.

The investigation was begun to examine the long-term effectiveness of clobazam, in the first instance, as an adjunct to existing anticonvulsant medication. Here we report the overall results of clinical experience with this compound and the preliminary findings of a continuing and more detailed study. In this, the effects of clobazam were assessed not only from the clinical and electroencephalographic standpoints, but in addition a variety of psychological tests were employed. These included established methods such as The Middlesex Hospital Questionnaire (Crown and Crisp, 1974) and the Stroop test (Klein, 1964), as well as visual analogue scales derived from another benzodiazepine study in epilepsy (Moffett and Scott, 1984) and a short questionnaire designed to indicate whether the patient had stress precipitated fits.

The long-term aim was to investigate a group of patients whose chronic seizure disorder had presented problems on conventional anticonvulsant regimens, and follow them up for at least two years. In order to determine the continuing usefulness or otherwise of clobazam, the appropriate dose level and any beneficial effects of its known psychotropic actions were also assessed.

Patients and Methods

Patients

The patients admitted to the study had almost invariably been under surveillance over several years in an epilepsy clinic and seen only by the present investigators. Therefore, the nature of the seizure disorder and other background factors were well documented. The diagnosis was as complete as possible, with EEG and other investigations such as CT scan, having been performed. Those receiving a complex drug regimen when first referred to the clinic had this simplified, but even so, no patient was receiving a single anticonvulsant. Carbamazepine and valproate was the commonest combination, though phenytoin with valproate was the other main alternative. The response to the medication with anticonvulsant blood levels in the accepted therapeutic range was poor. It was explained to the patient that an additional anticonvulsant compound would be added to the existing regimen, and only those who indicated their agreement to taking clobazam were included. Sixty patients have so far been treated (Table 1a). More than half had focal epilepsy, mainly partial complex seizures, with or without secondary generalized attacks, and the remainder primary generalized seizures. Their average age was 33 years and duration of epilepsy 15·5 years. They had been followed up from three to 20 months with an average of nine months.

Detailed study
Because of the obvious beneficial effects of clobazam in this large group of patients a more comprehensive schedule of assessment was prepared (see below). Twenty-three patients have been admitted so far and reached at least the four-month assessment point (the aim will be to obtain 30 patients to be followed up for a minimum two-year period). Eighteen of the 23 have focal epilepsy, mainly partial complex seizures, half of which had infrequent generalized attacks, the

remainder having primary generalized epilepsies (Table 1b). The ages range from 16 to 63 with an average age of 31 years and duration of epilepsy of 10·5 years.

Methods
When the patient was admitted to the long-term detailed study, baseline assessment was made (Table 2). This included recording of the fit type and frequency over the preceding three months (all had at least two attacks per month), and the completion of the prognostic study scale (Korgeorgos *et al.*, 1981). There are 11 parameters to be scored, which are based on Rodin (1968), and include such

Table 2

Test schedule

Baseline	Clinical assessment, including prognostic scale
	EEG
	Blood levels
	Psychological assessment
	Crown Crisp Questionnaire
	Stroop test
	Visual Analogue Scales
	Stress/Anxiety questionnaire
1 Week	Check of drug tolerance
1 Month	Clinical assessment and psychological tests
3 Months	Clinical assessment, EEG, blood levels and psychological tests
and *3-monthly thereafter*	

Table 1

Background to patients

	(a) All patients ($N=60$)		(b) Detailed study ($N=23$)	
	FE	GE	FE	GE
Males	27	12	11	2
Females	10	11	7	3
Total	37	23	18	5

Mean age 33 yr (range 16–63 yr)
Mean duration 15·5 yr
Mean follow-up 9 months
  (range 3–20 months)

Mean age 31 yr (range 16–63 yr)
Mean duration 10·5 yr

FE–Focal epilepsy, mainly complex partial; GE = primary generalized.

factors as duration of epilepsy, age of onset, length of seizure-free period, and presence of brain damage. The higher the score the greater the chance of poor control of seizures. A standard EEG including hyperventilation and photic stimulation was performed and blood taken for determination of anticonvulsant levels. Psychological assessment comprised the Middlesex Hospital Questionnaire (Crown and Crisp, 1974) and the Stroop test (Klein, 1964). Visual analogue scales (Moffett and Scott, 1984) were employed with a total of 15 items for self-assessment including seizure frequency, psychiatric state, and possible drug side-effects. In addition a stress/anxiety questionnaire was used to determine in numerical form whether the patients regarded their seizures as stress precipitated or not, as clobazam is known to have anxiety relieving properties.

The patients were then prescribed 20 mg clobazam at night in addition to their current medication, and the general practitioner informed, with emphasis, that this new substance had been added specifically for its anticonvulsant property rather than as a tranquillizer. (In our experience this was very important because some doctors early on during the studies had discontinued the medication unaware of the antiepileptic effects of the drug.) A check that clobazam was tolerated was made at one week and then one month after commencement, the baseline assessment with the exception of EEG and blood levels, was repeated. The complete battery was then administered again at approximately three-monthly intervals. Minor variations from this schedule were sometimes necessary, as the patients were assessed throughout only by the same two investigators.

If at follow-up the patients seizure frequency was not diminished an additional 10 mg of clobazam was given. This has been necessary for five patients so far, and two are now receiving a total daily dose of 40 mg. In two patients increase in dosage was begun because an initial response had been good, but seizures returned before the second assessment point following treatment. Side-effects as measured by clinical impression have been minimal, though more detailed information derived by self-rating with the visual analogue scales will be presented under "results". Only two patients had to be withdrawn because of unwanted effects, one because she reported that clobazam kept her

awake, the other, a male because it made him "dozy". This patient subsequently asked to recommence the therapy, and has done so, without recurrence of this problem. Four patients who were assigned to the study failed to attend for assessment according to the schedule and were withdrawn. However, in two cases subsequent follow-up showed that this was because of a beneficial effect of the drug, not because of side-effects. Serum levels of clobazam were not obtained during the study.

Results

All patients

Considering the total group of 60 patients treated with clobazam (Table 3), 29 showed marked improvement as defined by a reduction of 50% or more in fit frequency. A

Table 3

Clinical outcome in all 60 patients treated

	Focal			Generalized		
	MI	I	U	MI	I	U
Males	10	16	1	6	6	0
Females	8	2	0	5	4	2
Total	18	18	1	11	10	2

MI = markedly improved; I = improved; U = unchanged.

similar number, 28, were improved, showing definite beneficial effects on the control of attacks. Only three patients reported no change and none was worse after the addition of clobazam. The severity of individual fits, or other alterations in their pattern, were sometimes observed by the patients, but no systematic reports were obtained on these. An improvement in general "well being" was a feature commented on spontaneously by many patients but not confirmed on the tests. Benefit from the drug did not appear to be different, in terms of reduction in seizure frequency, for focal as distinct from generalized epilepsy or males versus females. However, when the patients were categorized as to whether they had "brain damage"* (none had evidence of progressive lesions), there was a tendency to show less effect with clobazam administration.

Detailed study

To date 23 patients have entered the long-term detailed investigation but only 12 patients have been seen for a period of four months or more. The results based on this group will be presented here.

Fit frequency
The findings are shown in three ways (Table 4a). First, with clinical assessment, five showed a reduction in fit frequency of 50% or greater, six were improved and one was unchanged. Three patients were seizure-free. The prognostic rating score for those with the best improvement was 5·0, for the others 7·1. Secondly, absolute seizure frequency before and after treatment was compared. A marked average decrease from 14·8 per three months to 5·1 for the same period after treatment was noted. Thirdly, the visual analogue scale scores on the patients' assessment of fits showed an obvious reduction corresponding to the clinical rating. The benefits from the addition of clobazam were not different for focal or generalized epilepsy.

---

*Patients with previous history of birth or head injuries, and known neurosurgical lesions such as aneurysms, with or without subarachnoid haemorrhage (n = 24).

EEG changes
The pre- and post-treatment recordings were compared for the same 12 patients (Table 4b). The latter was noted as "improved", i.e. reduction of paroxysmal features, in eight of the 12 patients (Fig. 1 shows an example). In none was the tracing more abnormal.

Psychological results
Changes were noted in the psychological tests. The Middlesex Hospital Questionnaire (Table 5a) indicates a decrease in free floating anxiety and concern about somatic symptoms, while other sub-tests were unchanged. The Stroop test (Table 5b) showed a decrease in the time taken for the interference patterns, as well as a decrease in error scores. The visual analogue scales (Table 6) indicated that there was an increase in alertness as well as a reduction in tension and anxiety. The patients considered that their thoughts had become clearer and they felt steadier after clobazam. There were no changes in symptoms such as sleep, vision and fear of attacks nor were there signs of heavy headedness after the drug had been prescribed. No patient reported that all their attacks were precipitated by stress but three felt that a considerable proportion, and three that a few, were thus triggered. Response to clobazam did not appear to be related to these observations by the patients.

Discussion

The findings reported here are in accord with those of other workers (Critchley et al., 1981;

Table 4

Clinical outcome in 12 patients

(a)	Seizures and clinical state			
	(1)	Marked improvement	Improvement	Unchanged
		5 (3 fit-free)	6	1
	(2)	Fit frequency	Baseline	After clobazam
		(mean per 3 months)	14·8	5·1
	(3)	Visual analogue	Before clobazam	After clobazam
		scales (mean scores)	5·3	2·3
(b)	EEG changes			
			Focal (n = 8)	Generalized (n = 4)
	Improved		5	3
	Unchanged		3	1

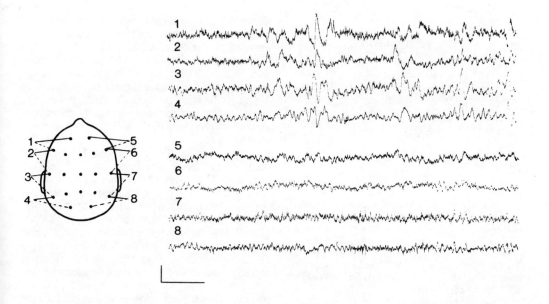

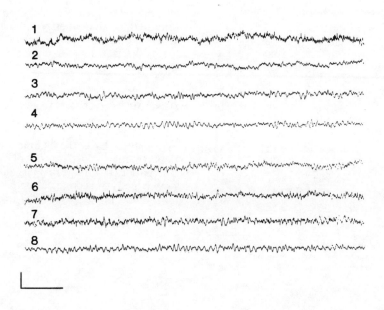

Figure 1. *Two samples of EEGs from a 42-year-old female patient with intractable partial complex seizures of unknown aetiology are shown. The upper trace (before) and lower trace (after) 20 mg clobazam daily, added to medication with valproate, and carbamazepine. A very marked decrease in seizure frequency resulted. Note the frequent high voltage complexes over the left temporal leads in the upper trace; this was characteristic of the whole recording. They disappeared completely in the post-treatment tracing, which also has an increase in fast components. Calibration: vertical line 50 mV, horizontal line 1 s.*

Table 5

Psychological tests

(a) Middlesex Hospital Questionnaire (means; $N = 12$)

	Baseline	4 weeks	12 weeks
FFA	5·2	4·7	3·8
PHO	3·6	3·4	3·1
OBS	5·5	5·6	5·3
SOM	4·9	3·8	3·8
DEP	3·5	3·9	3·7
HYS	5·5	5·3	5·1

(b) Stroop test

	Baseline	4 weeks	12 weeks
Mean time (s)	44·5	38·4	31·1
Errors	2·5	0·8	0·5

FFA, free-floating anxiety; PHO, phobic anxiety; OBS, obsessionality; SOM, somatic anxiety; DEP, depression; HYS, hysteria.

Table 6

Visual Analogue Scales
(means; N = 12)

	Baseline	4 weeks	12 weeks
Sleep	1·3	0·7	1·1
Alertness	2·5	1·5	1·2
Steadiness	2·9	2·9	1·5
Tension	3·9	4·4	2·6
Thoughts clear	3·1	2·7	2·1
Feel well	2·3	1·5	2·4
Headache	1·9	1·7	0·9
Heavy-headed	2·8	3·9	3·0
Afraid of fits	3·8	3·2	3·0
Sickness	1·8	1·8	2·7
Anxiety	3·3	4·1	2·3
Sadness	2·7	2·3	2·0
Vision	2·0	2·7	2·7
Dizziness	1·0	1·5	2·0

Note: (1) The symptoms listed are an abbreviated version of the statements used on the actual form given to the patient.

(2) The lowering of the score indicates lessening of the symptom.

Allen et al., 1983) who have used double-blind techniques. In the larger group of 60 patients, those having focal epilepsy, mainly partial complex seizures, or with the primary generalized disorder, responded equally well. Although no patients with known active brain disease were included, those with brain damage occurring from previous cerebral insults showed improvement, although not as marked as for those without.

In the more detailed investigation our aim was two-fold: first, to test clinically the long-term effect of clobazam, eventually studying 30 patients with intractable epilepsy over a period of two years; and secondly, to employ apart from routine EEG, a battery of psychological tests to check the positive and the negative aspects of the compound. So far the results have been gratifying and side-effects minimal. There have been positive benefits to the patients, according to their own reports; on the visual analogue scales, for example, increased alertness and reduction of fits occurred; and improved performance on Stroop test was reported. With the Middlesex Hospital Questionnaire, a decrease in free-floating anxiety and somatic anxiety was seen. So far, however, aims to predict which patients might respond to clobazam have yielded mixed results. Although the prognostic ratings (Kogeorgos et al., 1981) may suggest a good outcome, patients with stress-induced seizures do not show a particularly beneficial effect. On the positive side, the drug was well tolerated, no dependency arose and problems of breakthrough after a period on the treatment do not in our hands appear to be insuperable.

Acknowledgements

We wish to thank the technicians of the EEG department, who carried out recordings on our patients. Mrs Jean Held is warmly acknowledged for secretarial help.

References

Allen, J. W., Oxley, J., Robertson, M. M., Trimble, M. R., Richens, A. and Jawad, S. S. M. (1983). Clobazam as adjunctive treatment in refractory epilepsy. *British Medical Journal* **286**, 1246–1247.

Critchley, E. M. R., Vakil, S. A., Hayward, H. W., Owen, M. V. H., Cocks, A. and Freemantle, N. P. (1981). In "Clobazam" (I. Hindmarch and P. D. Stonier, eds), pp. 159–163. International Congress and Symposium Series, Number 43. Royal Society of Medicine, London.

Crown, S. and Crisp, A. H. (1974). The Middlesex Hospital Questionnaire in clinical research. In "Psychological Medicine and Psychopharmacology" (T. Pichot, ed.), pp. 111–124. Karger, Basle.

Klein, G. S. (1964). Semantic power measured through the interference of words with colour naming. *American Journal of Psychology* **77**, 576–588.

Kogeorgos, J., Evans, S. and Scott, D. F. (1981). Methods of quantification applicable to the assessment of progress and prognosis in epilepsy. In "Perspectives on epilepsy 1980/1981", pp. 71–77. British Epilepsy Association, Crowthorne, Berkshire.

Moffett, A. and Scott, D. F. (1983). Stress and epilepsy: the value of a benzodiazepine—lorazepam. *Journal of Neurology, Neurosurgery and Psychiatry* **47**, 165–167.

Rodin, E. A. (1968). "The Prognosis of Patients with Epilepsy." Charles C. Thomas, Springfield, Illinois.

Clobazam in Resistant Epilepsy—A Retrospective Survey

M. A. DALBY

Neurological University Clinic, Aarhus City Hospital, Aarhus, Denmark

Nine patients with severe resistant epilepsy have been treated with clobazam as adjunctive therapy for 1–7 months. Results have been very promising and the drug is now used frequently in cases of epilepsy that do not respond to conventional therapy.

Seven female and two male patients with ages ranging from 6–61 years were treated. The age of onset of epilepsy varied from birth to 20 years (average 9 years). The duration of epilepsy varied from 4–44 years with an average of 22 years. Seven patients had complex partial seizures in the form of automatisms with a frequency of 2–50 attacks per day for many years. These patients also had generalized tonic-clonic attacks at a frequency of 4–8 per month. There was one patient with a Lennox-Gastaut syndrome of 28-years duration and with atonic attacks occurring up to 100 times a day. The other patient, aged six, had a West syndrome with salaam attacks, absences, right- and left-sided motor attacks and generalized tonic-clonic seizures—from 50–100 attacks daily for four years.

All patients had been treated with available antiepileptic medication in varying combinations but without substantial change in the frequency of attacks. Clobazam was added to the patients current medication in doses varying between 30 and 100 mg/day or $\frac{1}{2}$–$1\frac{1}{2}$ mg/kg/day. Serum levels after 2–4 weeks of treatment varied from 50–390 μmol/l.

The treatment with clobazam was started during admission to the hospital and continued on an ambulatory basis with monitoring every 1–2 months. Four patients with complex partial seizures were completely seizure-free within 2–3 days after the start of clobazam and have remained so for the duration of the medication, 2–7 months. The patient with Lennox-Gastaut syndrome stopped having seizures one day after the start of clobazam and has remained seizure-free for seven months. Two patients had their seizures reduced by 75% or more. Two patients showed no effect of the drug after one month's treatment.

Side-effects were observed in three patients and consisted of muscular weakness, sedation, ataxia, tremor, and constipation. Side-effects subsided after reduction of dosage in two patients and in one patient the drug had to be withdrawn.

In patients who became seizure-free the prior medication was reduced or withdrawn, especially clonazepam and primidone, without detrimental results.

A distinct psychological improvement was observed in patients who were rendered seizure-free. The patient with Lennox-Gastaut syndrome has now been free from attacks for 208 days, having had daily atonic seizures for more than 20 years and has started learning a hand printers trade. A 61-year-old patient with daily automatisms for 44 years writes that he has not felt so well since his youth. This represents a profound change from his former obsessional compulsive behaviour when he had to describe each attack, and his bodily functions, which he registered meticulously in neatly ordered note-books.

Summary

Nine patients with chronic resistant epilepsy were treated with clobazam (30–100 mg/day) as adjunctive therapy for 1–7 months (study continuing). Five patients (four with complex partial seizures and one with Lennox-Gastaut syndrome) have been seizure-free since commencement of therapy (2–7 months). Two patients have had seizures reduced by 75% or more. In seizure-free patients, prior medication has been reduced or withdrawn without detriment and psychological and social improvement has been observed.

EEG Changes in Epileptic Children treated with Clobazam as Monotherapy

P. PLOUIN and C. JALIN

Laboratoire d'Explorations Fonctionnelles du Système Nerveux, Hospital Saint Vincent de Paul, 74 avenue Defert-Rochereau, 75014 Paris, France

Summary

The electroencephalographic (EEG) changes of 15 children treated with clobazam as monotherapy are reported. Normalization of the EEG is seen most often with good clinical control in benign partial epilepsy. In other cases, the EEG response was variable and did not predict the clinical response. In patients who lose control of their seizures following therapy, EEG abnormalities reappear before the clinical deterioration.

Introduction

All reports describing the effects of clobazam on the EEG have currently been in trials using clobazam in polytherapy. Gastaut (1981) first discussed these modifications as: a widespread fast activity, maximal in anterior areas; an increase of the frequency of background activity (mostly the alpha rhythm); a decrease or suppression of the slowest EEG components (theta or delta waves, spontaneous or induced by hyperpnoea); and a decrease or suppression of paroxysmal activity induced by intermittent light stimulation in photosensitive patients. All these changes were described in the first week of treatment in patients with a good clinical response.

Martin (1981) pointed out the possibility of EEG normalization in patients with a positive response to clobazam even if gross and persistent abnormalities had been present.

Pechadre *et al.* (1981), who studied patients with the Lennox-Gastaut syndrome and given clobazam as adjunctive therapy as opposed to other anticonvulsant drugs, were able to identify two groups: one with a good initial response and the other with an unfavourable response. They noted that among the good responders, spike and wave discharges disappeared immediately, and after two to three months of treatment a normalization of background activity could follow. The group with an unfavourable response was defined by an increase of slow waves on the EEG, which was clinically associated with drowsiness and, in one case, by an increase of seizure frequency.

Shimizu *et al.* (1982) saw a good EEG response in 18 out of 36 patients given clobazam as a combined treatment. In nine of these 18, the seizures disappeared, and in the other nine the frequency was reduced by more than 50%.

Recently Dulac *et al.* (1983) published a study concerning clobazam given in monotherapy to 25 children with benign or severe epilepsy. Of these, 15 had an EEG recorded in our laboratory, before and after the beginning of treatment with clobazam, and the results are presented here.

Materials and Methods

In these 15 cases, clobazam was given either because previous treatment was ineffective (12 cases), or because it was the drug of choice as first treatment in children who also needed an anxiolytic (three cases). Clobazam was given in increasing dosage over one or two weeks, at the daily dose of 1 mg/kg in infants, or 0·5 mg/kg in children.

Routine EEGs, including sleep records in younger children, were performed before introducing clobazam (patients being given another treatment in 12 cases and no treatment in three cases), and following clobazam after a variable delay (one week in two cases, two months in six cases, six months in five cases, and one year in two cases).

The age distribution of patients is shown in

Table 1a. The sex ratio showed no difference between boys ($n = 8$) and girls ($n = 7$).

The type of epilepsy is seen in Table 1b. Lesional partial epilepsies were defined by a clinically or radiologically patent cerebral lesion. Unclassifiable partial epilepsies did not have the criteria of the other two groups: benign and lesional. To define severe myoclonic epilepsy we took into account the criteria of Dalla Bernardina et al. (1978). In the Landau-Keffner syndrome, also called aphasia-epilepsy, atypical absences, and partial and generalized motor seizures can occur.

Treatments given before the introduction of clobazam are detailed in Table 1c. The three cases without any treatment before clo-

Table 1

Background of patients

	Number of patients
(a) Age distribution (yr)	
0–2	5
3–10	7
11–15	2
15+	1
(Range six months–23 yr)	
(b) Type of epilepsy	
Benign partial epilepsy (BPE)	7
Lesional partial epilepsy (LPE)	3
Unclassifiable partial epilepsy (UPE)	2
Severe myoclonic epilepsy (SME)	1
West syndrome	1
Landau-Keffner syndrome (LKS)	1
(c) Previous treatment	
None	3
Carbamazepine	7
Sodium Valproate	1
Phenobarbital	1
Ethosuccimide	1
Hydrocortisone	1
Hydrocortisone + clonazepam	1

bazam were one of benign partial epilepsy, one case of lesional partial epilepsy, and one case of severe myoclonic epilepsy.

Results

The clinical course of the patients on clobazam allowed differentiation into four groups (Table 2). In the first (six cases), the children were free from seizures for a follow-up period

Table 2

Clinical course on clobazam

	No. of patients	
Freedom from fits	6	(BPE, 4; LPE, 2 > 12 months)
Reduction in fits	4	(BPE, 2; UPE, 2)
Transitory freedom from fits	3	(SME, 1 week; LKS, 5 months; BPE, 8 months)
No change in fits	2	(West; BPE)

of at least one year. In the second (four cases), a reduction of more than 50% in the frequency of fits was observed. In the third group (three cases), children were transitorily free from fits during variable periods: one week for a child with severe myoclonic epilepsy, five months for the patient with the Landau-Keffner syndrome, and eight months for the child with a benign partial epilepsy. Finally, in the fourth group, two children had no change in their fit frequency.

The EEG changes were different in each group. In group one, i.e. those free from fits, we noted a complete disappearance of the spike focus and/or an increase of speed of the background activity in the four cases with benign partial epilepsy (Figs 1 and 2). In the two cases of lesional partial epilepsy, abnormalities persisted in one case, and in the other there was an improvement of the background activity, but spikes persisted.

In the second group, the reduction of seizure frequency was associated with a normalization of the EEG in two cases of benign partial epilepsy, and with the appearance of rapid rhythms in one of these two cases. In the children with unclassifiable partial epilepsy, one case had no EEG change, and the other had a transitory decrease of paroxysmal bursts.

In the third group, with a transitory period free from fits, the EEG changes were variable. In the case of Landau-Keffner syndrome there was a normalization of the EEG during the months without seizures, but a return of spikes and waves took place before the recurrence of clinical fits (Figs 3, 4, 5). In the case of severe myoclonic epilepsy, there was a transitory improvement of the background activity and a decrease of paroxysmal bursts during the period free from seizures. In the case of benign partial epilepsy, paroxysmal

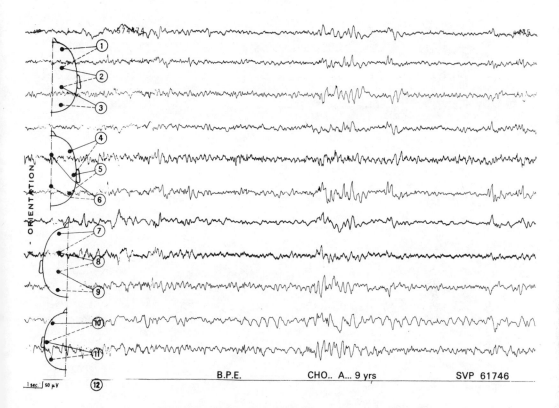

Figure 1. EEG before clobazam; group I, BPE.

bursts were more frequent on the EEG although the child was free from fits for eight months (Figs 6 and 7).

In the fourth group, with no change in fit frequency, the EEG remained unchanged in the case of benign partial epilepsy, but there was a transitory improvement in the case of West syndrome.

Discussion

Our results suggest that, in the first two groups, with a good clinical response to clobazam, normalization of EEG does not always occur. In benign partial epilepsy, we have observed it in all six cases, but in the other forms of partial epilepsy there was no change in the EEG in two cases and variable changes in the other two. In the groups with a transitory or an absent clinical response to clobazam, we found a transitory improve-

ment of the EEG in three cases, but a worsening in one case.

Normalization of EEG, suggested in the literature to accompany a good clinical response, is not a constant finding in our material, and was seen only in the cases of benign partial epilepsy. We consider that this effect must be due to clobazam since, in our study, the drug was used in monotherapy.

Two further points may be emphasized. First, when escape is seen, EEG abnormalities reappear before seizures. Hence repeated EEG records after the first weeks of treatment may help predict the return of seizures. Secondly, a worsening of EEG can be seen even where there is a transitory disappearance of seizures. This is similar to the report of Ohtsuka *et al.* (1982), who reported the occurrence of microseizures during slow sleep in patients treated by benzodiazepines (clobazam) for the Lennox-Gastaut syndrome.

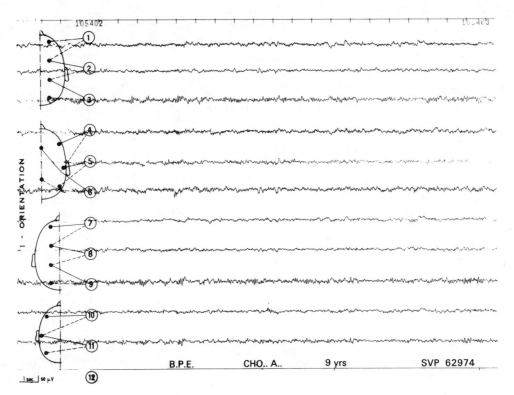

Figure 2. Same child, two months later; clobazam given for two months. Normalization of background activity.

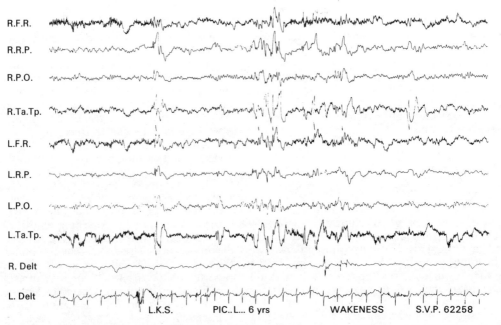

Figure 3. Landau-Keffner syndrome, before clobazam, group III EEG while awake.

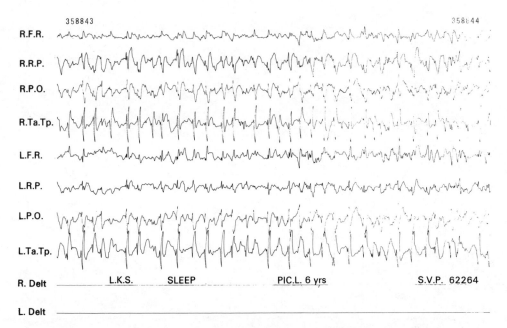

Figure 4. Same child during slow sleep: continuous spike and wave activity.

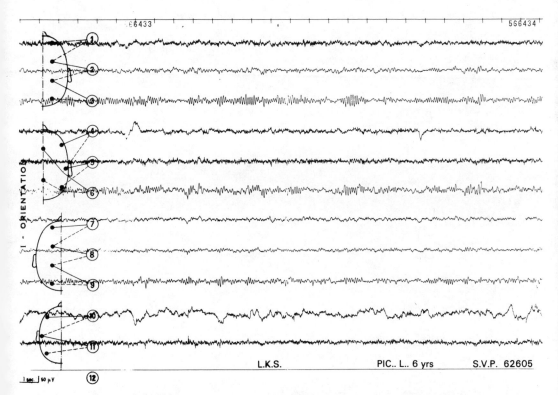

Figure 5. Same child; clobazam given for two months; EEG while awake. Normal background activity and no more spikes.

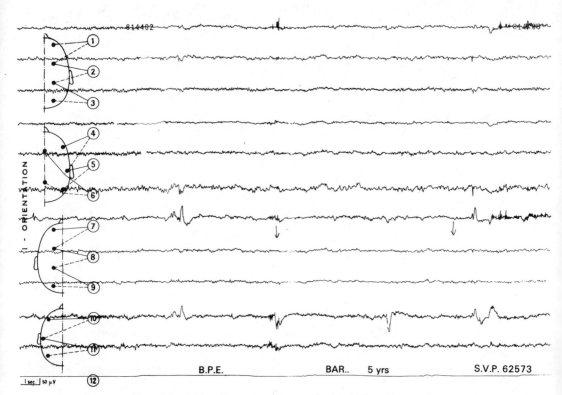

Figure 6. EEG before clobazam; group III, BPE, few spikes.

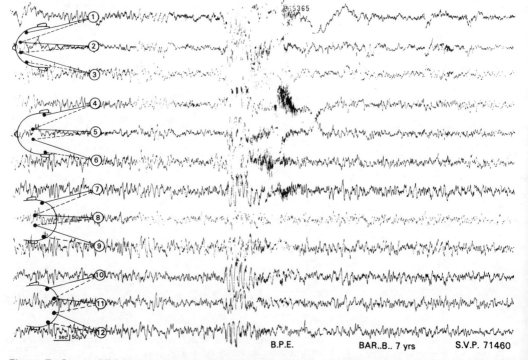

Figure 7. Same child two years later, transitory efficacy of clobazam; worsening of the EEG with generalized poly-spikes and waves.

References

Dalla Bernardina, B., Bureau, M., Tassinari, C. A., Roger, J. and Dravet, C. (1978). "Epilepsies et encéphalopathies épileptiques de l'enfant (limites et diagnostic différentiel)." 4é Réunion de la Société de Neurologie Infantile, La Baule.

Dulac, O., Figueroa, D., Rey, E. and Arthuis, M. (1983). Monothérapie par le clobazam dans les épilepsies de l'enfant. *La Presse Médicale* 12, 1067–1069.

Gastaut, H. (1981). The effects of benzodiazepines on chronic epilepsy in man (with particular references to clobazam). In "Clobazam" (I. Hindmarch and P.D. Stonier, eds), pp. 142–150. International Congress and Symposium Series, Number 43. Royal Society of Medicine, London.

Landau, W. M. and Keffner, F. R. (1957). Syndrome of acquired aphasia with convulsive disorders in children. *Neurology* (Minneap.) 7, 523–530.

Martin, A. A. (1981). The anti-epileptic effects of clobazam: a long-term study in resistant epilepsy. In "Clobazam" (I. Hindmarch and P. D. Stonier, eds), pp. 142–150. International Congress and Symposium Series, Number 43. Royal Society of Medicine, London.

Ohtsuka, Y., Yoshida, H., Miyake, S., Ichib, N., Inoue, H., Yamatogi, Y. and Ohtara, S. (1982). Induced Microseizures: a clinical and electroencephalographic study. In "Advances in Epileptology: XIIIth Epilepsy International Symposium" (H. Akimoto, H. Kanzamatsuri, M. Seino and A. Ward, eds), pp. 33–36. Raven Press, New York.

Pechadre, J. C., Beudin, P., Devoize, J. L. and Gibert, J. (1981). Utilisation du clobazam comme anti-épileptique dans le syndrome de Lennox-Gastaut. *Encéphale* 7, 181–190.

Shimizu, H., Futagi, Y., Onoe, S., Tagawa, T., Mimaki, T., Yamatodani, A., Kato, M., Kamio, M., Sumi, K., Sugita, T. and Yabuuchi, H. (1982). Antiepileptic effects of clobazam in children. *Brain and Development* 4, 57–62.

Benzodiazepines, Psychiatry and Epilepsy

M. R. TRIMBLE

*Department of Neuropsychiatry, National Hospitals for Nervous Diseases,
Queen Square, London, U.K.*

Summary

The historical links between certain psychiatric disorders and epilepsy are reviewed concluding with a consideration of behavioural phenomena common to both. Recent evidence relating to the actions of benzodiazepines on gabaminergic neurones and the benzodiazepine receptor complex provides a neuroanatomical and neurochemical substrate for a relationship between epilepsy, principally temporal lobe epilepsy, and psychiatric disorder, principally anxiety. Finally, the antiepileptic properties of benzodiazepines are discussed and the differences between sedative 1,4-benzodiazepines and non-sedative 1,5-benzodiazepines compared in terms of clinical application.

Introduction

The interrelationships between psychiatry and epilepsy have been reviewed extensively and will only briefly be highlighted here (Trimble, 1981; Trimble, 1983a). Although controversial, much of this has revolved around the concept of personality disorders and the so-called "epileptic personality". Thus, around the turn of the century, it was inevitably thought that patients with epilepsy would show intellectual deterioration, this either on account of recurrent seizures, or more ominously because of the hereditary degeneration that was thought to occur in patients with diseases such as epilepsy. The mid-twentieth century saw a reversal of the position, namely with the ideas of Lennox (Lennox, 1960), that patients with epilepsy were psychologically normal, although impairment of cognitive function and changes in behaviour could be noted on account of several factors secondary to seizures, for example, recurrent head injuries, or the conse-quences of toxic anticonvulsant drugs.

The introduction of the electroencephalogram in the 1950s led to a different viewpoint, namely that it was patients with "psychomotor" epilepsy who were most likely to suffer from psychiatric problems, the position being summed up perhaps best by the quotation of Gibbs and Stamps (1958) that: "the patient's emotional reactions to his seizures, to his family and to his social situation are less important determinants of psychiatric disorder than the site and type of the epileptic discharge."

Although this viewpoint is still a subject of controversy (e.g. see Trimble, 1983a), there is a growing literature on the interlinks between temporal lobe disturbances in epilepsy and behaviour changes stimulated by two main lines of evidence. The first of these relates to an understanding of those regions of the brain referred to as the limbic system, which are thought to be involved with the regulation and expression of emotions. The limbic system concept, ushered in by Papez (1937) and elegantly explored by MacLean (1970), has recently been the subject of much interest with the emergence of newer techniques for exploring neuroanatomical pathways in the central nervous system, and the realization that neurotransmitters that are closely interlinked with the regulation of mood (for example, the monoamines and peptides), are found in high concentrations in limbic structures (Trimble and Zarifian, 1984). The second has been an improved emphasis on classification in epilepsy, with an improvement of techniques for the assessment of psychopathology, particularly with the use of standardized and validated rating scales, both of which have led to a renewed interest in examining differences in psychiatric morbidity between patients with temporal lobe abnormalities in comparison with other epileptic and non-epileptic groups.

Temporal Lobe Epilepsy Revisited

The recommended international classification of epileptic seizures broadly divides them into two, namely generalized and partial (Gastaut, 1969). In generalized seizures there is no evidence, clinical or otherwise, to imply a local onset; and manifestations, usually loss of consciousness with motor changes, reflect bilateral disturbances of brain function. In contrast, partial seizures begin focally, the symptom pattern being dependent on the area of the brain from which the abnormality is arising. The term "complex partial seizure" has been introduced to refer to focal attacks that usually, but not always, arise within the temporal lobes, during which episodes consciousness is altered. This form of seizure has a long history going back to Hughlings Jackson and beyond. Thus, although partial epilepsy was probably first described by Pritchard (1822), who identified examples of epilepsy without convulsions, it was Hughlings Jackson's description of certain motor seizures, which were designated by Charcot as "Jacksonian", that clarified this distinction. Of particular importance in Jackson's work was the delineation of "dreamy states" as a manifestation of epilepsy, and the "uncinate group of fits". The latter could be associated with paroxysms of smell or taste, and were related to abnormal discharging lesions in the uncinate region of the temporal cortex. These early descriptions provided us with the coherent characterization of seizures which were re-named psychomotor by Gibbs. Thus the introduction of the concept of temporal lobe epilepsy in the 1940s following widespread investigations with the newly applied electroencephalogram was a reinstitution of Jackson's idea of "the uncinate groups of fits" (see Trimble, 1983b).

Psychiatric Disorders in Temporal Lobe Epilepsy

The extensive and continually expanding literature on the links between temporal lobe epilepsy and psychiatric disorder is not to be reviewed here (for further references see Trimble, 1981, 1983a). The point should be re-emphasized that the area is one of active research and considerable conflict, although most of the confusion surrounds the issue of personality disorder in relation to epilepsy. For the present, it can only be stated that some authors have found differences between matched patients with temporal lobe and generalized epilepsy on certain rating scales, which suggest a different profile of psychopathology in the former compared with the latter. Of particular interest here is the recent paper from Hermann et al. (1982) in which patients with temporal lobe epilepsy were compared to a group with generalized epilepsy using the Minnesota Multiphasic Personality Inventory (MMPI). Clinically they identified a group of temporal lobe patients who had an aura of ictal fear and they noted that those with this scored significantly higher on several of the MMPI scales than those without such fear or those who had generalized epilepsy. Now the phenomenon of ictal fear clearly leads us to the doorstep of psychiatry. Williams (1956) examined ictally related emotions and noted that they tended to be generally unpleasant and of a primitive nature. Fear was particularly common, occurring in 60% of cases who had ictally related emotional experiences, and ranged from a strange unnatural apprehension of fear without a clear object, to stark terror. Autonomic changes associated with the emotional experience occurred, and sometimes behavioural accompaniments, such as running were reported, so-called "cursive epilepsy". Three-quarters of those who experienced this fear had a focus of origin on the electroencephalogram which pointed to an abnormality in the anterior part of the temporal lobe, more commonly on the left-hand side. Gloor et al. (1982) have provided further evidence of a close link between the anterior temporal lobe and an experience of ictal fear. Patients with epilepsy undergoing investigation for potential surgery had electrodes implanted into various areas of their brain, including the temporal lobes. The latter placements were in both medial and lateral areas, and the patients ictal emotional experiences, or their feelings following stimulation through the electrodes, were recorded. They reported that fear was particularly common, occurring in nearly 60% of cases, and was nearly always associated with medial as opposed to lateral temporal excitation. In particular, limbic system stimulation and after discharges were associated with such feelings. These data from patients with epilepsy highlight the involvement of medial temporal structures in the mediation of anxiety, and provide further evidence of the close association between limbic system function and emotional expression.

Thus, anxiety, and its more severe manifestation, fear, may therefore be said to occur as an ictal experience more commonly in patients with temporal lobe epilepsy, especially those where limbic system function is disturbed, perhaps more commonly in the dominant hemisphere.

Benzodiazepines in Epilepsy

Benzodiazepines are traditionally used for the control and management of anxiety-related disorders. There is, however, considerable evidence that they possess useful clinical anticonvulsant activity, and their pharmacological profile emphasizes anticonvulsant potential. The clinical literature with regard to the anticonvulsant effects of the benzodiazepines has been extensively reviewed elsewhere (Browne and Penry, 1973; Woodbury *et al.*, 1982) and only a brief introduction will be given here. The use of diazepam, and more recently clonazepam intravenously for status epilepticus is well recognized. Absences status seems particularly sensitive, infantile myoclonic status responding poorly. Orally, however, diazepam has never found acceptance as an anticonvulsant and there are only a few trials of its use as the sole anticonvulsant. Chien and Keegan (1972) randomly divided 42 epileptic patients into two groups, one of which was taken off former drugs and started on diazepam at a dose of 10 mg three times a day. The trial was for six months, and although no differences in the number of patients having seizures was noted, the diazepam group had a significantly higher number of generalized tonic/clonic attacks, and the standard treatment group had more "minor seizures". In a further double-blind study, 32 patients were treated with either diazepam or pheneturide as adjunctive therapy in uncontrolled epilepsy (Hershon and Parsonage, 1969). Fifty per cent of those on the benzodiazepine and 31% on pheneturide had satisfactory improvement in seizure frequency over six months, and this was said to be best in "sub-cortical seizures". Additionally, one reviewer of the subject has reported that findings suggest there is some limited effectiveness of diazepam in the treatment of psychomotor epilepsy (Mattson, 1972).

Other benzodiazepines used in the management of epilepsy include chlordiazepoxide, chlorazepate, lorazepam, nitrazepam, oxazepam, and more recently, the newly introduced 1,5-benzodiazepine, clobazam. Few have been investigated in controlled or double-blind trials. Lon (1968) gave 15 mg of oxazepam or placebo to 11 patients with predominantly complex partial seizures in a cross-over design. The active drug was given as an adjunct to existing therapy for a period of two months. Three became seizure-free, and nine showed a reduction of seizures greater than 50%. Nitrazepam has been found effective in a variety of seizures but particularly in the treatment of infantile spasms with hypsarrhythmia, and in the myoclonic epilepsies of childhood. Reviewing the literature, Baruzzi *et al.* (1982) also commented that nitrazepam was of value in the Lennox-Gastaut syndrome in doses of up to 75 mg a day. Tolerance to its effects was noted in some 50% of patients within three months.

The literature on clonazepam has been well reviewed (Browne, 1978), and of all the benzodiazepines in current use, it has found the most acceptance as oral adjunctive therapy. It has been shown in double-blind trials to be as effective as ethosuccimide, and superior to placebo or diazepam in the management of generalized absence seizures (Chandra, 1973; Mikkelsen *et al.* 1976; Sato *et al.*, 1977). Doses of 3–6 mg a day are typical, and seizures seem controlled with serum concentrations up to 70 ng per ml. Double-blind studies have also confirmed its value in the management of myoclonic seizures (Nanda *et al.*, 1977). However, its potential in the management of generalized tonic/clonic seizures is less clear, and in a recent controlled trial it was shown to be ineffective (Feldman *et al.*, 1981).

There have been some double-blind trials of its use in partial seizures. It seems to be equivalent to sodium valproate in the control of petit mal absences and myoclonic jerking in cases where seizures are intractable, but superior to the latter drug in the management of partial seizures (Lance and Anthony, 1977).

With regard to the effects therefore of the 1,4-benzodiazepines in epilepsy, the limited data which has been collected in a controlled fashion would suggest that they are of value across a wide spectrum of epileptic seizures, but there is a hint that they are more effective against focal seizures than generalized attacks, and the tendency has been towards their acceptance as adjunctive rather than first line therapy in difficult cases of epilepsy. Little pharmacokinetic data is available, and most are reported in the clonazepam studies. In general, interaction with other anticonvulsants is minimal, although phenytoin levels may fall in patients on combined therapy as may the levels of phenobarbitone (Nanda *et al.*, 1977; Edie and Tyrer, 1980).

A limiting factor to their use has been the high frequency of side-effects, especially behaviour problems (see Browne, 1978). Drowsiness and ataxia are recorded in a high percentage of cases and interaction with barbiturates can be particularly severe. Other problems include nausea, headache, double vision, speech disturbance, loss of appetite, listlessness and hypotonia. Behaviour disorders are particularly frequent, especially irritability, restlessness, aggression, outbursts of violence and disinhibition, and more rarely, overt psychiatric illness, including psychotic episodes. Unfortunately, nearly all references to behaviour changes are anecdotal, but the findings bear a resemblance to similar statements that were made about phenobarbitone and behaviour when that drug was tried in epilepsy. In addition, several authors have commented on the role that "forced normalization" may play in the precipitation of behaviour problems in patients with epilepsy prescribed benzodiazepines (Livingstone and Paull, 1977). Thus, in the epilepsy literature, there has been discussed for many years the so-called antagonism theory of the link between psychiatry and epilepsy (for review see Trimble, 1981). At the turn of this century it was thought that seizures and psychosis were somehow mutually exclusive, a concept that led to the introduction of convulsive therapies in psychiatry. Later in time, Landolt (1958) recorded the electroencephalograms of patients with epilepsy who had psychotic episodes that lasted several days or longer, and noted an improvement in their previously abnormal records during the psychosis. On resolution of the psychosis, sometimes initiated by a seizure, the EEGs returned to abnormality leading Landolt to refer to the concept of "forced normalization" of the EEG as a possible mechanism for the development of the psychosis. Such observations have been noted by others, albeit in fewer cases than Landolt collected.

Clinically, while such phenomena are rare, their existence does raise the question of the effect of suddenly normalizing the EEG in epileptic patients with benzodiazepines. This is reported in the literature (Browne and Penry, 1973), and while it is more frequent with generalized discharges, focal abnormalities may be equally responsive. The relationship of such EEG changes to behaviour problems requires further investigation.

1,5-Benzodiazepines in Epilepsy

In contrast to the above literature on the 1,4-benzodiazepines, several authors have suggested that the 1,5-benzodiazepines may have effective anticonvulsant activity but provoke relatively fewer side-effects. Several papers are reviewed in this volume and refer to the early work of Gastaut and Low (1979) in which the authors refer to antiepileptic effects in a percentage of cases "never observed before with any antiepileptic medication". They also commented on a "psychomotor arousal with increased attention, energy and participation in everyday activities".

In a recent trial reported elsewhere (Allen *et al.*, 1983), 26 patients from the Chalfont Centre for Epilepsy with uncontrolled seizures at a rate of four a month were given clobazam or identically matching placebo tablets over a nine-week period using a cross-over design and an eight-week wash-out period between treatments. Half received the placebo first, and half clobazam, the dose of the latter being 30 mg at night with dosage adjustment being permitted if clinical indications required it.

In analysis of the results, the seizures were broadly classified into partial attacks with or without secondary generalization, and generalized episodes. Response to treatment was graded according to the percentage fall in seizures on the active treatment, a 50% or greater drop in frequency in those patients completing the trial being taken as a good therapeutic result. Tolerance to the effect of the drug was examined by comparing the seizure frequency in the first and second half of the active treatment epoch for those responding to the drug and those who had no change in clobazam dose. Withdrawal seizures were assessed by recording the number of attacks in a ten-day period following withdrawal of clobazam in comparison with a similar phase after placebo.

The results of this trial, summarized in Fig. 1 were as follows. Six patients dropped from the study, one during the placebo period. Two patients had the dose of clobazam lowered but completed the trial. A significant fall in seizure frequency during the active treatment period was noted, but most significantly with partial seizures. No tolerance to the effects of the drug was recorded for the nineweek trial period but significantly more seizures were seen in the clobazam withdrawal period when compared with placebo.

In addition to this double-blind trial, we have been collecting data on the long-term use of clobazam in patients with intractable seizures (Allen *et al.*, this publication p. 137). Although from these studies it is clear that tolerance develops in a high percentage of patients who initially respond, a proportion of previously intractable patients continue to benefit without side-effects for a period of at least eight months, similar experiences to those originally reported by Gastaut and Low (1979).

These data taken together indicate that benzodiazepines are effective anticonvulsants clinically, and some of the newly developed ones possess less in the way of sedative effects and possibly more potent anticonvulsant effects than the 1,4-benzodiazepines (Thomp-

son and Trimble, 1981). It is, in particular, partial seizures that respond, which includes of course patients with complex partial seizures arising from a temporal lobe focus.

The Benzodiazepine Receptor, Psychiatry and Epilepsy

Among the significant discoveries in biological psychiatry in recent years has been the characterization of benzodiazepine receptors. These high affinity binding sites on cell membranes from mammalian central nervous system structures seem to have relative potencies for the binding in relation to animal tests that predict anxiolytic properties (Iversen, S. 1983). Of most interest has been that the benzodiazepine and the GABA receptor are intimately linked, and that benzodiazepines enhance the inhibitory synaptic actions of GABA in various regions of the brain where GABAergic synapses are found (see Costa *et al.*, 1978). Further, both GABA and chloride interact with the benzodiazepine binding site to enhance benzodiazepine binding and increase the affinity for diazepam and related drugs (Iversen, L. 1983). It is widely accepted that GABA is involved in modulation of the seizure threshold and that drugs that enhance GABA activity are anticonvulsant (Meldrum, 1981). Further, drugs that enhance GABA transmission are anxiolytic and one of the mechanisms of the action of benzodiazepines in anxiety is through this GABA link (Gray *et al.*, 1983). Benzodiazepines, not only have a well-established role as anxiolytics, but also, as noted above, seem effective anticonvulsants, particularly clinically in patients with focal seizures arising from the temporal lobe. In addition, as emphasized above, temporal lobe structures seem intimately involved in the generation of anxiety, and indeed one current theory lays strong emphasis on links between the hippocampus and the septal area of the limbic system (Gray *et al.*, 1983).

Thus we have an interesting interrelationship between epilepsy, anxiety, benzodiazepines, and GABA, which lays heavy emphasis neuroanatomically on the medial temporal structures which, in particular, have direct limbic system connections, and are of course involved in the pathogenesis of temporal lobe epilepsy. Although benzodiazepine receptors are found all over the central

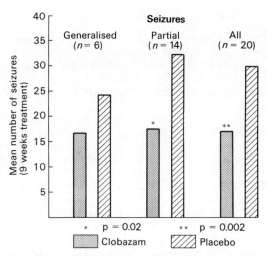

Figure 1. Double-blind controlled study of clobazam in patients with uncontrolled seizures.

nervous system, the high density in the amygdalla (Iversen, S., 1983) may be important in this scheme, particularly with the discovery of different sub-types of benzodiazepine receptors (Iversen, L., 1983).

We have then clinical interrelationships between a psychiatric phenomena, namely anxiety and a neurological problem, namely epilepsy, and laboratory and experimental evidence which hinges anxiolytic and anticonvulsant actions around the newly discovered benzodiazepine receptor. Similar comparisons may be noted with the fascinating interlinks between movement disorders and psychiatry, with the dopamine receptor as a potential theoretical link to explain the clinical phenomena. Thus, movement abnormalities are common in psychiatric patients, drugs which treat psychiatric illness can precipitate movement disorders, and primary movement disorders, such as Huntington's Chorea, are frequently associated with severe psychopathology (see Trimble, 1981). Thus the dopamine receptor has been related not only to control of movement, but the dopamine hypothesis of schizophrenia and related psychotic illnesses also invokes over-activity in at least one group of dopamine receptors in the central nervous system in such disorders. These ideas not only provide grounds for future research, but the finding of clinical phenomena such as a link between temporal lobe epilepsy and anxiety, which appear to have isomorphic representations in the central nervous system in the setting of benzodiazepine receptors, must be of great relevance for our understanding of neuropsychiatric relationships.

References

Allen, J. W., Oxley, J., Robertson, M. M., Trimble, M. R., Richens, A. and Jawad, S. S. M. (1983). Clobazam as an adjunctive treatment in refractory epilepsy. *British Medical Journal* **286**, 1246–1247.

Baruzzi, A., Michelucci, R. and Tassinari, C. A. (1982). Nitrazepam. In "Antiepileptic Drugs" (D. M. Woodbury, J. K. Penry and C. E. Pippenger, eds), pp. 753–769. Raven Press, New York.

Browne, T. R. (1978). Clonazepam. *New England Journal of Medicine* **299**, 812–815.

Browne, T. R. and Penry, J. K. (1973). Benzodiazepines in the treatment of epilepsy. *Epilepsia* **14**, 277–312.

Chandra, B. (1973). Clonazepam in the treatment of petit mal. *Asian Journal of Medicine* **9**, 433–438.

Chien, C. and Keegan, D. (1972). Diazepam as an oral long term anticonvulsant for epileptic mental patients. *Diseases of the Nervous System* **33**, 100–104.

Costa, E., Guidotti, A. and Tofano, G. (1978). Molecular mechanisms mediating the action of diazepam on GABA receptors. *British Journal of Psychiatry* **133**, 239–248.

Edie, M. J. and Tyrer, J. H. (1980). "Anticonvulsant therapy." Churchill Livingstone, Edinburgh.

Feldman, R. G., Hayes, M. K. and Browne, T. R. (1981). A double blind comparison of clonazepam with placebo for refractory tonic/clonic seizures. *Neurology* **31**, 159.

Gastaut, H. (1969). Clinical and electroencephalographic classification of epileptic seizures. International League against Epilepsy. *Epilepsia* **10** (Suppl.), S2–S13.

Gastaut, H. and Low, M. D. (1979). Antiepileptic properties of clobazam. A 1,5-benzodiazepine in man. *Epilepsia* **20**, 437–446.

Gibbs, F. A. and Stamps, F. W. (1958). "Epilepsy Handbook." Thomas, Springfield.

Gibbs, F. A., Gibbs, E. L. and Lennox, W. G. (1938). Cerebral Dysrhythmias of epilepsy. *Archives of Neurology and Psychiatry* **39**, 298–314.

Gloor, P., Olivier, A., Quesney, L. F., Andermann, F. and Horowitz, S. (1982). The role of the limbic system in experimental phenomena of temporal lobe epilepsy. *Annals of Neurology* **12**, 129–144.

Gray, J. A., Quintero, S. and Mellanby, J. (1983). GABA, the benzodiazepines and the septohippocampal system. In "Benzodiazepines Divided" (M. R. Trimble, ed.), pp. 101–127. John Wiley and Sons, Chichester.

Hermann, B. P., Dikmen, S., Schwartz, M. S. and Karnes, W. E. (1982). Interictal psychopathology in patients with ictal fear. A quantitative investigation. *Neurology* **32**, 7–11.

Hershon, H. I. and Parsonage, M. (1969). Comparative trial of diazepam and pheneturide in the treatment of epilepsy. *Lancet* **2**, 859–862.

Iversen, L. (1983). Benzodiazepine receptors. In "Benzodiazepines Divided" (M. R. Trimble, ed.), pp. 79–85. John Wiley and Sons, Chichester.

Iversen, S. (1983). Where in the brain do benzodiazepines act. In "Benzodiazepines Divided" (M. R. Trimble, ed.), pp. 167–185. John Wiley and Sons, Chichester.

Lance, J. W. and Anthony, M. (1977). Sodium valproate and clonazepam in the treatment of intractable epilepsy. *Archives of Neurology* **34**, 14–17.

Landolt, H. (1958). Serial EEG investigations during psychotic episodes in epileptic patients and during schizophrenic attacks. In "Lectures on Epilepsy" (A. M. Lorentz de Hass, ed.), pp. 91–133. Elsevier, London.

Lennox, W. G. (1960). Epilepsy and Related Disorders." J. and A. Churchill, London.

Livingston, S., Pauli, L. L. and Pruce, I. (1977). Clorazepate in epilepsy. *Journal of the American Medical Association* **237**, 1561.

Lon, H. O. C. (1968). Oxazepam in the treatment of psychomotor epilepsy. *Neurology* **18**, 986–990.

MacLean, P. D. (1970). The triune brain, emotion and scientific bias. In "The Neurosciences: Second Study Programme" (F. O. Schmitt, ed.), pp. 336–349. Rockefeller University Press, New York.

Mattson, R. H. (1972). The benzodiazepines. In "Antiepileptic Drugs" (D. M. Woodbury, J. K. Penry and R. P. Schmidt, eds), pp 497–516. Raven Press, New York.

Meldrum, B. S. (1981). GABA agonists as antiepileptic agents. In "GABA and Benzodiazepine Receptors" (E. Costa, G. De Chiara and G. L. Gessa, eds), pp. 207–217. Raven Press, New York.

Mikkelsen, B., Birket-Smith, E., Brandt, S., Holme, P., Lund, M., Thorn, I., Olsen, P. Z. and Vestermark, S. (1976). Clonazepam in the treatment of epilepsy. *Archives of Neurology* **33**, 322–325.

Mikkelsen, B., Berggreen, P., Joensen, P., Kristensen, O., Kohler, O. and Mikkelsen, B. O. (1977). Treatment of epilepsy with clonazepam and its effect on other anticonvulsants. *Journal of Neurology, Neurosurgery and Psychiatry* **40**, 538–543.

Nanda, R. N., Johnson, R. H., Keogh, H. J., Lambie, D. G. and Melville, I. D. (1977). Treatment of epilepsy with clonazepam and its effet on other anticonvulsants. *Journal of Neurology, Neurosurgery and Psychiatry* **40**, 538–543.

Papez, J. W. (1937). A proposed mechanism of emotion. *Archives of Neurology and Psychiatry* **38**, 725–743.

Pritchard, J. C. (1822). "A Treatise on Diseases of the Nervous System." Thomas and George Underwood, London.

Sato, S., Penry, J. K., Dreifuss, F. and Dyken, P. (1977). Clonazepam in the treatment of absence seizures. A double blind clinical trial. *Neurology* **27**, 371.

Thompson, P. and Trimble, M. R. (1981). Clobazam and cognitive functions. In "Clobazam." *Royal Society of Medicine International Congress and Symposium Series* **43**, 33–38.

Trimble, M. R. (1981). "Neuropsychiatry." John Wiley and Sons, Chichester.

Trimble, M. R. (1983a) Interictal behaviour and temporal lobe epilepsy. In "Recent Advances in Epilepsy" (T. A. Pedley and B. S. Meldrum, eds), Vol. 1, pp. 211–228. Churchill Livingstone, Edinburgh.

Trimble, M. R. (1983b). History of classification in epilepsy. In "Research Progress in Epilepsy" (F. Clifford Rose, ed.), pp. 1–7. Pitman, Bath.

Trimble, M. R. and Zarifian, E. (1984). "Psychopharmacology of the Limbic System." Oxford University Press, Oxford.

Williams, D. (1956). The structure of emotions reflected in epileptic experiences. *Brain* **79**, 29–67.

Woodbury, D. M., Penry, J. K. and Pippenger, C. E. (1982). "Antiepileptic Drugs." Raven Press, New York.

A Review of Clobazam Studies in Epilepsy

D. KOEPPEN

Klinische Forschung, Hoechst AG, D-6230 Frankfurt am Main 80,
W. Germany

Summary

Clobazam, a 1,5-benzodiazepine, was given to 1055 patients with epilepsy in daily doses of $0.1–2.5$ mg/kg in 21 open, one single-blind and three double-blind placebo-controlled studies.

Clobazam was used predominantly as adjunctive therapy to standard anticonvulsant medication in order to improve the treatment response. In the open studies, disappearance or a reduced incidence of seizures was observed in 69% of the patients. In 40% of those who initially improved, a relative or absolute loss of efficacy was observed over a period of time. The placebo-controlled studies have further demonstrated the anticonvulsant efficacy of clobazam, and a response was seen in all seizure types.

Side-effects occurred in one-third of patients and consisted mainly of sedation, muscular weakness and mood disturbances. Positive treatment benefits were reported in 19% of patients; usually improved vigilance, school and work performance and an elevation of mood.

The overall data show clobazam to be a potent and well-tolerated adjunctive medication for epileptic patients with all types of seizures. Possible tolerance after initial therapeutic response, withdrawal symptoms including seizures and pharmacokinetic interactions with standard anticonvulsants should be taken into account when assessing the risk-benefit ratio of clobazam treatment in individual patients.

Introduction

Benzodiazepines such as clonazepam, diazepam, and nitrazepam are "standard drugs in the treatment of epilepsy" (Schmidt, 1981) and are also accepted as "first-line antiepileptic agents" (Matthes, 1977). Their spectrum of action in the various types of seizures is relatively broad (Eadie, 1981; Glaser, 1980), however major problems when treating epileptic patients with benzodiazepines are a loss of efficacy after initial response and side-effects (Gastaut, 1981). The reasons for this loss of efficacy known as the "escape phenomenon" are unclear. Where it occurs, the effects either lessen considerably or subside completely after weeks or months of successful therapy which are not reversed by a further dose increase.

Side-effects of benzodiazepines in epilepsy are usually drowsiness, confusion, changes in mood, and impairment of motor performance. As with phenobarbital, primidone or phenytoin, withdrawal symptoms can be expected when benzodiazepines are discontinued; sleep disturbances, restlessness, tremor and an increase of seizures (Schmidt, 1981).

The benzodiazepines currently used in the treatment of epilepsy have a 1,4-structure, whereas clobazam is a 1,5-benzodiazepine (Kuch, 1979). The 2,4-dione structure of clobazam, present in several other antiepileptic drugs may be the chemical feature which is responsible for its anticonvulsant effects (Kruse, this issue, pp. 113–120).

Clobazam has shown marked anticonvulsant effects in animal studies (Ballabio *et al.*, 1981; Caccia *et al.*, 1980; Chapman *et al.*, 1978; Shenoy *et al.*, 1982) and its main metabolite, *N*-desmethylclobazam (Meldrum and Croucher, 1982) has one quarter the potency of clobazam. However, both substances have different pharmacokinetics, the elimination half-life of *N*-desmethylclobazam being 35–133 h, markedly longer than that of clobazam which is 10–55 h (Lüttkenhorst and Ochs, 1980; Marcia Divoll *et al.*, 1982; Rupp *et al.*, 1979). Therefore, during long-term treatment, steady-state levels of the metabolite become higher than those of clobazam itself.

With regard to psychomotor effects, animal studies suggest memory-protective

effects for clobazam in comparison to diazepam in electroshock induced amnesia (Hock
and Kruse, 1982). Further, clobazam showed
less pronounced effects on vigilance, psychomotor performance and memory in comparison to the 1,4-benzodiazepines at therapeutically equipotent doses in healthy volunteers
and anxious patients thus confirming the
animal studies (Hindmarch, 1979; Koeppen,
1983; Nicholson, 1979; Paes de Sousa et al.,
1981).

These results suggest that clobazam possesses antiepileptic activity and has less detrimental sedative and dysmnesic effects compared with the 1,4-benzodiazepines.

Patient Populations

Twenty-one open studies were performed
in 1055 epileptic patients (Bianchi et al., 1980;
Bonis, 1979; Bravaccio et al., 1979; Bunn et
al., 1983; Cano et al., 1981; Courjon, 1979;
Dehnerdt et al., 1981; Dulac et al., 1983;
Escobedo et al., 1978; Favel, 1980; Gastaut
and Low, 1979; Grappe, 1982; Loiseau,
1979a; Martin, 1981; Pechadre et al., 1981;
Ramos et al., 1981; Rucquoy-Ponsar et al.,
1979; Shimizu et al., 1982; Sorel et al., 1982;
Vakil et al., 1981; Wolf et al., 1981), one
single-blind study (del Pesce et al., 1979) and
three double-blind placebo-controlled studies
(Critchley et al., 1981; Feely et al., 1982;
Allen et al., 1983). In addition, the interaction of clobazam with standard anticonvulsants was followed-up in two pharmacokinetic studies in healthy volunteers (Loiseau,
1979b; Tedeschi et al., 1981).

The majority of studies were carried out in
France, England and Italy where five studies
each were performed, in Germany and Bel-
gium with two studies each and one study
each in Spain, Japan and Mexico.

Clobazam was given mainly to patients
(approximately $\frac{2}{3}$ of cases) of both sexes and
of ages from six months to 67 years, suffering
from various therapy-resistant epileptic disorders (Table 1).

Clobazam was administered mainly as
adjunctive therapy to standard anticonvulsants, but in one study clobazam was given as
monotherapy to epileptic children (Dulac et
al., 1983), and a further recent study included
15 children treated with clobazam as
monotherapy in which EEG changes were
studied (Plouin and Jalin, this issue). When

clobazam was prescribed by a mg/kg regimen, the daily doses varied from 0·1–2·5 mg/
kg/day [Dose Range 10–120 mg/day]. The
majority of clobazam daily doses were
30–80 mg (0·5–1·0 mg/kg).

Results

Open studies

A reduction in seizures was observed in
69% of the 793 epileptic patients from the 18
open studies which contained detailed reports
on efficacy data (Table 2). Clobazam pos-
sessed anticonvulsant activity for all types of
seizures. The EEG data tended to correlate
with clinical observations on improvement
and efficacy data showed a high degree
(17·7%) of total seizure reduction, which is of
significance considering that most patients
were therapy-resistant. The risk of worsening
epileptic states by adding clobazam seems to
be very low (2%).

In studies lasting longer than three months,
consistently positive effects with clobazam
were reported in 41·6% of the patients.

The rate of seizure recurrence was calculated in this sample as the number of patients
who, after the initial improvement, showed a
poorer response with further treatment compared with their initial response.

This rate not only includes patients where
the initial response completely disappeared,
but also patients in whom the long-term
effect was worse than the initial response.
Although the condition of the latter was still
better than that before taking clobazam,
these patients were included in the calculation
of those suffering from the escape phenomenon. The escape rate with clobazam was
39·8%. Tolerance was seen in some cases as
early as a few days after starting treatment,
but in others it did not occur until up to 27
months of therapy. The majority of escapes
were reported after 1–3 months.

Placebo-controlled studies

One single-blind and three double-blind
studies compared clobazam to placebo. The
single-blind study was carried out in 28
patients with either generalized ($N = 17$) or

Table 1

Seizure types in the patient population

Seizure type	Number of patients[a]
Partial (not specified)	201
Simple partial	26
Complex partial[b]	81
Complex partial evolving to GTC[b]	130
Sum of partial seizures	438
Generalized (not specified)	251
Absences	63
Myoclonic	23
Clonic	2
Tonic-clonic (Grand Mal)	84
Atonic, Lennox-Gastaut	80
Sum of generalized seizures	503
Partial and generalized	86
Mixed	19
Unclassified	118
Total sum	1164

[a]Patients with multiple seizures included, therefore the number of patients according to seizure type is greater than the overall number of patients investigated (1055).
[b]Known to be therapy resistant.
GTC = Generalized Tonic-Clonic.

Table 2

Anticonvulsant activity of clobazam (open studies)

Reduction of seizures	Number of patients	Percentage
Reduction (unspecified)	250	31·5
100%	140	17·7
>75%	72	9·1
50–75%	76	9·6
<50%	9	1·1
Sum: Improvement	547	69·0
No change	230	29·0
Worsening	16	2·0
Total	793	100·0

partial ($N = 11$) seizures. Clobazam was given as an adjunct to existing treatment in doses of 20–50 mg/day (del Pesce *et al.*, 1979). Based on patient preference ratings, the antiepileptic action of clobazam was judged to be significantly better than placebo.

The use of clobazam 20 mg (single evening dose) as co-medication was followed up in a double-blind placebo comparison in 28 therapy-resistant epileptic patients (Critchley *et al.*, 1981). The periods of medication lasted six weeks, interrupted by a one-week placebo washout period. The mean frequencies of generalized and partial seizures in the clobazam and placebo periods indicated a superior antiepileptic efficacy of clobazam (Fig. 1).

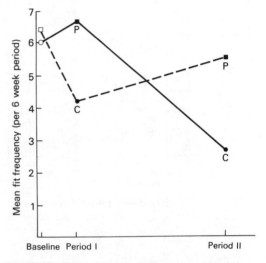

Figure 1. Mean seizure frequency with clobazam (20 mg/day) (C) and placebo (P) in 28 therapy-resistant epileptic inpatients (Critchley et al., 1981).

In a further double-blind study, daily doses of clobazam 30 mg/day were given to therapy-resistant patients with partial ($N = 14$) and generalized ($N = 6$) seizures (Allen *et al.*, 1983). Clobazam and placebo were administered adjunctively for nine weeks with an intermittent washout period of eight weeks. The follow-up withdrawal period lasted one week. The seizure frequency with clobazam was significantly better than placebo ($P < 0·01$), especially for that of partial seizures (Fig. 2).

Eighteen patients with catamenial epilepsy (a clustering of seizures during menstruation), suffering from generalized, simple, complex and absence seizures received daily doses of 20–30 mg clobazam or placebo for ten days during and around the menstrual period. Clobazam showed a significantly better reduction of seizures than placebo (Feely *et al.*, 1982) (Fig. 3).

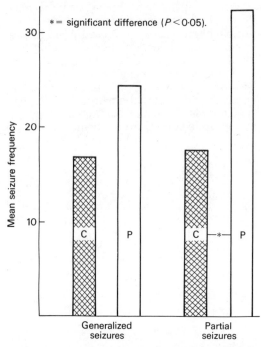

Figure 2. Generalized and partial seizures with clobazam (30 mg/day) (C) and placebo (P) (Allen et al., 1983).

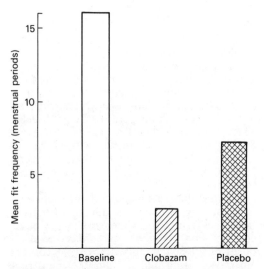

Figure 3. Clobazam (20–30 mg/day) and placebo in 18 outpatients with catamenial epilepsy (Feely et al., 1982).

Side effects

Open studies

Nineteen of the 21 open studies reported side-effect data with clobazam (Table 3), although often the reports did not specify their incidence. Where quantifiable data were given, the overall incidence was 33%. Sedative effects such as drowsiness, dizziness and fatigue, predominated in 19 studies. Further side-effects were muscular weakness, restlessness, aggression, ataxia, and unpleasant mood states. Weight increase was seen in five studies, although two studies reported no weight changes (Courjon, 1979; Grappe, 1982).

Placebo-controlled studies

In a brief report on the single-blind study, drowsiness ($N = 14$) and impairment of cognitive function (no incidence given) were reported as side-effects of clobazam (del Pesce et al., 1979).

Critchley et al. (1981) stated "side effects and behaviour monitored throughout the study did not indicate differences between clobazam and placebo". Allen et al. (1983) observed side-effects in six patients on clobazam (irritability, depression, and disinhibition) and two patients on placebo (not speci-

Table 3

Adverse reactions of clobazam
in epileptic patients

Adverse reactions (19 out of 23 open studies)	Number of studies
Drowsiness, dizziness, fatigue	19
Muscular weakness	7
Restlessness aggressiveness	7
Weight increase	5
Ataxic state	4
Unpleasant mood state	3
Atonic state	
Hyperkinetic symptoms	
Delusional state	
Psychotic symptoms	
Behaviour disturbances	2
Vertigo	
Hypersalivation	
Oedema	

fied) out of a total of 20 patients. The latter two studies also mentioned the occurrence of withdrawal seizures after cessation of clobazam.

Feely *et al.* (1982) reported sedation ($N=4$), depression ($N=2$), galactorrhoea ($N=1$) and nausea, diarrhoea, tightness in chest and throat ($N=1$) with clobazam.

In summary, these studies indicated that sedation, mood disturbances and muscular weakness were the most common side-effects of clobazam as adjunctive medication in epilepsy. Aggressiveness and restlessness are mentioned more frequently than in studies with anxious patients (Koeppen, 1981). Withdrawal symptoms including seizures were reported as important complications of therapy.

Neither physical examination (general, cardiac and circulatory function, neurological examination) nor laboratory measures showed any adverse changes with clobazam.

Positive Effects

In 13 out of the 21 open studies, beneficial effects in addition to anticonvulsant activity were reported. The incidence of these favourable side-effects was 18·7%. They were increased alertness, better school and job performance and improved social activity (ten studies). In eight studies, patients stated they felt better and in three studies there was a reduction of anxiety, aggressiveness, hyper-

Table 4

Blood levels of clobazam and N-desmethylclobazam during concomitant standard treatment with anticonvulsanmts

Author	Clobazam blood levels				N-desmethylclobazam blood levels			
	CBZ	DPH	PBT	VPA	CBZ	DPH	PBT	VPA
Cano	(↓)	(↓)	↓	↓	↑	↑	(↓)	
Loiseau	↓		↑					
Sorel	0	0	0	0	0	0	0	0

↑ or ↓: Increase or decrease of blood levels.
0: no change.
(↑) (↓): exceptional changes.
No indication of correlation therapeutic response/C and NDC blood levels (Dulac *et al.*, 1983).
Possible correlation sedation/C and NDC blood levels (Wolf *et al.*, 1981).
CBZ = carbamazepine, DPH = phenytoin, PBT = phenobarbital, VPA = sodium valproate, NDC = *N*-desmethylclobazam.

Table 5

Blood levels of standard anticonvulsants during clobazam treatment

Author	CBZ	DPH	PBT	PRM	VPA	Anticonvulsants (unspecified)
Bianchi	0	0	0			
Bonis	0	0	0		0	
Courjon						0
Dehnerdt						0
Pechadre			0			
Ramos						0
Sorel	0	0	0	0	↑	
Vakil	(↑)	(↑)	(↑)			
Wolf	(↑)					

0: No change; ↑: increase of blood levels; (↑): exceptional increase of blood levels.
CBZ = carbamazepine, DPH = phenytoin, PBT = phenobarbital, PRM = primidone, VAP = sodium valproate.

kinesis or restlessness. In one study, improvement of vertigo, enuresis and psychomotor performance was reported.

Pharmacokinetics

Two studies with healthy volunteers (Loiseau, 1979b; Tedeschi *et al.*, 1981) and 11 clinical studies reported on pharmacokinetic interactions between clobazam and standard anticonvulsants (Bianchi *et al.*, 1980; Boris, 1979; Cano *et al.*, 1981; Courjon, 1979; Dehnerdt *et al.*, 1981; Pechadré *et al.*, 1981; Ramos *et al.*, 1981; Sorel *et al.*, 1982; Allen *et al.*, 1983; Vakil *et al.*, 1981; Wolf *et al.*, 1981). The findings suggest that clobazam blood levels tend to decrease with concomitant standard anticonvulsants (Table 4) as did blood levels of *N*-desmethylclobazam with concomitant phenobarbitone. However, if carbamazepine or phenytoin were taken as concomitant medication, blood levels of the metabolite increased.

Blood levels of standard anticonvulsants tended to increase with concomitant clobazam. However, these trends were not consistent and require further confirmation (Table 5).

Discussion

When considering the efficacy and safety of clobazam in epileptic patients it must be borne in mind that in most of the 25 studies reviewed it was usually co-prescribed for therapy-resistant patients as adjunctive medication to existing standard anticonvulsants.

The efficacy of anticonvulsant medication in general (single *and* combined drug therapy) is such that one-third show a disappearance of seizures, one-third a reduction and the remaining third exhibit no change, or a deterioration in the overall condition (Christiani, 1982; Schmidt, 1981; Wolf, 1979).

In 42% of patients treated for more than three months with clobazam, seizures disappeared or decreased. While this percentage is lower than that with standard anticonvulsants (approximately 66% over 2–3 years), it must be considered, that the reports for clobazam are for therapy-resistant cases, and that the overall result for clobazam represents a notable additional therapeutic benefit.

Matthes (1977) mentions a seizure rate of recurrence of 10–20% for clonazepam. Browne and Penry (1973) cite rates of recurrence of between 8 and 52% (median 26%) in their review article on benzodiazepines. The rate of recurrence with clobazam was 40% in refractory patients already undergoing treatment with other anticonvulsant agents.

The overall incidence of side-effects was almost the same as that of patients with anxiety (Koeppen, 1981). With respect to specific types of side-effects, there were similarities to those seen in patients with anxiety who were treated with clobazam. In both indications, drowsiness was the most frequent problem, however muscular weakness, ataxia, atonia, restlessness, and aggression are more frequent in epileptic than anxious patients. In epilepsy, the effects of an interaction between clobazam and standard anticonvulsants should be considered, especially with respect to the predominance of sedative effects.

Compared with the other benzodiazepines prescribed in epilepsy, it is likely that clobazam leads to less sedation. Browne and Penry (1973) cite seven out of 23 studies reporting an incidence of drowsiness with 1,4-benzodiazepines higher than 40%. Such a rate of drowsiness was found in only two out of 16 studies (12·5%) with clobazam. These weaker sedative effects of clobazam are also in keeping with reported improvements in performance at school and work.

Symptoms of withdrawal are known to occur with other benzodiazepines as well as clobazam and the non-benzodiazepine anticonvulsants (Schmidt, 1981). A possible explanation for these rare but important withdrawal effects which are seen with clobazam may be related to enzyme induction by standard anticonvulsant medication and might lead to accelerated elimination of the adjunctive medication (clobazam) after a rapid termination of therapy.

There was no correlation between clobazam dose, blood levels and side-effects. However, it is possible that sedation and confusion might occur with high blood levels of clobazam and *N*-desmethylclobazam (Wolf *et al.*, 1981).

From the data available an absolute dose recommendation cannot be determined. However, the following dosage regimens are efficacious and safe; low initial doses (5–10 mg/day) should gradually be increased to daily doses of about 40 mg. Fixed medium doses (20 mg/day) and intermittent treatment, with re-prescribing of clobazam after clobazam-free intervals are the regimens of choice in those patients who exhibit the escape phenomenon.

As with other anticonvulsant medication particular attention must be paid to possible withdrawal reactions (including seizures), especially after abrupt cessation of clobazam (Schmidt, 1981). In addition, the pharmacokinetic data suggest that when establishing patients on supplementary anticonvulsant therapy and during the course of treatment generally, routine assessments of blood levels of other anticonvulsants are necessary when giving clobazam, especially if toxicity is suspected.

In summary, clobazam can be characterized as a useful adjunctive medication in therapy resistant patients. Its usefulness as monotherapy, and in patients generally responding to alternative anticonvulsant treatment remains to be investigated further.

References

Allen, J., Oxley, J., Robertson, M., Trimble, M., Richens, A., and Jawad, S. (1983). Clobazam as adjunctive treatment in refractory epilepsy. *British Medical Journal* **286**, 1246–1247.

Ballabio, M., Caccia, S., Garattini, S., Guiso, G., and Zanini, M.G. (1981). Antileptazol activity and kinetics of clobazam and *N*-desmethylclobazam in the guinea pig. *Archives of International Pharmacodynamics and Therapeutics* **253**, 192–199.

Bianchi, A., Bollea, A., and Sideri, G. (1980). L'Emploi du Clobazam dans l'Epilepsie: Experience d'un An de Traitement. Canger, R./Avanzini, G./Tassinari, C.A. (Hrsg.). *Progressi in Epilettologia. Boll Lega Italiana contro l'Epilepsia* **29–30**, 215–218.

Bonis, A. (1979). A clinical investigation into the usage of clobazam in the treatment of severe chronic epilepsy. Unpublished report on file.

Bravaccio, F., Tata, M.R., Ambrosio, G.D., De Rosa, A., and Volpe, E. (1979). Sulle Proprieta Antiepilettiche di un Diazepinico (Clobazam). *Acta Neurologica* **39**, 58–64.

Browne, T.R., and Penry, K.J. (1973). Benzodiazepines in the treatment of epilepsy. *Epilepsia* **14**, 277–310.

Bunn, H., Iliadis, A., Bruno, R., Cano, J.P., Dravet, C., and Roger, J. (1983). Contribution of simulation in the study of the time-dependence and clinical response of clobazam. Internal report, Faculte de Pharmacie Marseille, Frankreich.

Caccia, S., Carli, M., Garattini, S., Poggesi, E., Rech, R., and Samanin, R. (1980). Pharmacological activities of clobazam and diazepam in the rat: relation to drug brain levels. *Archives of International Pharmacodynamics and Therapeutics* **243**, 275–283.

Cano, J.P., Bun, H., Iliadis, A., Dravet, A., Roger, J., and Gastaut, H. (1981). Influence of anti-epileptic drugs on plasma levels of clobazam and desmethylclobazam: application of research on relations between doses, plasma levels and clinical efficacy. International Congress and Symposium Series, No. 43 (I. Hindmarch and P. D. Stonier, eds), pp. 169–174. Royal Society of Medicine, Lodon.

Chapman, A.G., Horton, R.W., and Meldrum, B.S. (1978). Anticonvulsant action of a 1,5-benzodiazepine, clobazam, in reflex epilepsy. *Epilepsia* **19**, 293–299.

Christiani, K. (1982). Klinik der epilepsien. *Nervenheilkunde* **1**, 1–5.

Courjon, J. (1979). Rapport sur l'action du clobazam sur l'epilepsie. Lyon. Unpublished report on file.

Critchley, E.M.R., Valil, S.D., Hayward, H.W., Owen, M.V.H., Cocks, A., and Freemantle, N.P. (1981). Double-blind clinical trial of clobazam in refractory epilepsy. International Congress and Symposium Series No. 43 (I. Hindmarch and P. D. Stonier, eds), pp. 159–163. Royal Society of Medicine, London.

Dehnerdt, M., Boenick, H.E., and Rambeck, B. (1980). Clobazam (Frisium^R) zur Behandlung komplizierter Epilepsien? "Epilepsie" (H. Remschmidt, R. Rentz and J. Jungmann, eds), pp. 172–175. G. Thieme Verlag, Stuttgart.

Dulac, O., Figueroa, D., Rey, E., and Arthuis, M. (1983). Monotherapie par le clobazam dans les epilepsies de l'enfant. *La Presse Médicale* **12** (17), 1067–1069.

Eadie, M.J. (1981). Anticonvulsant therapy: Present and future. *TIPS* **2**, 37–39.

Escobedo, F., Otero, E., Chaparro, H., Flores, T., and Rubio-D, F. (1978). Experience with clobazam as another antiepileptic drug. Epilepsy International Symposium, Vancouver.

Favel, P. (1980). Experimentation du Clobazam dans le traitement de l'epilepsie. Tai-L'Hermitage. Unpublished report on file.

Feely, M., Calvert, R., and Gibson, J. (1982). Clobazam in catamenial epilepsy. A model for evaluating anticonvulsants. *The Lancet* **2**, 71–73.

Gastaut, H. (1981). The effects of benzodiazepines on chronic epilepsy in Man (with particular reference to clobazam). *In* "Clobazam" (I. Hindmarch and P. D. Stonier, eds), pp. 141–150. International Congress and Symposium Series No. 43. Royal Society of Medicine, London.

Gastaut, H., and Low, M. (1979). Antiepileptic properties of clobazam, a 1,5-benzodiazepine in man. *Epilepsia* **20**, 437–446.

Glaser, G.H. (1980). Mechanisms of antiepileptic drug action: clinical indicators. *In* "Antiepileptic Drugs: Mechanisms of Action" (G. H. Glaser, J. K. Penry, and D. M. Woodbury, eds), p. 11. Raven Press, New York.

Grappe, G. (1982). Resultats du traitement de 61 epilepsies graves par le clobazam (thesis). University of Nancy.

Hindmarch, I. (1979). Some aspects of the effects of clobazam on human psychomotor performance. *British Journal of Clinical Pharmacology* **7** (Suppl. 1), 77S–82S.

Hock, F.J., and Kruse, H.J. (1982). Differential effects of psychotropic drugs on ECS-induced amnesia in a passive avoidance task. Anxiolytic drugs: diazepam versus clobazam. *IRCS-Medical Science* **10**, 3, 221–222.

Koeppen, D. (1981). Clinical experience with clobazam (1968–1981). *In* "Clobazam" (I. Hindmarch and P. D. Stonier, eds), pp. 193–198. International Congress and Symposium Series No. 43. Royal Society of Medicine, London.

Koeppen, D. (1983). Memory and benzodiazepines. Animal and human studies with 1,4-benzodiazepines and clobazam (1,5-benzodiazepine). World Congress of Psychiatry, Vienna.

Kruse, H.J. (1982). Clobazam: induction of hyperlocomotion in a new nonautomatized device for measuring motor activity and exploratory behaviour in mice: comparison with diazepam and critical evaluation of the results with anautomatized hole-board apparatus. *Drug Development Research* **2** (Suppl. 1), 145–151.

Kuch, H. (1979). Clobazam: chemical aspects of the 1,4- and 1,5-benzodiazepines. *British Journal of Clinical Pharmacology* **7** (Suppl. 1), 17S–21S.

Loiseau, P. (1979a). Essai Clinique du clobazam, I. 3 mois. II. 1 an. Bordeaux.

Loiseau, P. (1979b). Clobazam interaction with carbamazepine in normal man. Bordeaux.

Lüttkenhorst, M., and Ochs, H.R. (1980). Untersuchungen zur Kinetik von clobazam (Frisium). 86. Tagung der Dtsch. Gesellschaft für innere Medizin, Wiesbaden.

Marcia Divoll, B.S., Greenblatt, D., Ciraulo, D., Surendra, K., Ho, I., and Shader, R. (1982). Clobazam kinetics: Intrasubject variability and effect of food on absorption. *Journal of Clinical Pharmacology* **22**, 69–73.

Martin, A.A. (1981). The anti-epileptic effects of clobazam: A long-term study in resistant epilepsy. *In* "Clobazam" (I. Hindmarch and P. D. Stonier, eds), pp. 151–157. International Congress and Symposium Series No. 43. Royal Society of Medicine, London.

Matthes, A. (1977). Epilepsie. Diagnostik und Therapie für Klinik und Praxis. G. Thieme Verlag, Stuttgart.

Meldrum, B.S., and Croucher, M.J. (1982). Anticonvulsant action of clobazam and desmethylclobazam in reflex epilepsy in rodents and baboons. *Drug Development Research* Suppl. 1, 33–38.

Nicholson, A.N. (1979). Differential effects of the 1,4- and 1,5-benzodiazepines on performance in healthy man. *British Journal of Clinical Pharmacology* 7 (Suppl. 1), 83S–84S.

Paes de Sousa, M., Figuiera, M.-L., Loureiro, F., and Hindmarch, I. (1981). Lorazepam and clobazam in anxious elderly patients. *In* "Clobazam" (I. Hindmarch and P. D. Stonier, eds), pp. 119–123. International Congress and Symposium Series No. 43. Royal Society of Medicine, London.

Pechadre, J.C., Beudin, P., Devoize, J.L., and Gilbert J. (1981). Raport sur les effets antiépileptiques dans le syndrome de Lennox et Gastaut. *L'Encéphale* VII, 181–190.

Del Pesce, M., Fua, P., Giuliani, G., Provinciali, L., Pigin, P., and Gamba, G. (1979). Clobazam as an antiepileptic drug. 11th Epilepsy Intern. Symposium Florench, Abstract 423.

Ramos, P.R., Diez-Cvervo, A., Caro, J.S., Manrique, M., Serrano, J.P., and Coullaut, J. (1981). Pharmacological action of clobazam in serious epileptic patients. *In* IIIrd World Congress of Biological Psychiatry (G. Struwe, ed.). Stockholm, Abstract F395.

Rucquoy-Ponsar, M., Harmant, J., and Sorel, L. (1979). Etude Préliminaire des Effets antiépileptiques du Clobazam (Frisium) vortrag BCNBP, Lüttich 11.

Rupp, W., Badian, M., Christ, O., Hajdu, P., Kulkarni, R., Taeuber, K., Uihlein, M., Bender, R., and Vanderbeke, O. (1979). Pharmacokinetics of single and multiple doses of clobazam in humans. *British Journal of Clinical Pharmacology* 7 (Suppl. 1), 51S–57S.

Schmidt, D. (1981). "Behandlung der Epilepsien medikamentös, psychosozial, operativ." Georg Thieme Verlag, Stuttgart, New York.

Shenoy, A.K., Miyahara, J.T., Swinyard, E.A., and Kupferberg, H.J. (1982). Comparative anticonvulsant activity and neurotoxicity of clobazam, diazepam, phenobarbital, and valproate in mice and rats. *Epilepsia* 23 (4), 399–408.

Shimizu, H., Abe, J., Futagi, Y., Onoe, S., Tagawa, T., Nimaki, T., Yamatodani, A., Kato, M., Kamio, M., Sumi, K., Sugita, T., and Yabuuchi, H. (1982). Antiepileptic effects of clobazam in children. *Brain and Development* 4 (1), 57–62.

Sorel, L., Kittirath, S.H., Rucquoy-Ponsar, M., and Harmant, J. (1982). Etude de l'action antiepileptique du clobazam (Frisium). Ottingnies.

Paes de Sousa, M., Figuiera, M.L., Loureiro, F., and Hindmarch, I. (1981). Lorazepam and clobazam in anxious elderly patients. *In* "Clobazam" (I. Hindmarch and P. D. Stonier, eds), pp. 119–123. International Congress and Symposium Series No. 43. Royal Society of Medicine, London.

Tedeschi, G., Riva, R., and Baruzzi, A. (1981). Clobazam plasma concentrations: pharmacokinetic study in healthy volunteers and data in epileptic patients. *British Journal of Clinical Pharmacology* 11, 619–621.

Vakil, S.D., Critchley, E.M.R., Cocks, A., and Hayward, H. (1981). The effect of clobazam on blood levels of phenobarbitone, phenytoin and carbamazepine (preliminary report). *In* "Clobazam" (I. Hindmarch and P. D. Stonier, eds), pp. 165–167. International Congress and Symposium Series No. 43. Royal Society of Medicine, London.

Wolf, P. (1979). Verlaufsprognose von Epilepsie. *Aktuelle Neurologie* 6, 197–203.

Wolf, P., Beck-Mannagetta, G., Meencke, J., Röder, U.U., Rohland, C., and Schmidt, D. (1981). Erfahrungen mit der Anwendung von Clobazam (Frisium) als Antiepileptikum. *In* "Epilepsie 1980" (H. Remschmidt, R. Rentz and J. Jungmann, eds), pp. 164–171. Thieme, Stuttgart and New York.